Mental Health Service Evaluation

STUDIES IN SOCIAL AND COMMUNITY PSYCHIATRY

Volumes in this series examine the social dimensions of mental illness as they affect diagnosis and management, and address a range of fundamental issues in the development of community-based mental health services.

Series editor
PETER J. TYRER
Professor of Community Psychiatry, St Mary's Hospital Medical School, London

Also in this series
IAN R. H. FALLOON AND GRAINNE FADDEN *Integrated Mental Health Care*
T. S. BRUGHA *Social Support and Psychiatric Disorder*
M. PHELAN, G. STRATHDEE AND G. THORNICROFT *Emergency Mental Health Services in the Community*
J. PARIS *Social Factors in Personality Disorders*
R. J. BARRETT *The Psychiatric Team and the Social Definition of Schizophrenia*

With the emerging international consensus towards deinstitutionalisation and community care of the mentally ill, there comes a growing need for evaluation of mental health services. Redressing the current lack of guidance on conducting this research, this book comprehensively reviews the most recent developments in research design, method and measurement. At the level of both whole systems and individual programmes within mental health services, the issues are adeptly illustrated with practical descriptions of comprehensive evaluation projects.

The book is divided into six parts. Part I introduces the background to community services and provides an overview of research levels and designs which are further illustrated in Part II. Part III focuses on technical measurement issues and new developments in statistical applications. Special problems and system-level research are highlighted in Part IV. Parts V and VI then address programme-level evaluation-projects, including user outcomes and needs assessment, and finally consider the health economic implications.

All those involved directly in mental health services research or who wish to learn from its evaluation will find this book of importance.

Mental Health Service Evaluation

edited by

HELLE CHARLOTTE KNUDSEN
Institute of Preventive Medicine, City Hospital of Copenhagen, Denmark

GRAHAM THORNICROFT
PRiSM, Institute of Psychiatry, London, UK

Foreword by NORMAN SARTORIUS

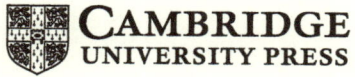

CAMBRIDGE
UNIVERSITY PRESS

CAMBRIDGE UNIVERSITY PRESS
Cambridge, New York, Melbourne, Madrid, Cape Town,
Singapore, São Paulo, Delhi, Tokyo, Mexico City

Cambridge University Press
The Edinburgh Building, Cambridge CB2 8RU, UK

Published in the United States of America by Cambridge University Press, New York

www.cambridge.org
Information on this title: www.cambridge.org/9780521283113

© Cambridge University Press 1996

First published 1996
First paperback edition 2011

A catalogue record for this publication is available from the British Library

Library of Congress Cataloguing in Publication data
Mental health service evaluation / [edited by] Helle Charlotte
Knudsen, Graham Thornicroft ; foreword by Norman Sartorius.
    p.   cm. – (Studies in social and community psychiatry)
Includes index.
ISBN 0 521 46088 3 (hc)
1. Community mental health services – Evaluation. 2. Community
mental health services – Research. 1. Knudsen, Helle Charlotte.
[DNLM: 1. Community Mental Health Services – organization &
administration. 2. Program Evaluation – methods. 3. Research
Design. WM 30 M553162 1996]
RA790.5.M46 1996
362.2′2′0685–dc20
DNLM/DLC
for Library of Congress   95–20757   CIP

ISBN 978-0-521-46088-0 Hardback
ISBN 978-0-521-28311-3 Paperback

Contents

Contributors

CLIVE ADAMS,
Dept of Psychiatry, Warneford Hospital, Oxford OX3 7JX, UK

LEONA L. BACHRACH
19108 Annapolis Way, Gaithersburg, MD 20879, USA

JENNIFER BEECHAM
Personal Social Services Research Unit, Cornwallis Building, The
University of Kent at Canterbury, Kent CT2 7NF, UK

WILLIAM W. EATON
Johns Hopkins University, Department of Mental Hygiene, School
of Hygiene and Public Health, 624 N. Broadway, Baltimore, MD
21205-1999, USA

NICK FREEMANTLE
NHS Centre for Reviews and Dissemination, University of York,
York Y01 DD, UK

GAIL M. GAMACHE
Akademisch Ziekenhuis bij de Universiteit van Amsterdam,
Meibergdreef 9, 1105 AZ Amsterdam Zuidoost, the Netherlands

HEINZ HÄFNER
Central Institute of Mental Health, J5, 68159 Mannheim, Germany

LARS HANSSON
Department of Psychiatry, University of Lund, University Hospital,
22185 Lund, Sweden

WOLFRAM AN DER HEIDEN
Zentralinstitut für Seelische Gesundheit, Postfach 12 21 20, 68072 Mannheim, Germany

PETER HUXLEY
Department of Psychiatry, University of Manchester, Mathematics Tower, Oxford Road, Manchester M13 9PL, UK

BRIAN JARMAN
Department of General Practice, St Mary's Hospital Medical School, Lisson Grove Health Centre, Gateforth Street, London NW8 8EG, UK

BIRGIT JESSEN-PETERSEN
Department of Psychiatry, Copenhagen Health Services, City Hospital of Copenhagen, 1399 Copenhagen K, Denmark

HERMAN KLUITER
Department of Social Psychiatry, State University of Groningen, WHO Collaborating Center, Akademisch Ziekenhuis, Oostersingel 59, PO Box 30.0001, 9700 R.B. Groningen, the Netherlands

MARTIN KNAPP
Personal Social Services Research Unit, Cornwallis Building, The University of Kent at Canterbury, Kent CT2 7NF, UK

HELLE CHARLOTTE KNUDSEN
Institute of Preventive Medicine, Copenhagen Health Services, City Hospital of Copenhagen, Øster Farimagsgade 5, 1399 Copenhagen K, Denmark

ALLAN KRASNIK
Department of Social Medicine, University of Copenhagen, Panuminstitute, Blegdamsvej 3, 2200 Copenhagen N, Denmark

SVEND KREINER
Department of Sociology, University of Copenhagen, Linnesgade 22, 1361 Copenhagen K, Denmark

GLYN LEWIS
London School of Hygiene and Tropical Medicine, Keppel Street, London WC1E 7HT, and Institute of Psychiatry, De Crespigny Park, London SE5 8AF, UK

MERETE NORDENTOFT
Psychiatric Department E, Copenhagen Health Services, Bispebjerg Hospital, Bispebjerg Bakke, 2400 Copenhagen NV, Denmark

TINEKE OLDEHINKEL
Department of Social Psychiatry, State University of Groningen, WHO Collaborating Center, Akademisch Ziekenhuis, Oostersingel 59, PO Box 30.0001, 9700 R.B. Groningen, the Netherlands

MICHAEL PHELAN
PRiSM (Psychiatric Research in Service Measurement), Institute of Psychiatry, De Crespigny Park, London SE5 8AF, UK

MIRELLA RUGGERI
Servizio di Psicologia Medica, Instituto di Psichiatria, Ospedale Policlinico, 37134 Verona, Italy

HENRIK SÆLAN
Social Welfare Department, City of Copenhagen, Bernstorffsgade 17–21, 1577 Copenhagen V, Denmark

AART H. SCHENE
Akademisch Ziekenhuis bij de Universiteit van Amsterdam, Meibergdreef 9, 1105 AZ Amsterdam Zuidoost, the Netherlands

CLAES-GÖRAN STEFANSSON
Psychosocial Research Unit, Karolinska Institute, Ektorpsvägen 2, 13147 Nacka, Sweden

GERALDINE STRATHDEE
PRiSM (Psychiatric Research in Service Measurement), Institute of Psychiatry, De Crespigny Park, London SE5 8AF, UK

FRANK J. SULLIVAN
Department of Health and Human Services, Substance Abuse and
Mental Health Services Administration, Rockville, MD 20857, USA

SJOERD SYTEMA
Department of Social Psychiatry, State University of Groningen,
WHO Collaborating Center, Akademisch Ziekenhuis, Oostersingel
59, PO Box 30.0001, 9700 R.B. Groningen, the Netherlands

MICHELE TANSELLA
Servizio di Psicologia Medica, Instituto di Psichiatria, Ospedale
Policlinico, 37134 Verona, Italy

RICHARD C. TESSLER
Akademisch Ziekenhuis bij de Universiteit van Amsterdam,
Meibergdreef 9, 1105 AZ Amsterdam Zuidoost, the Netherlands

GRAHAM THORNICROFT
PRiSM (Psychiatric Research in Service Measurement), Institute
of Psychiatry, De Crespigny Park, London SE5 8AF, UK

DURK WIERSMA
Department of Social Psychiatry, State University of Groningen,
WHO Collaborating Center, Akademisch Ziekenhuis, Oostersingel
59, PO Box 30.0001, 9700 R.B. Groningen, the Netherlands

JOHN K. WING
College Research Unit, Royal College of Psychiatrists, 11 Grosvenor
Crescent, London SW1X 7EE, UK

Foreword

The veracity of the statement that mental illnesses are frequent and can have severe consequences has now been accepted in most developed and many developing countries. The notion that mental health services can offer the mentally ill more than asylum and protection is also becoming accepted; but just how much health services can do, at what cost and how remains a matter of debate and uncertainty because information about the issue is insufficient in quality and quantity. In part, this is due to the methodological difficulties arising in any attempt to measure changes in human behaviour, quality of life and levels of functioning in social roles. In part, the lack of data is due to a reluctance to carry out detailed (and often tedious) measurements and to provide sufficient resources to make assessment in a scientifically and ethically acceptable manner. It is still rare to find that research on service evaluation receives as much recognition in academic circles and among decision-makers as its complexity and importance deserve. In part, data are difficult to obtain because those who operate services fear that the data will be used to reduce budgets, personnel or both, or to induce changes in the operation of services. In part also, there is insufficient awareness about the existence of methods that can be used in the evaluation of services and about the advantages that those who are involved in providing them can have if valid and relevant data are made available without delay.

The authors and editors of this book have every reason to be proud of its appearance. They have brought together many of the elements which have to be available if evaluation of mental health services is to happen and be useful to all concerned. The book contains lucid reviews of epidemiological issues arising in evaluation programmes, clear and straightforward descriptions of methods which can be used to evaluate programmes and health service systems, and fine examples which illustrate the issues raised.

It is my sincere hope that this volume will serve not only as a repository of knowledge but also as a tool box which its authors and readers will use in making evaluation an integral part of practice. If it does become that, evaluation will not be an act done by third persons for reasons external to the goals of the service and of the people employed in it, hated and eventually useless or harmful: it will be as much a part of work that satisfies and helps as are the other components of mental health care. There are hundreds of millions of people in the world who could benefit from mental health care: rational evaluation will make our resources go further in providing them with the help they need.

Norman Sartorius

Preface

Since the beginning of the nineteenth century, society has struggled to meet the ever-growing needs for psychiatric services from an ever-growing population with ever-growing demands for better standards of care. During the nineteenth century, mental hospitals were built outside the urban areas; these hospitals were organised in accord with the best standards of care of that time. But because of progressive overcrowding and understaffing, the care of the patients in these hospitals became inhumane and humiliating. These conditions led to an ideological movement intending to give back to patients their dignity and autonomy. This movement has been encouraged by changed perceptions of an individual's rights and dignity which have blossomed during the twentieth century.

At the present time the ideological assumptions guiding the development of policy in the care of the mentally ill have been joined with economic considerations. As a consequence, the reduction in the availability of psychiatric beds has not been sufficiently balanced by an increase in community services for the mentally ill. Among the most visible social consequences of these changes are the homeless mentally ill wandering the streets of metropolitan areas and the unacceptably high numbers of people with mental illness who remain in prisons. To address these deficits, changes in service must both improve standards of care and at the same time be cost-effective. It is no longer acceptable for well-intentioned, humanitarian professionals alone to be involved in planning decisions; the caregivers, the service users and their relatives must also be involved. Consequently it is now necessary to set clear goals for services, to develop new, more effective treatments, and to develop services which are based on evidence.

But research and practice in mental health are not straightforward.

The complexity of society must be reflected in the complexity of the research. The care of the severely mentally ill patient involves more than the patient, his or her relatives and the psychiatrist. The social welfare system, volunteer organisations, primary health care staff and the criminal justice system all play key roles in the pattern of care. Their joint impact must be a part of the overall assessment of the effectiveness of the care of the patient.

The strengths and weaknesses of the newly evolving ways of organising mental health services and institutions have been subjects of growing concern in the last 30 years. The early 1970s saw an enthusiastic wave of research efforts in the evaluation of community mental health services. The focus of these studies was evaluation of changes in the use of services. We are now witnessing a new wave of research activities in this area. This new work continues the original lines of investigation and also stresses meeting the needs of the mentally ill and the health economic consequences of structural changes in the mental health system. These new investigations have been supported by developments in the areas of epidemiology and statistics. Equally important is the growing concern of national health authorities with the improvement of mental health services, which is expressed in many countries by setting mental health services research as a high priority.

Even though there is an emerging international consensus that mental health services should be increasingly decentralised away from central hospital sites, and that community mental health services should be sensitive to the needs and views of their users, there is still a lack of guidance on how relevant research should be conducted. This book provides a relevant and timely contribution to this rapidly developing field. The authors are both directly concerned with the planning, implementation, delivery, evaluation and modification of community-based mental health services, and have outstanding research qualifications in health sciences, social science, statistics and epidemiology.

The book addresses those researchers, research assistants, ancillary staff, public health physicians and research workers, and mental health service staff who are producing, or wish to learn from, the results of mental health service evaluations. We also intend to reach planners, mental health managers, finance directors, public policy staff, and politicians who wish to be informed by the results of research projects in their judgements, and who wish to use this information to commission higher-quality research in future. We also wish to reach students of these various disciplines who wish to upgrade their technical knowledge of mental health service evaluation during their training years.

The book is divided into six parts. Part I introduces the history, background and goals of deinstitutionalisation and community mental health services and provides an overview of research designs and the levels of research. In particular it addresses the interrelationship between evaluative research and public policy. Part II (Comprehensive Service Evaluation Projects) illustrates these issues with practical descriptions of three comprehensive evaluation projects: the Copenhagen Community Psychiatric Project (Denmark), the Mannheim Project (Germany) and the Nacka-Värmdö (Stockholm) Project (Sweden). Part III (Methods: Measurement, Strategies and New Approaches) focuses on more technical measurement issues and on new developments in statistical applications. Part IV (System-Level Research) highlights special problems and opportunities in research at the level of the mental health system. Part V (Programme-Level Research) considers the special circumstances of programme-level evaluation projects including patients' and caregivers' outcomes and the assessment of needs. The volume concludes with Part VI (Health Economics in Mental Health) that contains a chapter on health economics at programme and system levels and a conclusion.

The inspiration for this book was lectures given at a NATO Advanced Research Workshop on Research Evaluation of Community Psychiatric Services held in Il Ciocco, Italy, on 3–7 September, 1993, where contributions from many outstanding research experts in related fields were presented. We wish to thank NATO (the North Atlantic Treaty Organization) for the grant which facilitated that workshop. It is refreshing that an international body dedicated to military purposes can also find the resources to contribute to issues of health. We owe especial thanks to the Institute of Preventive Medicine, the Copenhagen Health Services, and especially to Ms Vibeke Munk, the administrative director of the Institute, for their outstanding contribution to the organisation and coordination of both the NATO workshop and this book. We wish also to thank Professor Sarnoff Mednick, Social Science Research Institute, University of Southern California, for his considerate and inspiring contribution as a member of the organisation committee and in his guidance in the development of the book. Finally we wish to thank the discussants and participants at the workshop for their inspiring and expert contributions and their warm encouragement.

Helle Charlotte Knudsen
Graham Thornicroft
Copenhagen and London

PART I

INTRODUCTION

1

Deinstitutionalisation: promises, problems and prospects

Leona L. Bachrach

Introduction

Over the past several decades many nations have embarked upon dedicated efforts to reduce, if not to eliminate, the role of psychiatric hospitals in the treatment of mentally ill persons. This movement, popularly known as 'deinstitutionalisation', has greatly altered the lives of psychiatric patients throughout the Western world. This chapter will examine the history and current status of the deinstitutionalisation movement and identify some specific problems that may be traced directly to the implementation (often incomplete or faulty) of deinstitutionalisation policy. A 'new chronic' patient population will be described, and the positive legacy of deinstitutionalisation will be noted. The chapter will conclude with a plea for a new, more realistic understanding of what successful deinstitutionalisation must entail. This discussion is based largely on service delivery trends in the United States. However, both the popular and professional literature (Thornicroft & Bebbington, 1989; Schmidt, 1992; Thornicroft et al., 1993), as well as extensive personal observation, suggest that other countries are encountering similar circumstances. Precisely why this is so is an intriguing question that merits serious consideration, in view of vast differences in nations' health care philosophies and service delivery practices. One may speculate that there are common issues in serving psychiatric patients in the community that transcend national boundaries, and that these must be frankly examined for their broader implications.

Deinstitutionalisation: definition and background

Deinstitutionalisation, which refers to a complex series of interrelated events and policy decisions, may be defined as *the replacement of long-stay psychiatric hospitals with smaller, less isolated community-based service alternatives for the care of mentally ill individuals.* In theory it consists of three component processes: the release of patients residing in psychiatric hospitals to alternative facilities in the community; the diversion of potential new admissions to the alternative facilities; and the development of special community-based programmes, combining psychiatric and support services, for the care of a non-institutionalised patient population (Bachrach, 1976). The last of these processes is held to be particularly important, for it is assumed that patients' altered life circumstances will inevitably result in new configurations of service need.

In the United States the depopulation of psychiatric hospitals began in the mid-1950s with the introduction and rapid spread of psychoactive medications. However, official policy supporting deinstitutionalisation was not articulated until 1963, when President John Kennedy, prompted by numerous disclosures of inhumane conditions inside psychiatric hospitals, called for a 'bold new approach' in mental health service delivery. In response, the federal government undertook to replace the country's psychiatric hospitals, which were largely administered by state governments, with some 1500 community mental health centres. About half of these were eventually funded and built before the federal initiative ended in the early 1980s. Community mental health facilities exist today in both the private and non-federal public sectors, and they constitute the most highly utilised psychiatric service sites (Manderscheid & Sonnenschein, 1992). The effects of pursuing deinstitutionalisation policy are dramatically portrayed in service utilisation statistics. In 1955, the resident patient count in American state psychiatric hospitals stood at a record high of 560 000. That number has declined in each successive year and stands today at 101 000, a reduction of 82%. Even more striking is the drop of 88% in the resident patient rate, from 339 per 100 000 population in 1955 to 41 per 100 000 today (Manderscheid & Sonnenschein, 1992). The rationale for pursuing deinstitutionalisation, combining elements of idealism and pragmatism, reflected justifiable concern for the well-being of psychiatric patients, many of whom were living miserable lives inside the state hospitals (Bachrach, 1993a). It encompassed several critically important assumptions. First, it was widely, even passionately, assumed that community-based care would be instrinsically more humane than hospital-based care. Second, it was similarly assumed that community-based care would be intrinsically more therapeutic than hospital-based care. And, third, it was further assumed that community-based care would be more cost-effective than hospital-based care (Bachrach, 1976, 1978; Thornicroft & Bebbington, 1989).

These assumptions had, however, not been tested empirically, and there has been cause over the years to question their validity. We have, for example, begun to realise that community care may indeed hold the potential for being more humane and more therapeutic than hospital care; however, this promise cannot be realised unless comprehensive services for the most severely disabled patients have been mandated, and adequate resources have been provided to ensure their implementation. We have also begun to understand that if one considers all the hidden costs associated with responsible programming, it is generally not accurate to conclude that community services will result in substantial savings over hospital care (Aldrich, 1985; Kovaleski, 1993; Okin, 1978, 1993).

We have learned as well that we are not ready to close all our psychiatric hospitals, although their imminent demise was often predicted in the optimism of the 1960s. Many planners who continue to harbour the hope that we will some day eliminate these facilities increasingly acknowledge the difficulty of establishing alternative sites where patients can be admitted for intensive hospital-based observation or comprehensive care.

Issues in deinstitutionalisation

Since deinstitutionalisation began in the United States, the first two of the three component processes mentioned above – releasing patients from and reducing admissions to psychiatric hospitals – have proceeded apace. However, the critical third process, that of developing a full array of services in the community to meet the unique needs of a non-institutionalised patient population, has often lagged. This has resulted in a variety of serious service delivery problems in many communities.

One such problem is related to the fragmentation of the patient population, for a once relatively stable hospital cohort has been splintered as long-stay patients have been released to the community. Although some individuals have been successfully placed in community-based facilities, others have been shunted to 'mini-institutions' where the quality of their lives has actually deteriorated. Other patients have become homeless (Bachrach, 1992b), or been incarcerated in jails and other correctional facilities (Anon; 1993). And still other patients have demonstrated a persistent dependency on institutional care and developed 'revolving door' patterns of repeated admission and discharge (Cohen, 1993; Geller, 1993). However, not all long-stay patients have been released; for some, considered to be poor risks for discharge, remain inside psychiatric hospitals. Many more recently admitted individuals have become 'short-stay' hospital residents, staying for only days or weeks before their release; but others have become 'new long-stay' patients. Still other mentally ill individuals, many of them severely symptomatic or disabled, have avoided admission altogether and spent no time at all in hospital. Indeed, some American communities report that the number of never-hospitalised mentally ill people now exceeds the number who have ever been hospitalised (Bachrach, 1978).

This diversity in patients' histories represents a major change in service utilisation patterns. Before deinstitutionalisation most mentally ill people entered psychiatric hospitals and generally stayed for extended periods, often for the rest of their lives. There was relatively little variation in their treatment histories, and individual differences among them were easily overlooked. Today in the community, however, those differences have become difficult to ignore. It is increasingly apparent that patients vary not only in their diagnoses and functional levels, but also in their symptomatologies, available support systems, and treatment needs. And although the acknowledgement of such diversity may be considered a major positive outcome of the deinstitutionalisation movement (Bachrach, 1993b), it also holds certain disadvantages from a service planning perspective. Our imagination and our creativity, to say nothing of our financial resources, have not always been equal to the challenge of responding to the varied treatment needs of mentally ill people living in the community.

A second problem revolves around difficulties inherent in achieving continuity of care for long-term patients outside the hospital setting – an issue that was easily overlooked in the early years of deinstitutionalisation when many proponents believed that, absent the negative effects of institutional residence, chronicity would disappear. Programme planning today frequently focuses on patients' immediate requirements and ignores the future, even though their service needs tend to endure no matter where they live. Indeed, all aspects of continuity of care, including patients' access to needed programmes over time and their ability to establish therapeutic relationships with caregivers, have been jeopardised (Bachrach, 1993c).

Third, attempts to provide comprehensive care have similarly met with difficulty. Long-term mental patients, precisely because of their illnesses and related disabilities, generally require a wide variety of psychiatric, medical, social, rehabilitative, residential, vocational, and quasi-vocational services (Belkin, 1992). Some also need sanctuary or asylum: an escape from the pressures and threats of the world (Bachrach, 1984; Wasow, 1993). Some may require such asylum temporarily, until a crisis can be resolved, although others may need it indefinitely.

In the past, providing comprehensive care to psychiatric patients, including responding to their need for asylum, was relatively easily accomplished, since virtually all services could be arranged within the single physical setting of the psychiatric hospital. And although we may not always have liked what happened inside some hospitals in those years, particularly in the large and isolated 'warehouse' facilities, centralisation carried certain practical advantages.

Today, by contrast, the authority for providing services is typically divided among many separate health and human service agencies in the public and private sectors, and successful programming depends upon the fine tuning of initiatives that orginate with separate, and sometimes competing, authorities. To use a cliche, our service systems are often hopelessly fragmented.

A fourth major problem attending deinstitutionalisation in many communities is related to patient selection and gatekeeping. In the early years of the movement there was a clear intention that the new community mental health programmes would serve the most severely mentally ill individuals – i.e. those who would otherwise be hospitalised. However, with increased 'boundary busting' in the selection of patients for care (Dinitz & Beran, 1971), many agencies came to favour individuals who were less symptomatic and disabled; and they overlooked, either unintentionally or sometimes quite by design, those who were originally intended to be the major beneficiaries of deinstitutionalisation (Bachrach & Lamb, 1989). Thus, many needy persons have been left to fend for themselves, although they may lack the skills and confidence, and almost certainly the resources, that would enable them to seek out services on their own.

Fifth, we have generally not developed the kinds of information and communication links that are essential in fragmented systems of care where services are housed in administratively and geographically separated agencies. In fact, we require ready access to at least three varieties of information if our deinstitutionalisation efforts are to prove successful. We must, first, have simple, descriptive, and timely data about the people whom we serve. We must, for treatment planning purposes, know who they are, where they have been sent, and what happened to them after they arrived at their destinations – if, in fact, they ever arrived.

We also need reliable programme evaluations so that we can establish whether the services we promote are living up to their promise. And, in this connection, we must have meaningful and valid measures by which to assess programme outcome, including indices of incremental progress for those patients who appear to proceed slowly or who, as part of their illnesses, experience episodic reversals (Bachrach, 1987b; NASMHPD, 1993).

In contradistinction to programme evaluation, we must also have system-level assessments that tell us whether services are actually reaching those whom the system is meant to serve; or whether, alternatively, there are numbers of potential service recipients who are routinely overlooked (Neigher & Schulberg, 1982). However, all three data bases tend to be poorly developed (Graham & Birchmore-Timney, 1989; Thornicroft & Bebbington, 1989; Johnson & Thornicroft, 1993; New York State, 1993). Information about patients, for example, is frequently ill-suited to clinical use, for it tends to be incomplete, difficult to access, and slow to retrieve. Programme data are also less than ideal, for our evaluations often focus on questions that lack relevance to the clinical process. For example, we generally fail to inquire about the small but critical kinds of progress that many patients make, or about the quality of their care or the quality of their lives in the community. We tend instead to employ gross measures of hospital utilisation and are often discouraged from focusing on the more subtle variables by funding agencies that prefer uncomplicated and politically popular questions.

In fact, this tendency has spawned a preoccupation with statistical analysis and experimental design in programme evaluation that is irrelevant or at least premature much of the time. It sometimes appears that an investigator's ability to demonstrate technical competence in these areas, and not his or her appreciation of clinical reality, has become the major criterion for research support, at least in the United States (Brand, 1983).

As for comprehensive system-level information, that too is often compromised, for we frequently settle for circumscribed programme evaluations instead of attempting to assess the effects of our gatekeeping. There are, unfortunately, mentally ill individuals who, at best, remain on the fringes of our care systems and whose experience cannot be captured in programme evaluations because, very simply, they are not enrolled in any programmes. Many are homeless and sleeping rough, and I regret to report that I have seen them in every country that I have visited in recent years. Not to include them in our system assessments is both diversionary and deceptive.

The new chronic patient population

It is within this paradoxical service delivery climate, with its idealism and its problems, that a population of new chronic psychiatric patients has become increasingly evident in deinstitutionalised service systems (Bachrach, 1982; Pepper *et al.*, 1981). I use the term 'new chronic patient' with misgiving, for many individuals so labelled find the title to be objectionable. Nevertheless, the term is descriptive and can serve a useful function by providing a new perspective from which to view contemporary service delivery problems. It can thus be regarded as a metaphor for long-term patienthood in an era of deinstitutinalisation; and just as other metaphors do, it serves the purpose of refining our understanding of reality.

Diagnostically, new chronic patients have the same range of psychiatric illnesses as other severely mentally ill individiuals. Most have been diagnosed with schizophrenia, and many others with bipolar disorders. In some communities, substantial numbers have been diagnosed with personality disorders, often in addition to other major diagnoses. Thus, what distinguishes them from long-term psychiatric patients of the past is not their illnesses *per se*, but rather their aggregate demand for services and their unique impact on the service system.

Those new chronic patients who are enrolled in psychiatric services tend to be pervasive users of the system. They regularly appear in psychiatric hospitals, general hospitals, community mental health centres, and all kinds of outpatient psychiatric facilities. However, at any given time, substantial numbers of these patients are enrolled in no psychiatric services whatever and are essentially unserved by the system of care.

Those who utilise the service system tend to do so in a 'revolving door' manner and frequently move among facilities. They often appear in the criminal justice system in addition to, or else in place of, the mental health service system. In many communities, new chronic patients become general hospital emergency room regulars, but their referral out tends to be problematic for they generally lack an established niche within the system of care.

Other characteristics of these patients as they are described in the American literature are their high risk for suicide, their fragile ego development, and their vulnerability to stress and personal rejection (Ely, 1985). In addition, practically every reference to them comments as well on the high prevalence of alcohol or other substance use within the population.

Thus, new chronic patients tend to present for treatment in ways that puzzle and discourage service providers; and clinicians and administrators are often confused and frustrated in their attempts to engage and serve them. Harris & Bergman (1979) have written, 'After several rounds of bouncing between hospital and community, no one expects these patients to change. They are treated perfunctorily by a staff that is too discouraged to do more than go through the motions.' Similarly, an article by Robbins and his associates (1978) describes these patients as surly individuals whom staff perceive as 'negativistic, difficult, and frightening'.

Although these fairly typical descriptions come from inner city service settings, new chronic patients are found in suburban and rural places as well (Bachrach, 1982; Claiborne, 1993). A particularly revealing account documents new chronic patients who migrate into rural Montana, a relatively remote and isolated part of the United States (Bachrach, 1988). There they are admitted to the state psychiatric hospital for brief stays, during which they receive food and temporary shelter before they leave to wander again. In fact, patterns of gross geographical mobility characterise the lives of many new chronic patients. Their apparent restlessness often makes them difficult to find and serve; and, not surprisingly, they have contributed materially to homeless populations in many parts of America (Bachrach, 1992b). Although this portrait of a patient population is necessarily an abbreviated one, it is sufficient to underscore a significant reality. New chronic patients represent a *truly deinstitutionalised population*. They constitute the first generation of psychiatric patients who, since the onset of their illnesses, have lived exclusively in an era of deinstitutionalisation. Their problems in receiving adequate care thus reflect all the major issues described above – and others, as well – that have come to be identified with the deinstitutionalisation movement.

Mixed messages and social realities

It is essential to emphasise that not all of today's psychiatric patients fit this general and somewhat depressing description. In fact, many appear to respond favourably to the programmes offered in our deinstitutionalised service systems. But even as we rejoice that some fare well, we must acknowledge those new chronic patients who are difficult to place in the community: those who are characterised by volatility and non-compliance; and who often seem to insist upon receiving, but then regularly and vociferously reject, whatever the system offers. We must thus attempt to understand the forces that this population's presence reflects. Dunham (1976) observed that the sociology of patient care changed dramatically with deinstitutionalisation. In the past, the psychiatric hospital provided clearly outlined rules of behaviour for both patients and staff, and patients knew precisely who they were and what was expected of them. By contrast, today's new chronic patients have poorly defined social roles, for the prescriptions and proscriptions associated with patienthood have become blurred in community-based service systems (Estroff, 1981).

In fact, behavioural clues have largely been supplanted by mixed messages (Bachrach, 1990). We tend to remind patients that they are 'very sick' and should 'behave like patients'. However, we often fail to provide the structure or milieu in which such an admonition holds real meaning. We ask the individual to accept the role of mental patient voluntarily – a role filled with ambiguity, stigma, and diminished opportunity – and are then surprised when the person resists.

We are also ambiguous in the messages we give patients about their place in society. An early goal of deinstitutionalisation was to 'mainstream' or 'normalise' psychiatric patients by making their lives as much like the lives of other people as possible. Yet, such encouragement has not consistently served these individuals well.

For example, outside the protected environment of the psychiatric hospital, behaving like everybody else might imply geographical mobility. Moving to a new place is an accepted and expected social pattern throughout the United States, particularly among young adults; and when we instruct mentally ill people to behave like their age peers, we may be promoting gross migration patterns among people who are desperately in need of continuity in their care and who might potentially profit from staying in one place where they might establish a therapeutic relationship (Bachrach, 1987a).

Again, doing what everybody else does might mean, particularly for young adults, using alcohol and street drugs recreationally. As a result, the prevalence of substance use is sufficiently marked within the population that it has become necessary to plan special services for dually diagnosed new chronic patients in the community (Bergman & Harris, 1985; American Psychiatric Association, 1993).

Thus, although moving around and using alcohol and street drugs recreationally might in some sense be regarded as normalising activities, they are not highly recommended for mentally ill people. And we may conclude that the philosophy of normalisation, whatever benefits it might confer on some patients, has also created major difficulties for others. It appears that there are some patients who must have their ideas about life in the community tempered. These individuals require more structure and support than we have ordinarily been prepared to offer in community-based programmes, and their special needs must be acknowledged (Bachrach & Lamb, 1989; Lamb, 1993).

The positive legacy

It is because the problems noted here are so critical that I have devoted the major portion of this chapter to the negative aspects of deinstitutionalisation: these are circumstances that absolutely require remediation. Yet it is equally important to note the positive effects of that movement, for there are, in fact, a number of excellent community-based service programmes that have responded with success to the challenges of deinstitutionalisation. I have seen examples of these 'model' programmes in every country I have visited, although within any country they tend to be rare, localised, and dependent upon the existence of aggressive and dedicated leadership (Bachrach, 1989).

Apart from these excellent programmes, deinstitutionalisation has also fostered a critical 'paradigm shift' that has begun to influence service planning today. Our experience of several decades has now demonstrated the need for an orientation that is patient-focused and essentially positive in its direction. This is increasingly stressed in contemporary service plans, and it constitutes the positive legacy of the movement (Bachrach, 1993b).

During the 1970s and 1980s Wing (1978a, b; Wing & Morris, 1981) authored several articles that articulated this legacy that today, decades later, we are finally beginning to exploit. According to Wing, psychiatric patients are affected by multiple sources of disability. Not only do they experience a variety of disabling primary symptoms directly attributable to their mental illnesses; they are additionally disabled by certain adverse personal reactions that result from their unique responses to the experience of being mentally ill. Wing wrote that the secondary reactions sometimes engender greater problems in engaging and treating patients than do the primary symptoms themselves.

In addition, psychiatric patients also experience what Wing called 'social disablements' that result from such external social forces as stigma, discrimination, poverty, unemployment, and unequal access to entitlements. These events carry with them a distinct social disadvantage that further increases the range of their disabilities.

Now, in proposing this trichotomy of disabilities – primary symptoms, adverse personal reactions, and social disablements – Wing essentially urged us to look beyond the psychiatric condition itself to understand the treatment needs of mentally ill people. Only when we are able to view mental illness as having psychological and sociological components can we respond sensitively to patients as people. Deinstitutionalisation, by increasing patients' visibility and sensitising us to their needs, has effectively opened the door to our acceptance of this reality, for we appear more nearly ready today than ever before to adopt the holistic thinking that is part and parcel of a comprehensive service approach.

Deinstitutionalisation's legacy is actually manifested in a variety of developments. It is illustrated in the United States in a growing insistence on combining psychosocial rehabilitation interventions with psychiatric care in the treatment of mental illness (Bachrach, 1992a). It is also reflected in newly developing outreach efforts that alter clinicians' traditional concepts of time and space by requiring them to go wherever patients are, in order to meet them on their own ground both physically and psychologically (Cohen, 1990; Zealberg et al., 1993).

Deinstitutionalisation's legacy is documented as well in a growing literature that underscores the necessity for professionals to respond to patients as people with uniquely personal hopes, fears, frustrations, and ambitions; and to involve those patients and their relatives in the treatment planning process to the fullest extent possible (Bachrach, 1993b). And although these developments are in themselves not new, they have come into their own in this era of deinstitutionalisation. It is now widely acknowledged that patients and family members possess unique insights and important knowledge to share with professional caregivers, even though, before deinstitutionalisation, these individuals were rarely viewed as active contributors to the treatment planning process.

There is, of course, still much damage from inappropriately conceived and executed interventions that service systems must undo, and this suggests the need for an altered view of deinstitutionalisation today – one that departs from the simplistic ideology of the 1960s (Minkoff, 1987; Sartorius, 1992; Bell, 1993). Deinstitutionalisation, if it is to be effectively implemented, must be realistically approached. It is not all glamour; nor is it the elimination of chronicity, nor communities' reaching out to welcome psychiatric patients. It encompasses more subtle, and sometimes less appealing, circumstances as well.

Deinstitutionalisation means providing care in the community to people whom we once locked away because, in all candour, we did not want to see them. It means becoming advocates for these people even when the community rejects them. It means acknowledging the possibility of chronicity and the need to provide longitudinal and comprehensive services, including care, when indicated, inside psychiatric hospitals.

Beyond this, deinstitutionalisation implies that we must recognise and support the diversity of the patient population and the individuality of its members, some of whom fare well in community-based service systems but many of whom get lost in the cracks and require special attention and programmes (Cohen, 1990). It means that we must appreciate the stresses, disappointments, and failed hopes of these individuals.

Finally, our experience reveals the necessity for refined techniques for evaluating deinstitutionalisation efforts, so that we may more effectively assess not only individual patients and selected programmes but also the exclusory gatekeeping practices that sometimes serve to ration care in our service systems.

The American philosopher, Santayana (1905), wrote at the beginning of this century that, 'Those who cannot remember the past are condemned to repeat it.' In the United States, at least, we have probably reached the point of no return with deinstitutionalisation, for it is unlikely that we will ever go back to totally hospital-oriented systems of care. Thus, as we approach the beginning of a new century, we must look to the past for the lessons that deinstitutionalisation has bestowed. The difficulties of service planning for long-term psychiatric patients in the future will almost certainly be exacerbated by a scarcity of resources and, in many places, a wavering dedication to serving those in need (Robinson, 1993). At the same time, however, planning can be facilitated by appreciating and capitalising upon deinstitutionalisation's positive legacy.

References

Aldrich, C.K. (1985). Deinstitutionalization. *Newsletter of the University of Virginia Institute of Government*, 1–5 September.

American Psychiatric Association (1993). *Dual Diagnosis of Mental Illness and Substance Abuse: Collected Papers from H&CP*. Washington: American Psychiatric Association H&CP Service.

Anon. (1993). Penal institutions said to be this country's newest asylums. *Psychiatric News*, 2 July, pp. 10, 22.

Bachrach, L.L. (1976). *Deinstitutionalization: An Analytical Review and Sociological Perspective*. Rockville, Maryland: National Institute of Mental Health.

Bachrach, L.L. (1978). A conceptual approach to deinstitutionalization. *Hospital and Community Psychiatry*, **29**, 573–8.

Bachrach, L.L. (1982). Young adult chronic patients: an analytical review of the literature. *Hospital and Community Psychiatry*, **33**, 189–97.

Bachrach, L.L. (1984). Asylum and chronically ill psychiatric patients. *American Journal of Psychiatry*, **141**, 975–8.

Bachrach, L.L. (1987a). Geographic mobility and the homeless mentally ill. *Hospital and Community Psychiatry*, **38**, 27–8.

Bachrach, L.L. (1987b). Measuring program outcomes in Tucson. *Hospital and Community Psychiatry*, **38**, 1151–2.

Bachrach, L.L. (1988). Transient patients in a western state hospital. *Hospital and Community Psychiatry*, **39**, 123–4.

Bachrach, L.L. (1989). The legacy of model programs. *Hospital and Community Psychiatry*, **40**, 234–5.

Bachrach, L.L. (1990). Afterword: deinstitutionalization and the future: the past as prologue. In *Psychiatry Takes to the Streets*, ed. N.L. Cohen, pp. 273–93. New York: Guilford Press.

Bachrach, L.L. (1992a). Psychosocial rehabilitation and psychiatry in the care of long-term patients. *American Journal of Psychiatry*, **149**, 1455–63.

Bachrach, L.L. (1992b). What we know about homelessness among mentally ill persons: an analytical review and commentary. *Hospital and Community Psychiatry*, **43**, 453–64.

Bachrach, L.L. (1993a). American experience in social psychiatry. In *Principles of Social Psychiatry*, ed. D. Bhugra & J. Leff, pp. 534–48. Oxford: Blackwell Scientific Publications.

Bachrach, L.L. (1993b). The biopsychosocial legacy of deinstitutionalization. *Hospital and Community Psychiatry*, **44**, 523–4, 546.

Bachrach, L.L. (1993c). Continuity of care: a context for case management. In *Case Management for Mentally Ill Patients*, ed. M. Harris & H.C. Bergman, pp. 183–97. New York: Harwood Academic Publishers.

Bachrach, L.L. & Lamb, H.R. (1989). What have we learned from deinstitutionalization? *Psychiatric Annals*, **19**, 12–21.

Belkin, L. (1992). Treating the sick can mean clothing them too. *New York Times*, 24 November, pp. B1, B2.

Bell, C.C. (1993). The new community psychiatry in 2000 A.D. *Hospital and Community Psychiatry*, **44**, 815.

Bergman, H. & Harris, M. (1985). Substance abuse among young adult chronic patients. *Psychosocial Rehabilitation Journal*, **9**, 49–54.

Brand, P.W. (1983). Comments on the article, 'The effectiveness of preventive management in reducing the occurrence of pressure sores'. *Journal of Rehabilitation R & D*, **20**, 78.

Claiborne, W. (1993). 'Quaint' Maine battles urban problems as facilities release mentally ill patients. *Washington Post*, 9 March, p. A9.

Cohen, N.L. (ed.) (1990). *Psychiatry Takes to the Streets*. New York: Guilford Press.

Cohen, N.L. (1993). Stigmatization and the 'noncompliant' recidivist. *Hospital and Community Psychiatry*, **44**, 1029.

Dinitz, S. & Beran, N. (1971). Community mental health as a boundaryless and boundary-busting system. *Journal of Health and Social Behavior*, **12**, 99–108.

Dunham, H.W. (1976). *Social Realities and Community Psychiatry*. New York: Human Sciences Press.

Ely, A.R. (1985). Long-term group treatment for young male 'schizopaths'. Social Work, **30**, 5–10.

Estroff, S.E. (1981). *Making It Crazy: An Ethnography of Psychiatric Clients in an American Community*. Berkeley, California: University of California Press.

Geller, J.L. (1993). Treating revolving-door patients who have 'hospitalphilia':

compassion, coercion, and common sense. *Hospital and Community Psychiatry*, **44**, 141–6.

Graham, K. & Birchmore-Timney, C. (1989). The problem of replicability in program evaluation. *Evaluation and Program Planning*, **12**, 179–87.

Harris, M. & Bergman, H. (1979). *Coordination of Inpatient Hospitalization and Community Support Programs*. Washington, DC: St Elizabeth's Hospital.

Johnson, S. & Thornicroft, G. (1993). The sectorisation of psychiatric services in England and Wales. *Social Psychiatry and Psychiatric Epidemiology*, **28**, 45–7.

Kovaleski, S.F. (1993). DC mental health plan raises ire. *Washington Post*, 9 July, pp. D1, D5.

Lamb, H.R. (1993). Lessons learned from deinstitutionalisation in the US. *British Journal of Psychiatry*, **162**, 587–92.

Manderscheid, R.W. & Sonnenschein, M.A. (eds.) (1992). *Mental Health, United States, 1992*. Washington, DC: US Government Printing Office.

Minkoff, K. (1987). Beyond deinstitutionalization: a new ideology for the postinstitutional era. *Hospital and Community Psychiatry*, **38**, 945–50.

NASMHPD (1993). *Developing Outcome Measures for Programs Serving Homeless People with Mental Illnesses*. Arlington, Virginia: National Association of State Mental Health Program Directors.

Neigher, W.D. & Schulberg, H.C. (1982). Evaluating the outcomes of human service programs. *Evaluation Review*, **6**, 731–52.

New York State (1993). *Discharge Planning Practices of General Hospitals: Did Incentive Payments Improve Performance?* Albany, New York: Commission on Quality of Care for the Mentally Disabled.

Okin, R.L. (1978). The future of state mental health programs for chronic psychiatric patients in the community. *American Journal of Psychiatry*, **135**, 1355–8.

Okin, R.L. (1993). Brewster v. Dukakis. Presented at the Annual Meeting of the American Psychiatric Association, San Francisco, 25 May.

Pepper, B., Kirshner, M.C. & Ryglewicz, H. (1981). The young adult chronic patient: overview of a population. *Hospital and Community Psychiatry*, **32**, 463–9.

Robbins, E., Stern, M., Robbins, L., *et al.* (1978). Unwelcome patients: where can they find asylum? *Hospital and Community Psychiatry*, **29**, 44–6.

Robinson, E. (1993). East and west, a gloomy forecast: Europeans see an end to long-guaranteed social welfare 'rights'. Washington Post, 12 April, pp. A1, A14.

Rossi, P.H. (1978). Issues in the evaluation of human services delivery. *Evaluation Quarterly*, **2**, 573–99.

Santayana, G. (1905). *Reason in Common Sense*. New York, Dover Publications edition, 1980, p. 284.

Sartorius, N. (1992). Rehabilitation and quality of life. *Hospital and Community Psychiatry*, **43**, 1180–1.

Schmidt, W.E. (1992). Across Europe, faces of homeless become more visible and vexing. *New York Times*, 5 January, pp. 1, 8.

Thornicroft, G. & Bebbington, G. (1989). Deinstitutionalisation: from hospital closure to service development. *British Journal of Psychiatry*, **155**, 739–53.

Thornicroft, G., Bisoffi, G., DeSalvia, D., *et al.* (1993). Urban–rural differences in associations between social deprivation and psychiatric service utilization in schizophrenia and all diagnoses: a case register study in Northern Italy. *Psychological Medicine*, **23**, 487–96.

Wasow, M. (1993). The need for asylum revisited. *Hospital and Community Psychiatry*, **44**, 207–8, 222.

Wing, J.K. (1978a). The social context of schizophrenia. *American Journal of Psychiatry*, **135**, 1333–9.

Wing, J.K. (1978b). Who becomes chronic? *Psychiatric Quarterly*, **50**, 178–90.

Wing, J.K. & Morris, B. (1981). Clinical basis of rehabiliation. In *Handbook of Psychiatric Rehabilitation Practice*, ed. J.K. Wing & B. Morris, pp. 3–16. Oxford: Oxford University Press

Zealberg, J.J., Santos, A.B., & Fisher, R.K. (1993). Benefits of mobile crisis programs. *Hospital and Community Psychiatry*, **44**, 16–7.

2

Background and goals of evaluative research in community psychiatry

HEINZ HÄFNER AND WOLFRAM AN DER HEIDEN

Introduction

Evaluative research in community psychiatry is one of the most difficult areas of psychiatric research. This is due to: (1) multiple conditions of care and complex measures of intervention; (2) difficulties in finding appropriate criteria and indicators of outcome (especially in assessing quality of life); (3) difficulties in measuring and controlling for relevant intervening variables; and (4) different methods and practices of data collection. As a result, it is hard to ensure both internal and external validity of the results obtained, that is, to isolate the reasons for observed changes and also to apply the results to other populations, services or community care systems. Indeed, many reviews and attempts at a meta-evaluation of studies on the effectiveness of community care (Renshaw *et al.*, 1988; Häfner & an der Heiden, 1989) have been faced with the following problems: the patient groups studied differed in their profiles of needs for care, the underlying social and institutional conditions of the programmes and services were hardly comparable and intervening variables, such as severity of illness and the patients' skills levels, were not taken sufficiently into account.

An additional hindrance to transnational comparative studies is the lack of comparable national databases or health information systems providing background information for a given structure of mental health care. In addition, there are differences in the organisation of health care, social and welfare systems as well as in the level of implementation of community care. As a consequence, the WHO Regional Office for Europe in its transnational comparative 10-year assessments of mental health care in the European member states included only a few crude indicators of community psychiatric care, such as number of psychiatric units in general hospitals, bed capacity and number of outpatient and day-care units (May, 1976; Freeman *et al.*, 1985). Such an approach naturally harbours fewer errors, but also narrows the range of relevant results.

The present chapter deals with some core questions of evaluative research in psychiatry. In the first part the objectives of psychiatric care and treatment will be discussed. Rather than providing a list of operational criteria for assessing effectiveness in the evaluation of outcome, the chapter focuses on the objectives explicitly determined or merely implied by the changed assumptions, principles and value judgements in the field of community care.

The second part of the chapter deals with the general conditions of mental health care. They include the prevailing social, political, administrative and economic conditions of a service area. These general conditions not only crucially influence the success or failure of rehabilitative measures, but also have to be taken into account in establishing the external validity of research results.

Goals of evaluative research in community psychiatry

Evaluative research in general aims to find out whether certain interventions applied to a selected group of individuals help to achieve or make progress towards defined goals set in a defined period of time (Milne, 1987).

From an epidemiological point of view J.K. Wing (1973) identified the reduction and containment of mental morbidity as the aim of mental health care. A WHO scientific group on the evaluation of methods for the treatment of mental disorders termed a treatment effective if patients 'who receive it recover and do so more rapidly than without it' (World Health Organization, 1991, p. 7). The analysis and specification of recovery, however, led to multiple and fairly complex outcome criteria, such as reduction of symptoms, so that the patients 'no longer fulfil the criteria for the illness in question; impairment and disability produced by the disorder are prevented or lessened; and there is an improvement in the ability to do productive work or to carry out important social roles such as being a parent. Even when the nature of the underlying illness makes complete resolution of the underlying pathology unlikely, "good" treatment enhances the quality of life of the patient, the patient's family, and carers, and facilitates the work of the health service concerned' (World Health Organization, 1991, p. 7).

It is obvious that these general goals have to be translated into more specific and measurable objectives in order to serve as a standard to weigh the results of an intervention against. Conceptual goals, such as those formulated by the WHO experts, need to be specified by operational goals. Operational goals, like conceptual goals, can be formulated at comprehensive or fairly detailed levels. The conceptual goal 'community based' in establishing mental health services, for example, involves immediate help in emergency cases, maintenance of social contacts during inpatient treatment and re-integration of socially disabled patients after discharge from hospital.

Visionary goals

E. Murphy has called a particular category of objectives of community mental health care 'visions', by analogy with the modern strategic and motivational techniques of large enterprises. She gives as an example of a visionary main aim of a service that it 'aspires to provide individuals with as fulfilling and rewarding a life as possible and provides for the ordinary needs of life – a home, daily occupation, emotional support through friendships and social contacts – and recognises individuals' rights as citizens' (Murphy, 1992, p. 125). It is a statement that contains 'legitimate principles in which services can be rooted' (Murphy, 1992, p. 125). The principles stem from social ethics. An entire social-policy programme could be based upon them. For decision makers and the staffs of psychiatric services ethical principles should be a source of motivation and provide guidelines for their action. As criteria for quality assessment or the evaluation of the effectiveness and efficiency of services they need to be translated into measurable or assessable realities.

Quality of life as a goal of community mental health services

Some aspects of these visionary goals are included in the concept of quality of life as a standard for service evaluation. Today there is an increasing movement towards evaluating services also in terms of the quality of life of service users. According to O'Brian (1987) the construct can be measured according to five components:

1 Community presence has to do with an individual's location within a community setting. Access to other people in a range of settings, such as shops, leisure facilities and places of education and employment, is a prerequisite for a satisfactory quality of life.
2 Relationships constitute a second component of quality of life. Most people rely heavily on a range of relationships with friends, family members, colleagues and peers.
3 A third component – choice – includes small, everyday decisions such as what to eat or what to wear, and extends to major life decisions such as where to live and where to work and with whom. A major part of social existence involves the exercise of rights, for example a citizen's right to vote and the right to refuse to engage in particular activities.
4 Another component may be labelled competence and requires basic activities in communication, mobility, self-help, and social and leisure skills in order to participate fully in everyday activities.
5 The dimension of respect is dependent on the attainment of each of the other components.

In addition, a subjective aspect of the quality of life of the service users, their life satisfaction, must be taken into account as a relevant measure at least in comparative evaluative studies of services working under the same goals. The preconditions for the first two components – community presence and relationships – seem to be realised with the establishment of treatment facilities according to the principles of community mental health care *per se*. But the inclusion of quality of life variables as outcome measures in evaluation research is still in its infancy.

Community care is not superior in every single case. The needs of certain groups, such as some chronic and severe alcoholics, drug addicts and mental patients requiring long-term inpatient care or secure accommodation, are probably met at a higher standard and lower costs in a remote public hospital providing good residential care and proper rehabilitative opportunities. Suitable alternatives in the community are medically supervised homes with 24-hour nursing care, as suggested by Wing *et al.* (1992a). The two alternatives can fully be weighed against each other only by taking into account needs and local conditions.

Accessibility of services

Assuming a hierarchy of operational goals, a higher-order objective might be that a community mental health service must be freely accessible to the whole population of its catchment area and provide optimal care meeting that population's needs.

Subordinate to this overall objective are operational goals pertaining to priority of needs, organisation and delivery of services. The issue of 'needs-led' care involves at least four aspects: (a) epidemiological data on and appropriate assessment of needs, (b) setting priorities when resources are limited (Murphy, 1992), (c) provision of effective and efficient care for special target groups, such as children and substance-abusers, and (d) monitoring under-, mis- or overprovision.

The goal of free access involves (1) a financial aspect, covering necessary medical and social measures at least for those unable to pay. (2) The geographical aspect of free access depends on several factors: population density, transportation and need for emergency care. An investigation of access to the 24-hour emergency care and crisis intervention service operating at the Central Institute of Mental Health in Mannheim showed that the main factor influencing utilisation was proximity. Only a minority of users lived outside a 10-kilometre zone, corresponding to about 30 minutes by road (own car, taxi or ambulance) (Häfner-Ranabauer & Günzler, 1984). Evaluating nine model communities in Baden-Württemberg revealed a similar geographical utilisation pattern among chronic patients (Rössler *et al.*, 1987). Hence, the crucial factor for most patients with acute needs and patients with reduced help seeking due to disabilities appears to be that services are within easy reach. (3) The goal of needs-led provision implies adequate capacities of services in both quantitative and qualitative terms. However, needs in a catchment area do not remain stable. Considerable quantitative and qualitative changes occur as a result of various factors, such as increasing unemployment or a high influx of immigrants and refugees from other countries. In this context Wing *et al.* (1992b) have stressed the necessity for services to be flexible in order to be able to meet changing needs. (4) Finally, the symbolic term 'community' in community mental health care must be specified. If 'community' is operationalised as a catchment population or sector (Paumelle, cited after Walsh, 1987; Strathdee & Thornicroft, 1992), pronounced differences will appear (Lindholm, 1983): sector sizes of 250 000 according to the recommendations of the Expert Commission on

Mental Health in 1975 in Germany and according to the Community Mental Health Centers Act of 1963 in the United States, as well as of 300 000 in the Netherlands, contrast with sizes of 100 000 in Finland, 40 000 in Norway and about 25 000 in Sweden.

Strathdee & Thornicroft (1992) recommend sectors with some 50 000 inhabitants 'as workable units for planning, provision and evaluation of community mental health services'. They have listed 17 factors concerning population characteristics, the organisation of services and locality influencing the size and location of a catchment sector. Most of the demographic, social and morbidity variables are more relevant to the assessment of needs, whereas the administrative and service variables are more important in determining the size and boundaries of a catchment area and the location of services. Of the three levels of mental health care in general – (1) acute, emergency and crisis care, (2) intermediate-term care and rehabilitation and (3) long-term care – the in- and outpatient services at levels 1 and 2 have to be within easy reach, which has implications for the optimal size of a catchment area. As with level 3 and specialist services (such as inpatient services for psychogeriatric patients and children, advanced diagnostic equipment like CCT) it should be considered whether they will be sufficiently used and thus efficiently operated within a catchment area. For this reason many countries have hierarchically organised multi-level systems of health care sectors.

It should also be asked whether the psychiatric-care community or catchment area should be identical with the political or administrative community. The question has considerable implications for planning and financing services and cooperation with or integration into medical and social services. A final aspect is ethical in nature: Should the utilisation of mental health services be limited to those in the catchment area or should the patients have a choice?

Which of these sector sizes and models are more practicable, effective and acceptable to the patients is an issue that has so far been addressed more ideologically than by research.

Integration and coordination of mental health care

The diversity and complexity of the needs and services provided make further operational goals of mental health care necessary:

1 Community mental health services should coordinate their programmes and capacities as specialist contributors to a needs-based
network of care.
2 As far as possible the individual community mental health services
should be integrated into existing systems of health and social care
to ensure their efficiency.
3 In order to meet the complex needs of individual patients the work
of individual community mental health services must be coordinated
to ensure needs-matched rehabilitation programmes. In Great
Britain and the United States the task has been allocated to case
managers, in Germany to social-psychiatric services (Rössler *et al.*,
1993). The cost-effectiveness aspects of these solutions are still
rather obscure.

Before evaluating a service, one has to decide how the service is
defined. Many services in the mental health field are complex
mixtures of such components as treatment, therapy and case
management. As these different tasks may imply different objectives,
it is important to decide whether the evaluation should be concerned
with the service as a whole or with particular components (Blunden,
1991).

In recurring and chronic disorders only limited relief can at present
be achieved by a purely psychiatric treatment. Therapy interventions
hence represent only one component of the complex goals of
community mental health care. Non-psychiatric interventions are
additionally required, especially in this particular field of community
mental health care.

Background of evaluative research in community psychiatry

Besides the direct goals of psychiatric treatment, such as symptom
reduction, the aforementioned WHO definition also includes indirect
goals, such as the ability to do productive work and to fulfil important
social roles.

Social-role functioning depends on the effectiveness of therapy and
some external prerequisites, such as availability of the roles and
reciprocity of the social network. The ability to do productive work,

for instance, depends on the availability of proper employment. But this is precisely what is currently lacking in many countries. Accepting the targets defined means that mental health care in many cases has to face the difficult task of improving the external conditions.

A pragmatic response to the demand for help in several areas of life that lie beyond the actual competence of psychiatry has been a multidisciplinary team. Through the cooperation of various professions – psychiatrists, psychologists, social workers, psychiatric nurses – a wide range of problems beyond the repertoire of psychiatric therapy interventions has successfully been addressed. With the multidisciplinary team a new field of evaluative research was created: the study of its tasks and functions and the assessment of its effectiveness regarding appropriate goal criteria (Braff & Lefkowitz, 1979; McKechnie et al., 1981; Freeman et al., 1985; Mosher & Burti, 1989).

The goal attainment of a multidisciplinary mental health service depends on the prevailing health, economic and social conditions of the catchment area. The dependence on the social conditions became particularly plain in connection with mass discharges and hospital closures. In the United States, with its poorly developed social-security system, discharge from hospital frequently ended in poverty and homelessness (Torrey, 1988).

The past attempts of some NIMH-funded community mental health centre programmes in the USA not only to provide psychiatric care but also to improve the social and living conditions of the slum populations of large cities were most instructive. After initial successes it soon turned out that the extent of deprivation – poverty, high unemployment, racial conflicts, insecurity and crime – was such that the community mental health workers had to give up and declare the failure of the programmes. Kaplan & Roman (1973) have given an impressive account of the Lincoln Mental Health Center programme at the Albert Einstein College in the Bronx (New York).

From the US experience three basic preconditions for the stability and success of community mental health programmes can be derived: (1) it is necessary to preserve political neutrality; (2) the goals must be oriented to what can realistically be done; and (3) the services offered must be adjusted to the available resources of the programmes and the competence of the staff. The socio-ethical vision of a better society is not achievable by a multidisciplinary mental health care programme.

Social deprivation was also the consequence in some Italian communities lacking complementary services on a sufficient scale. In

Great Britain, Scandinavia and the Benelux countries cuts in available psychiatric hospital beds led to better alternative care thanks to a more tightly woven social security net (Giel & ten Horn, 1982; Häfner & Klug, 1982; Freeman *et al.*, 1985; Thornicroft & Bebbington, 1988).

Finding out needs for mental health care

Comprehensive documentation of all psychiatric contacts of a defined population in psychiatric case registers allows continuous monitoring of needs satisfaction (Wing *et al.*, 1992b) by structural indicators (Häfner & an der Heiden, 1991). But unmet needs cannot be discovered by utilisation data. Population studies are very expensive and therefore practicable in model areas only and not continuously. An approximation, though unsatisfactory, is the assessment of mental health needs in the clientele of general practitioners (Goldberg & Huxley, 1980; Weyerer & Dilling, 1984; Goldberg, 1991). Great differences in judging the need for psychiatric treatment between general practitioners and psychiatrists illustrate the problems of validity of such assessments.

Changes in the demographic and social composition of a population aside, continuous monitoring of unmet needs can only be accomplished by studying functional indicators such as waiting lists to psychiatric services or accumulation of psychiatric diagnoses in adjacent medical and social services, including homes for the homeless and those 'on the street'. An investigation commissioned by the largest social insurance company in the German Free State of Bavaria showed that of 27 238 patients with a psychiatric diagnosis who had received inpatient care in 1983, 49% were treated in mental hospitals but as many as 51% in units or hospitals of other medical disciplines, primarily internal medicine (Hospital Management, 1985). This finding reflects a substantial underuse of psychiatric inpatient services.

Chances of putting the results of evaluative research into effect

It was the moving descriptions by social scientists such as Goffman's *Asylums* in 1961 and coverage in the mass media, rather than research results, that led to the emergence of the community mental health movement. Against this background the studies by Wing & Brown (1970), showing that lack of social stimulation in long-stay patients causes secondary impairments, gave an impetus to reform processes in psychiatry.

In this historical context the avoidance of long-term hospitalisation emerged as the leading operational goal. E. Murphy (1992) has stated what the plans for community mental health services developed against this historical backdrop had in common: '... the policy of community care was ... adopted' as the new philosophy linking two themes, firstly, 'a plan for short-term treatment ... in district general hospital units, out-patient clinics, day hospitals, and community mental health centers ...' and, secondly, 'a network of hostel and home accommodation, social-work support, day care, and sheltered work for chronically disabled people, to provide a real alternative to the back wards of the mental hospital' (Murphy, 1992, p. 120).

Murphy complains that in England and Wales considerable deficits in the implementation of hostels, home accommodation and sheltered work exist. This applies to a far greater extent in many other countries, for instance a majority of the WHO European member states, as stated in the report by Freeman *et al.* (1985). Obviously, the reasons do not lie in the basic philosophy, but in social, political and financial constraints.

At present, results of evaluative studies revealing deficits in care delivery have a chance of being translated into better financial resources only under particularly favourable conditions. Nevertheless, they are as urgently needed as in more affluent times, in order to create an awareness of the problem amongst the public, to place demands with decision makers and to justify prioritising against other goals.

Setting priorities

In health care in general and in psychiatry in particular numerous attempts have been made at setting priorities in service provision. To give an example, E. Murphy, who has given a profound description of the issue, has proposed eight target groups in the following order of preference, assuming that setting priorities 'is an explicit rationing and control procedure aimed at containment of costs and getting better value for money' (Murphy, 1992, p. 125):

1 people with life-threatening acute disorders;
2 people with acute disorders posing a threat to other people's health or safety;
3 people detained under the Mental Health Act legislation and their aftercare;
4 adults with severe chronic mental disorders;
5 elderly people with dementia living at home and in institutions;
6 adolescents and young people with severe behavioural problems;
7 mentally abnormal offenders in need of secure accommodation;
8 people with markedly distressing long-term neurotic symptoms.

Implicit in the above list of priority groups, as in all comparable compilations, are value judgements and discretionary elements.

Financial constraints in many countries permit only costs-neutral changes such as the transfer of National Health Service hospital budgets to local authorities for alternative facilities in connection with the closures of Friern and Claybury Hospitals in London (Beecham & Knapp, 1992) or mobilising voluntary services such as patients' clubs and self-help groups, which play a very important role in promoting social integration and organising leisure activities for the socially disabled mentally ill.

In times of lean budgets the humanitarian aspect must be taken very seriously, namely that the mentally ill should be provided residential care corresponding to the standard of living of the healthy population, as J.K. Wing has stressed. In poor countries and large urban areas this goal is very hard to attain. Here psychiatry should come in as a lobby for the mentally ill, who themselves are unable to push their claims and consequently are easily forgotten when limited resources are being allocated.

Preconditions for the external validity of evaluative studies

From the history of community mental health care it is understandable why chronic mental patients with cognitive and social disabilities are the category most frequently subjected to the evaluation of their community care. Their needs are located at five levels (Table 2.1). In a community mental health service care is provided at various levels, corresponding to the living conditions of the healthy, no longer by a

Table 2.1. *Levels of needs for care of the socially disabled mentally ill*

1. Psychiatric treatment
   (a) Neuroleptic medication
   (b) Training of deficits and compensatory skills
   (c) Promotion of individual coping strategies
   (d) Family education and therapy

2. Accommodation and support in activities of daily living

3. Work and occupation

4. Social integration

5. Leisure activities

single large institution such as mental hospital but by a number of relatively small services with different programmes tailored to different needs.

To ensure the applicability of the results of evaluative studies to the mental health care systems of other localities, the following requirements must be fulfilled:

(1) The profiles of needs of the target groups must be sufficiently homogeneous and reliably assessed. In order to obtain homogeneous profiles of needs for evaluative purposes, Wing *et al.* (1992a) have proposed that so-called case mix groups with common needs should be used instead of diagnosis-related groups (DRG; Mitchell *et al.*, 1987). The only group that case mix has so far been applied to successfully are disabled chronic patients requiring intensive psychiatric and social care. Looking at Strathdee & Thornicroft's (1992) set of criteria for impairments, disabilities and handicaps, developed for the purpose of evaluating community mental health services, it is fairly obvious that the majority of the criteria apply to schizophrenics (Table 2.2).

(2) Programmes must be standardised or, for the purpose of comparison or replication, at least adequately described and based on clearly stated hypotheses about needs-based effectiveness. The standardisation of complex care packages and the categorisation of services is a difficult task. R. Giel in collaboration with WHO has developed an instrument for the description and classification of mental health care facilities, the International Classification of

Table 2.2. *A framework for inter-agency definition of severely mentally ill*

Impairments	Disabilities	Handicaps
Cognitive		
Difficulties in thinking	Inefficient problem solving	Lack of friends
Interference with thought processes	Slowed learning	Unemployment
Distressing experiences of sight, sound or touch		
Affective		
Unusual, strange beliefs	Severe anxiety and fear	Limited leisure activities
Difficulty in movements and actions	Feelings of inadequacy	Poor housing and self-care
Decreased concentration		
Behavioural		
Loss of energy and drive	Low rate of constructive actions	Carers' burden
Reduced ability to solve problems		

From Strathdee & Thornicroft, 1992.

Mental Health Care (ICMHC; de Jong *et al.*, 1989). It comprises eight levels of assessment (Table 2.3). Although the instrument is still marred by considerable qualitative shortcomings and problems of practicability, it is an important first step on a path that no one has trod before.

(3) The complex patterns of care actually provided must be mapped. A study on the utilisation of mental health care facilities of a cohort of 148 schizophrenic patients in Mannheim (an der Heiden *et al.*, 1989) provided some insight into the patterns of care after discharge from hospital. The patients were followed up at four cross-sections over a period of 18 months. The data were obtained by interviewing the patients and their relatives, and information was accumulated on the basis of 2-week intervals for the whole period. In almost half of all intervals the patients used more than one institution at the same time, mostly a combination of outpatient medical treatment and sheltered accommodation. But there were also a few patients who were in contact with up to five facilities at the same time.

In view of the multiplicity and parallel usage of services it is reasonable to ask to what extent individual services and facilities contribute to the attainment of which goals.

Table 2.3. *International Classification of Mental Health Care (ICMHC)*
(de Jong et al., 1989)

Instrument for the description and classification of care available for the care of
groups of patients and individual patients

Assessment period covered: 1 month prior to interview

Areas assessed: highest levels of care available to a category of needs versus care
actually provided to a group of patients or to a single patient

Dimensions:
PROP   (diagnostic and problems assessment)
CRIS   (crisis management at short notice)
SOCI   (attendant and supportive – social – interventions directed to the
            environment of patients)
PSYC   (psychological intervention, individual group, focused on changes in the
            patient's behaviour – psychotherapy, psychomotortherapy, creative
            therapy, etc.)
BIOL   (biological-psychiatric interventions – medications)
MEDI   (general medical care including medical and nursing directed towards
            the general medical care carried out in the framework of mental
            health care)
ADLF   (activities of daily living – self-management)
ACCO   (residence and accommodation within the framework of mental health
            care)

Each dimension is rated: 3, intensive; 2, moderate-intensive; 1, minimally
    intensive; 0, no or only incidentally occurring activities.

Acceptance of patients and services in the community

Last but not least the implementation of community mental health
programmes and the social re-integration of mental patients depends
on acceptance by the local population and the community at large. In
1963, when two houses for alternative facilities were being looked for
in Heidelberg, restaurant owners brought their case to the State
Parliament, fearing that tourists would stay away from Heidelberg, if
'the mad in striped clothing strolled in the Castle Gardens'. The
neighbours threatened to sue for the decreased value of their
property. Since then acceptance in the population has increased
through growing experience and information.

In Mannheim, with a population of 300 000 the Central Institute
of Mental Health serves as a counsellor to five homes, five of nine
group homes with 21 places in supervised apartments, one sheltered

workshop operated on two sites and five patient clubs. A telephone poll among persons living at different distances from the homes and differing in their knowledge of the mentally ill (Rössler & Salize, 1994) revealed that those who had come in contact with mentally ill persons had very realistic and therefore positive, but not unreservedly favourable opinions. In contrast, we were still confronted with vigorous protests quite recently when establishing the first psychiatric home in a small German town.

Conclusion: What should and what can be evaluated?

To sum up the tasks and possibilities of evaluative research in community psychiatry, a long list of open questions is matched by an equally long list of problems and hindrances. These difficulties, the short history of mental health services research and the more rapid output of publications and fruition of research careers in biological psychiatry are the reasons why the number of researchers working in the field of mental health care evaluation is so small and the state of knowledge so incomplete. It therefore seems necessary to set priorities in psychiatric research according to the importance of the issues studied for the outcome and quality of life of as many groups of patients as possible. It is also necessary to do everything possible to raise the number of qualified research workers dealing with these questions in order to increase research capacities in this extraordinarily important field, which has so far been dominated by programmes and activities based on ideologies and rough estimates.

References

Beecham, J. & Knapp, M. (1992). Costing psychiatric interventions. In *Measuring Mental Health Needs*, ed. G. Thornicroft, C. Brewin & J.K. Wing, pp. 163–83. London: Gaskell/Royal College of Psychiatrists.

Blunden, R. (1991). Assessing the quality of community mental health services. In *Mental Health Services in the United States and England: Struggling for Change*, ed. V.E. Fransen, pp. 83–90. Princeton, NJ: The Robert Wood Johnson Foundation Office.

Braff, J. & Lefkowitz, M. (1979). Community mental health treatment: what works for whom? *Psychiatric Quarterly*, **51**, 119–34.

Freeman, H.L., Fryers, T.H. & Henderson, J.H. (1985). *Mental Health Services in Europe: 10 Years On.* Copenhagen: World Health Organization, Regional Office for Europe.

Giel, R. & ten Horn, G.H.M.M. (1982). Patterns of mental health care in a Dutch register area. *Social Psychiatry*, **17**, 117–23.

Goffman, E. (1961). *Asylums: Essays on the Social Situation of Mental Patients and Other Inmates.* Garden City: Anchor/Doubleday.

Goldberg, D. (1980). *Mental Illness in the Community: The Pathway to Psychiatric Care.* London: Tavistock.

Goldberg, D. (1991). Integrating mental health in primary health care. In *Evaluation of Comprehensive Care of the Mentally Ill,* ed. H. Freeman & J. Henderson, pp. 115–24. London: Gaskell/Royal College of Psychiatrists.

Goldberg, D.P. & Huxley, S. (1980). *Mental Illness in the Community: The Pathway to Psychiatric Care.* London: Tavistock.

Häfner, H. & an der Heiden, W. (1989). The evaluation of mental health care systems. *British Journal of Psychiatry*, **155**, 12–17.

Häfner, H. & an der Heiden, W. (1991). Evaluating effectiveness and cost of community care for schizophrenic patients. *Schizophrenia Bulletin*, **17**, 441–51.

Häfner, H. & Klug, J. (1982). The impact of an expanding community mental health service on patterns of bed usage: evaluation of a four-year period of implementation. *Psychological Medicine*, **12**, 177–90.

Häfner-Ranabauer, W. & Günzler, G. (1984). Entwicklung und Funktion des psychiatrischen Krisen- und Notfalldienstes in Mannheim. *Fortschritte der Neurologie und Psychiatrie*, **52**, 83–90.

an der Heiden, W., Häfner, H. & Krumm B. (1989). *Die Wirksamkeit ambulanter psychiatrischer Versorgung. Ein Modell zur Evaluation extramuraler Dienste.* Berlin: Springer.

Hospital Management (1985). *Patientenstrukturanalyse Psychiatrie Bayern.* Scientific evaluation by Prof. Dr Böcker (Bayreuth), Munich.

de Jong, A., Giel, R., ten Horn, G.H.M.M., Brook, F.G. & van der Ende, P.C. (1989). *The International Classification of Mental Health Care (ICMHC): A Tool for Classifying Services Providing Mental Health Care.* Groningen: Collaborative Centre for Research and Training in Mental Health, University of Groningen.

Lindholm, H. (1983). Sectorised psychiatry. *Acta Psychiatrica Scandinavica*, **67** (Suppl. 304).

Kaplan, S.R. & Roman, M. (1973). *The Organization and Delivery of Mental Health services in the Ghetto: The Lincoln Hospital Experience.* New York: Praeger.

May, A.R. (1976). *Mental Health Services in Europe: A Review of Data Collected in Response to a WHO Questionnaire.* Geneva: World Health Organization.

McKechnie, A.A., Philip, A.E. & Ramage, J.G. (1981). Psychiatric services in primary care: specialised or not? *Journal of the Royal College of General Practitioners*, **31**, 611–14.

Milne, D. (1987). *Evaluating Mental Health Practice: Methods and Applications.* London: Croom Helm.

Mitchell, J., Dickey, B., Liptzin, B. & Sederer, L.I. (1987). Bringing psychiatric patients into the medicare prospective payments system: alternatives to DRG's. *American Journal of Psychiatry*, **144**, 610–15.
Mosher, L.R. & Burti, L. (1989). *Community Mental Health: Principles and Practice*. New York: Norton.
Murphy, E. (1992). Setting priorities during the development of local psychiatric services. In *Measuring Mental Health Needs*, ed. G. Thornicroft, C.R. Brewin & J.K. Wing, pp. 118–39. London: Gaskell/The Royal College of Psychiatrists.
O'Brian, J. (1987). A guide to lifestyle planning. In *A Comprehensive Guide to the Activities Catalogue: An Alternative Curriculum for Youth and Adults with Severe Disabilities*, ed. B. Wolcox & G.T. Bellamy, pp. 43–52. Baltimore: P.H. Brookes.
Renshaw, J., Hampson, R., Thomason, C., *et al.* (1988). *Care in the Community: The First Steps*. Aldershot: Gower.
Rössler, W. & Salize, H.J. (1994). Gemeindenahe Versorgung braucht eine Gemeinde, die sich sorgt: Die Einstellung der Bevölkerung zur psychiatrischen Versorgung und zu psychisch Kranken. *Psychiatrische Praxis*, **22**, 58–63.
Rössler, W., Häfner, H., Martini, H., an der Heiden, W., Jung, E. & Löffler, W. (1987). *Landesprogramm zur Weiterentwicklung der ausserstationären psychiatrischen Versorgung Baden-Württemberg; Analysen, Konzepte, Erfahrungen. Schlussbericht des Zentralinstituts für Seelische Gesundheit im Auftrag des Ministeriums für Arbeit, Gesundheit, Familie und Sozialordnung Baden-Württemberg*. Weinheim: Deutscher Studienverlag.
Rössler, W., Fätkenheuer, B. & Löffler, W. (1993). *Soziale Rehabilitation Schizophrener: Modell sozialpsychiatrischer Dienst* (Forum der Psychiatrie). Stuttgart: Enke.
Strathdee, G. & Thornicroft, G. (1992). Community sectors for needs-led mental health services. In *Measuring Mental Health Needs*, ed. G. Thornicroft, C.R. Brewin & J.K. Wing, pp. 140-62. London: Gaskell/ Royal College of Psychiatrists.
Thornicroft, G. & Bebbington, P. (1988). Deinstitutionalisation: from hospital closure to service development. *British Journal of Psychiatry*, **155**, 739–53.
Torrey, E.F. (1988). *Nowhere To Go: The Tragic Odyssey of the Homeless Mentally Ill*. New York: Harper & Row.
Walsh, D. (1987). Mental health service models in Europe. In *Mental Health Services in Pilot Study Areas: Report on a European Study*, ed. WHO. Copenhagen: WHO.
Weyerer, S. & Dilling, H. (1984). Prävalenz und Behandlung psychischer Erkrankungen in der Allgemeinbevölkerung: Ergebnisse einer Feldstudie in drei Gemeinden Oberbayerns. *Nervenarzt*, **55**, 30–42.
Wing, J.K. (1973). Principles of evaluation. In *Roots of Evaluation, ed. J.K. Wing & H. Häfner, pp. 3–12. London: Oxford University Press*.
Wing, J.K. & Brown, G.W. (1970). *Institutionalism and Schizophrenia: A Comparative Study of Three Mental Hospitals 1960–1968*. London: Cambridge

University Press.

Wing, J.K., Brewin, C.R. & Thornicroft, G. (1992a). Defining mental health needs. In *Measuring Mental Health Needs*, ed. G. Thornicroft, C.R. Brewin & J.K. Wing, pp. 1–17. London: Gaskell/Royal College of Psychiatrists.

Wing, J.K., Thornicroft, G. & Brewin, C.R. (1992b). Measuring and meeting mental health needs. In *Measuring Mental Health Needs*, ed. G. Thornicroft, C.R. Brewin & J.K. Wing, pp. 308–16. London: Gaskell/Royal College of Psychiatrists.

World Health Organization (1991). *Evaluation of Methods for the Treatment of Mental Disorders: Report of a Scientific Group on the Treatment of Psychiatric Disorders*. WHO Technical Report Series 812. Geneva: World Health Organization.

3

Research designs for the evaluation of services

JOHN K. WING

Introduction

The intention of the chapter is to show that research highly relevant for the evaluative comparison of alternative patterns of service can be successfully carried out even though strictly controlled designs are rarely applicable. Such research would be based firstly on the routine application of methods of clinical audit, secondly on routine monitoring using high-quality data recorded during ordinary clinical practice, and finally on the sampling frames provided by the resulting epidemiologically based mental health information systems. A range of more closely comparable and controlled experiments, which in the past would have required intensive data collection and long-term analysis and write-up, could be carried out at relatively little extra cost by using such systems either directly or as sampling frames.

A combined epidemiological and clinical strategy for evaluating the effectiveness and efficiency of mental health services is outlined. Examples are taken mainly from the United Kingdom where the National Health Service, in spite of the creation of an internal market, still has the opportunity to implement a strategy for mental health informatics that meets top-down managerial needs for information by using bottom-up clinical recording.

The three overlapping methods of evaluation (clinical audit, monitoring and partially controlled experiments) are considered, first separately and then in combination. Recent uncoordinated evaluative studies of acute and medium-term hospital care are considered. They illustrate current designs and methods, which provide useful but limited conclusions.

In summary, the planning of services could be both improved and speeded up by the adoption of an audited recording system based on a minimum of routinely collected clinical data collected once only by the clinicians themselves. Such systems would also support more practically applicable evaluative research.

Designs for evaluative studies

Knowledge of three broad and overlapping kinds provides a basis for planning and evaluating services. The first is recognition of the characteristics, epidemiology and causes (biological, psychological, social) of mental disorders and any associated social disablement.

The more knowledge of this kind accumulates, the easier it becomes to acquire the second, which is concerned with effective methods of primary, secondary and tertiary prevention.

Both kinds of knowledge facilitate the accumulation of the third, which is efficient and economical delivery of prophylaxis, treatment and care; including enough properly trained staff, enough settings where staff and users can interact to best advantage, and cost-effective planning and administration.

The following discussion is principally concerned with the acquisition of the third kind of knowledge, but in order to acquire all three kinds it is necessary to design studies that will make crucial comparisons. The eventual goal is to provide knowledge that can be used to minimise disablement and optimise autonomy.

Designs for evaluative studies of services must therefore apply knowledge of the first two kinds from two perspectives: public health and epidemiology is population-based (top-down); clinical work with patients/clients and their immediate social environment is person-based (bottom-up).

All such designs must contain the following statements:

- objectives of the research, which should be wider than the aims of the service under study;
- hypotheses to be tested;
- methods of sampling to achieve meaningful comparisons;
- techniques of measurement and data collection including needs assessment and costs;
- methods of analysis.

For convenience of exposition and discussion, designs are grouped into three kinds, elements of which are often combined in one project:

- Clinical audit is usually restricted to comparing clinical procedures for individual patients against normative standards such as agreed guidelines or peer review, though this does allow before and after comparisons (completing the audit cycle).
- Monitoring involves routine or special collection of data that can subsequently be used as part of comparative hypothesis-testing, though with less control of key variables. Such databases can be used as sampling frames for clinical audit or for more focused research.
- Focused research uses controlled, or partially controlled (quasi-experimental), comparisons to test specified hypotheses.

A rational plan of research to elucidate service problems in a given population would include studies of all these types.

Clinical audit

Clinical audit is the basis for good clinical practice. Well-educated health workers audit their own work according to professional guidelines, with regular peer review. The clinical audit cycle comprises assessment of problems, formulation of needs, interventions to meet needs, and assessment of outcomes in order to re-assess and re-formulate needs.

Clinical audit is regarded as being a separate kind of activity from research. But when focused on consecutive cases involving the same clinical problems, all from a defined population and using similar assessment procedures and standard guidelines, it can come close to meeting the criteria for a research project. The crucial distinction is that comparison is made against the guidelines, rather than against a control group with the same sampling but a specifically different pattern of care.

Clinical audit is most effective when based on continuing education, a tradition of critical peer review using agreed guidelines, and good-quality routine data recorded by all health workers in all relevant services within a defined population area. Such (audited) routine clinical records could form the basis for a systematic bottom-up mental health information system under clinical supervision.

Designs for monitoring

Most mental health information systems are based on data collected by clerks from routine paper records, usually concerned with activities (admission rates, length of stay, etc.) rather than with clinical problems, treatments and outcomes. Diagnosis is often the only clinical item but is of limited practical value for use on its own in a mental health record.

Case registers

Local cumulative psychiatric case registers provide a model for data collection in defined geographical areas, because dated contacts with designated services are stored in a linked and cumulative file so that the care of any individual or group can be followed over time, no matter how complex the pattern of service attendance. Statistics can therefore be based either on people or on service events. The problem of defining episodes can be operationalised. Register staff ensure that high-quality data are collected.

Case registers therefore provide a useful tool both for local and for comparative (including international) health services research, which fills some of the gaps left by national systems (Bahn *et al.*, 1966; L. Wing *et al.*, 1967; Wing & Hailey, 1972; ten Horn *et al.*, 1986; Wing, 1989; Tansella, 1991). However, they have usually been clumsy, labour intensive and limited in coverage. Getting information out of them is complicated and requires experts. The advent of desktop and portable computers did not come quite in time to save many of them. But the pace of technological advance continues to be fast enough to envisage the creation of far more powerful and comprehensive systems, capable of providing for most local and national information needs.

Mental health information systems

The main problems now remaining to be resolved are not technological, but the motivation of users and the quality of recording. In the United Kingdom, advance has been most rapid in general practice, where information systems are often integrated into both the administrative and the clinical work of local health centres. Nearly half of general practitioners have a terminal on the desk of their consulting room. Thus the professionals who deliver the clinical service also manage the business.

Apart from a few pioneer applications, developed by a few clinical workers for their own use on small local networks (Lelliott *et al.*, 1993), there is a dearth of such systems for specialist hospital or community care. The national information system has been created by managers with little clinical input. It is not much used by clinicians because they see no reward in it for patient care. By extension, they tend to regard all data collection systems as top-down and unrewarding.

The Information Management Group (IMG) of the National Health Service Management Executive has recognised the problem. Its strategy includes the statement that 'data will be derived from systems used by healthcare workers in their day-to-day work. There should be little need for different systems to capture information specifically for management purposes' (Information Management Group, 1992). However, most systems created so far provide activity data for management and purchasing, with little support for clinical care.

Nevertheless, it is acknowledged that a better system is required; one that will comprehensively serve clinical, management, public health and research purposes. The most basic drive to ensure a clinical input is through the creation of a national nomenclature of terms commonly used in clinical records, each with a unique identifier or 'Read' code. A first specialist version for application in local 'customised' systems, including mental health information systems, is to be released in October 1995 (NHS CCC, 1994; Wing & Rix, 1994).

Other central initiatives that have led to the commissioning of bottom-up studies in order to meet top-down requirements include the specification by government of a mental health target: 'To improve significantly the health and social functioning of mentally ill people'. In order to measure progress towards the target, a brief set of 12 scales, covering severity of behaviour, disability, symptoms and social environment, is now being extensively tested (Department of Health, 1993). If feasibility, sensitivity, reliability and performance against more complex instruments of good provenance are satisfactory, the Health of the Nation Outcome Scales (HoNOS) will be introduced for routine use to measure outcomes, as an interim measure before the introduction of computerised systems.

A further initiative from IMG is intended to create Health Related Groups (HRGs), defined as clusters of diagnoses and procedure codes which, when assigned to inpatient episodes and day cases, produce groups of patients whose hospital stays can be judged to have cost similar amounts in terms of the resources that they have consumed. As noted above, diagnoses are not ideal predictors of service use and further studies are now under way to discover whether extra clinical items (e.g. from HoNOS) will enhance their value substantially (Horn *et al.*, 1989).

If these techniques are successful, it is intended that they will become part of minimum clinical data sets (eventually to be computerised) for routine use throughout the health services.

Minimum clinical data sets

A clinical data set, the essential basis for a mental health information system includes:

- personal and other identifiers
- history items
- onset data (e.g. referral letter)
- date, setting and staff involved at each contact
- legal status
- types of problem at each contact
- preferred intervention for each problem specified
- termination of episode/spell (e.g. discharge letter)

When repeated over time the data set also measures outcomes, multi-agency contacts, episodes, etc., for individual patients. When aggregated for a district, with a proper regard for confidentiality, such data sets could form the clinical basis for a local mental health information system to which management data such as costs can be added and statistical records maintained. Data quality control should be the responsibility of the Public Health Director for the district.

In effect, these would be case registers in a new guise, substantially more comprehensive geographically and richer in content, and with wide-reaching practical uses, including comparative evaluation of aspects of the services. *Ad hoc* surveys, based on samples, provide rich additional data to test hypotheses derived from local experience.

Controlled and partially controlled (quasi-experimental) designs

Double-masked designs are difficult to apply in service evaluation for many reasons. The practitioner administering the care is part of the service being evaluated. Different practitioners (as well as different settings and modes of care) are therefore required for the experimental and control groups. The differences between these practitioners, their forms of treatment and care, and the resources and milieu of the settings in which they work, must be specified in advance and independently monitored. Measurement of the target problems in the two groups before, during and following care, should be independent of the practitioners and not influenced by knowledge of the type of care given.

These requirements are in addition to the adoption of strict rules for ensuring that samples are representative both clinically and socio-demographically of the target population. Also allocation to the comparison groups should be unbiased, and prior decisions made for dealing with premature termination of care.

Finally, the extent to which experimental services attract resources of staff, expertise and enthusiasm that cannot be matched in routine practice requires careful consideration when generalising from positive results.

It is rarely possible to mount controlled studies of mental health services that meet all these criteria. However, studies that include checks to minimise the disadvantages of partial control do have value, particularly if several of them (conducted by reputable teams) come up with the same answers. Such work is easier when starting from a specifiable sampling frame such as a case register or mental health information system (MHIS). Generalisability to a wider population remains suspect (depending in part on the epidemiological character- istics of the area) but, so long as the decisions of gatekeepers who control access to sampling points are specifiable and reasonably constant, useful conclusions can be drawn from comparisons of different patterns of service. The results of independent studies with similar objectives, designs and methods can then be compared and, in time, it should be possible to draw reasonably hard conclusions.

Alternatives to residential care in hospital

Partially controlled designs have most commonly been used recently in studies of alternatives to residential care in hospital; in particular, alternatives to acute inpatient care. Because the relevant mental disorders have a high incidence at relatively early ages and tend to a chronic course, the long-term costs, both direct and indirect, are considerable. Both cross-sectional and longitudinal approaches are therefore necessary. Most follow-up, however, has been short term. A caveat that applies to all studies of residential settings is that the influence of care should be separated as far as possible from that of staff and settings.

Different designs have been used. Early studies compared patients admitted to District General Hospitals with those admitted to large mental hospitals (Jones & Goldberg, 1980; Jones et al., 1980). An obvious problem arose as to whether the sampling could be equivalent.

A second group of studies was concerned with the results of decreasing the use of either type of inpatient care for acute psychotic disorders, e.g. by rapid transfer to day or domiciliary care (Endicott et al., 1978; Dick et al., 1985; Creed et al., 1991; Wiersma et al., 1991).

A third group involved attempts to avoid admission altogether by providing a dedicated programme of community care (Stein & Test, 1980; Weisbrod et al., 1980; Hoult et al., 1984; Burns & Raftery, 1991; Burns et al., 1993a, b).

Some general conclusions can be drawn. Admission cannot be avoided altogether. Clinical outcomes are not unequivocally improved by staying longer out of hospital, particularly in the long term. However, non-hospital care is more acceptable in the short term and possibly cheaper. In deprived areas (with higher rates of emergency admission and greater social isolation) the only acceptable alternatives are hostels with staff awake at night, which are more costly than family care. Such areas find it difficult, even in experiments, to maintain staff continuity. In all areas, the question of how long improvement is maintained and whether positive research results can be replicated in routine practice, remains open.

There is a further note of caution: the most comprehensive costing, which included some indirect costs (Weisbrod et al., 1980), showed the alternative to be more expensive. There is often a transfer of cost to patient, family, and society more generally, that is not openly acknowledged.

Three partially controlled studies have been made of alternative accommodation for people in hospital for between 6 months and 3 years. The smallest of these (Hyde et al., 1987) was the best controlled. It underpinned the results of the others (Gibbons, 1986; Wykes, 1982) in suggesting that residents found the accommodation acceptable and mostly preferable. But if the hostel was situated away from a hospital site, admission policy had to be selective.

Interrelationships between the three methods of evaluation

Each of these three ways of evaluating services contains elements of the others; they are not pure categories. Ideally, the strengths of each should be combined in such a way as to compensate for the weaknesses of each.

Insofar as it is based on an assessment of a particular case or event, by peers using 'state of the art' guidelines, the concept of clinical audit cannot be regarded as 'research' except in the sense that 'every treatment is a clinical experiment'. However, the routine practice of external and self-administered audit is intended to lead to a gradual improvement in the average general standard of practice. It should also include and improve the standards of clinical recording. Thus auditing a series of similar clinical events or situations provides a basis for systematic descriptive clinical research. The same analysis can be applied to the skills and training of staff and to the suitability, convenience, social milieu and accessibility of the settings in which clinical transactions are carried out. Systematic clinical audit is therefore as relevant to the evaluation of services as it is to that of assessment and the prescription of treatment.

The idea behind the testing of a set of simple, but reasonably reliable and outcome-sensitive, scales for the routine collection of medical, psychological and social information (HoNOS) is being extended to the creation of instruments covering most aspects of clinical work. HoNOS would be part of the top (i.e. routine) level of a hierarchical mental health information system that offered opportunities for collecting more detailed and specialised clinical and service data. In this way, the principles and methods of clinical audit would be linked to those of routine monitoring. Such routine collection of high-quality audited information would enhance the administrative usefulness of the system and its potential for the implementation of more powerful research designs.

The value of readily available high-quality routinely collected and population-based data about health services is immediately evident when the sampling and data collection methods of earlier partially controlled research projects are examined. A 5-year follow-up study of patients with schizophrenia admitted to three hospitals in 1956 is highly relevant in this context. The hypothesis was tested that patients in the district that had the best developed aftercare services would have fewer clinical and social problems than those in the other two districts. The results showed no difference between districts, possibly because the most intensive community service was found not to be engaging patients with the most severe problems (Brown *et al.*, 1966). The conclusions were based on a design and methodology that could have been applied to routinely collected data had the clinical and technological expertise been available at the time. The results might have had a more substantial impact on the planning of services had it been possible to produce and replicate them as part of a routine monitoring system, accepted by patients, healthcare workers and managers.

Conclusion: Use evaluative designs systematically

The three kinds of evaluative method (which actually overlap and can be combined in various ways) provide the opportunity for a multi-dimensional approach to care planning; one that draws on clinical practice, public health appraisal and managerial requirements to provide tried and tested data of good quality on which, eventually, political decisions could also be based.

Such research also provides instruments that can be used to monitor progress throughout the whole range of services, including those not in the public eye.

This concept of 'epidemiologically based audit' is the logical way to pursue excellence in socio-medical services. It has long been pointed out that, if national health systems allocated the same percentage of their turnover to research as do successful commercial companies there would be no difficulty in funding such a multi-faceted information base, or in setting up experimental services worthy of test.

The analysis of the interrelationship that could exist between the three types of evaluative method depends on a clinically based and controlled data collection system in which most of the data needed for both bottom-up and top-down research purposes are collected only once, at the time of contact with the patient.

At the moment, there are separate collection systems for each kind of information. This exposes their separate weaknesses. Written records rarely supply standard research data. Much information gathered in audit sessions is not recorded or is anonymised. Routine monitoring is based on items that can be collected clerically, such as length of stay or number of beds occupied or attendances at an outpatient department, which cannot be linked to clinical problems and outcomes. Partially controlled research projects usually have to rely on *ad hoc* methods of sampling and data collection, which make comparison and generalisation of the results difficult.

All three methods therefore enhance and benefit from each other. The advantages of an acceptable health information system for patient care are evident. The opportunities for undertaking services research within such a system would greatly improve both the quality and the likely implementation of the results.

References

Bahn, A.K., Gardner, E.A., Alltop, L., *et al.* (1966). Comparative study of rates of admission and prevalence for psychiatric facilities in four register areas. *American Journal of Public Health*, **56**, 2033.

Brown, G.W., Bone, M., Dalison, B. & Wing, J.K. (1966). *Schizophrenia and Social Care*. London: Oxford University Press.

Burns, T. & Raftery, J. (1991). Cost of schizophrenia in a randomised trial of home-based treatment. *Schizophrenia Bulletin*, **17**, 407–10.

Burns, T., Beadsmoore, A., Bhat, A.V., *et al.* (1993a). A controlled trial of home-based acute psychiatric services. I. Clinical and social outcome. *British Journal of Psychiatry*, **163**, 49–54.

Burns, T., Raftery, J., Beadsmoore, A., *et al.* (1993b). A controlled trial of home-based acute psychiatric services. II. Treatment patterns and costs. *British Journal of Psychiatry*, **163**, 55–61.

Creed, F., Black, D., Anthony, P., *et al.* (1991). Randomised controlled trial of day and in-patient psychiatric treatment. *British Journal of Psychiatry*, **158**, 188–9.

Department of Health (1993). *The Health of the Nation. Key Area Handbook.* Mental illness, pp. 44–5. London: DoH.

Dick, P., Cameron, L., Cohen, D., *et al.* (1985). Day and full-time psychiatric treatment: a controlled comparison. *British Journal of Psychiatry*, **147**, 246–50.

Endicott, J., Herz, M. & Gibbon, M. (1978). Brief versus standard hospitalisation: the differential costs. *American Journal of Psychiatry*, **135**, 707–12.

Gibbons, J.S. (1986). Care of 'new' long-stay patients in a DGH psychiatric unit: the first two years of a hospital-hostel. *Acta Psychiatrica Scandinavica*, **73**, 582–8.

Gibbons, J.S. & Butler, J.P. (1987). Quality of life for 'new' long-stay psychiatric in-patients: the effects of moving to a hostel. *British Journal of*

Psychiatry, **151**, 347–54.

ten Horn, G.H., Giel, R., Gulbinat, W. & Henderson, J.H. (1986). *Psychiatric Case Registers in Public Health*. Amsterdam: Elsevier.

Horn, S.D., Chambers, A.F., Sharkey, P.D. & Horn, R.A. (1989). Psychiatric severity of illness: a case mix study. *Medical Care*, **27**, 69–84.

Hoult, J., Rosen, A. & Reynolds, I. (1984). Community oriented treatment compared to psychiatric hospital oriented treatment. *Social Science and Medicine*, **18**, 1005–10.

Hyde, C., Bridges, K., Goldberg, D., *et al.* (1987). The evaluation of a hostel ward: a controlled study using modified cost–benefit analysis. *British Journal of Psychiatry*, **151**, 805–12.

Information Management Group of the NHS Management Executive (1992). *An Information Management and Technology Strategy for the NHS in England*. London: HMSO.

Jones, R. & Goldberg, D. (1980). The costs and benefits of psychiatric care. In *The Social Consequences of Psychiatric Illness*, L. Robins, P. Clayton & J.K. Wing, pp. 50–70. New York: Brunner/Mazel.

Jones, J., Goldberg, D. & Hughes, B. (1980). A comparison of two different services treating schizophrenia: cost–benefit approach. *Psychological Medicine*, **10**, 493–505.

Lelliott, P., Flannigan, C. & Shanks, S. (1993). *A Review of Seven Mental Health Information Systems*. Research Unit Publication no. 1. London: Royal College of Psychiatrists.

NHS Centre for Coding and Classification (1994). *Read Codes and the Clinical Terms Projects: A Brief Guide*. London: Department of Health.

Stein, L.J. & Test, K.A. (1980). An alternative to mental hospital treatment: a conceptual model, treatment program and clinical evaluation. *Archives of General Psychiatry*, **37**, 392–7.

Tansella, M. (ed.) (1991). Community-based psychiatry: long-term patterns of care in South-Verona. *Psychological Medicine. Monograph Supplement 19.* Cambridge: Cambridge University Press.

Weisbrod, B.A., Test, M.A. & Stein, L.I. (1980). Alternative to mental hospital. II. Economic cost benefit analysis. *Archives of General Psychiatry*, **37**, 400–5.

Wiersma, D., Kluiter, H., Nienhuis, F.J., *et al.* (1991). Costs and benefits of day treatment with community care for schizophrenic patients. *Schizophrenia Bulletin*, **17**, 411–19.

Wing, J.K. (ed.)(1989). *Contributions to Health Services Planning and Research*. London: Gaskell.

Wing, J.K. & Brown, G.W. (1970). *Institutionalism and Schizophrenia*. Cambridge: Cambridge University Press.

Wing, J.K. & Hailey, A.M. (1972). *Evaluating a Community Psychiatric Service. The Camberwell Register 1964–1971*. London: Oxford University Press.

Wing, J.K. & Rix, S. (1994). Read codes for the mental health professions: an update. *Psychiatric Bulletin*, **18**, 234–5.

Wing, L., Wing, J.K. & Hailey, A.M. (1967). The use of psychiatric services in three urban areas: an international case register study. *Social*

Psychiatry, **2**, 158–67.

Wykes, T. (1982). A hostel-ward for 'new' long-stay patients: an evaluative study of a ward in a house. In *Long-term Community Care: Experience in a London Borough, ed. J.K. Wing. Psychological Medicine Monograph Supplement 2.* Cambridge: Cambridge University Press.

4

Evaluation and public policy

FRANK J. SULLIVAN

Introduction

Sound public policy should rest on sound information, and analysis of that information from a policy perspective. A statement of the obvious? Not if you ask policy-makers about the availability of useful information! In fact, determinations of emphases for research and evaluation generally are not made with an eye to the interests and needs of policy-makers. On the contrary, there is some degree of intellectual resistance to examining a research and evaluation agenda according to criteria relating to the needs of public policy. But public resources for mental health depend to a great extent on how well the evaluation and research community interacts with the public policy community.

The aim of this chapter is to describe the information needs and interests of the public policy community, and the importance of the political process in maintaining and enhancing mental health programmes. The role outcome data – reflecting a full array of measures – is discussed. The complexity of organising systems of care in the context of both multiple levels of government and multiple sources of support for services is described, along with several examples of State planning activities. The chapter concludes with a discussion of advocacy in the political process with a focus on mental health consumers' and families' interests, and the role of the research and evaluation communities.

Information for policy-makers

To meet the interests and needs of policy-makers, data must be timely, pertinent to the policy-level decisions, and analysed and presented in the context of other relevant information so that their implications are clear both to the policy-makers and to the policy-makers' constituents. The policy-maker will want to understand the extent to which results are replicable, statistically robust, and relevant to the issue at hand. But neither a policy-maker nor a politician is in a position to engage in a detailed analysis of the technical aspects of information used to support a recommended course of action. Hence, communication must be so clear that the facts, and their implications, can be accepted at face value by decision-makers and the constituencies they must respond to. Thus, information should also address the points that advocacy and other groups that impinge on public policy are likely to raise. The concerns of advocacy groups, budget analysts, zoning commissioners, health providers, civil rights advocates and legislators are not necessarily the concerns that the academic and professional worlds view as most significant. But to be useful, information must be clear and address the full range of perspectives of the user.

Miles Shore and Martin Cohen, directors of the Robert Wood Johnson Foundation Program for Chronic Mental Illness, have summarised the Program's experiences. All the nine Robert Wood Johnson cities made progress towards the aim of systems integration over a 5-year period, but none successfully achieved full integration of community care and State hospitals. In analysing the factors that influenced the success of the programmes, Shore & Cohen (1992) underscored the importance of the policy and political communities, noting that the process of creating systems of care for people with serious mental illness is as much a matter of applied political science as it is of mental health.

The current debate in the United States concerning health care reform illustrates the types of issues which must be addressed by policy-makers and then decided by politicians. A critical question has been the inclusion of substance abuse and mental health benefits in health insurance coverage, and the type and extent of benefits that should be provided. Some of the information needs related to this debate include:

- definitions of 'mental illness' and 'substance abuse';
- determination of numbers and socio-demographic characteristics of affected individuals and those at risk;
- the degree of illness that should trigger eligibility for coverage;
- determination of existing treatment capacity for these illnesses, as well as the cost of expanding capacity;
- estimation of likely demand for services;
- identification of effective treatments, including the special treatment needs resulting from differences in language or ethnic culture;
- identification of effective treatment systems;
- identification of appropriate quality assurance mechanisms;
- syntheses of treatment outcome via appropriate measures, including patient and family satisfaction with those outcomes;
- determination of the numbers and types of providers of services that are required;
- identification of barriers to accessing treatment;
- strategies for overcoming the stigma associated with these illnesses;
- strategies for dealing with these illnesses as chronic and recurring, with reasonable expectations of improvement following intervention but with recovery rates that are in line with other illnesses that can be chronic;
- cost; at each and every stage of discussion, cost is a pivotal question.

These information needs are staggering. In attempting to develop information and arguments in support of major systems-level changes, it becomes clear that many important areas have not been the subject of research or services demonstration and evaluation, and that there are broad areas essential to the decision-making process with little or no associated data or reliable information.

Developing outcome data

Fundamental to most policy and resource debates is the issue of impact and cost. As health and mental health programmes seek simultaneously to contain costs, increase access and increase quality, better measures of outcome and satisfaction will be needed. It is essential to develop valid, reliable and obtainable outcome measures which reflect the effectiveness of our systems of care. These outcome measures need to be meaningful and understandable and, above all, provide the policy and advocacy communities with a measure of performance for systems of care.

To date, the mental health field can be faulted for insufficient attention to the development, standardisation and use of such measures. The challenge is all the greater when we recognise that within the health care system, the provision of care for mental illnesses is held to a higher 'standard of proof'. There is overt scepticism about the capacity of the mental health field to characterise and understand mental disorders, and to treat and care for persons with mental illness. Despite advances in our knowledge about the aetiology of mental illness and how systems can be put in place to serve persons with a mental disorder, this perception continues to plague the mental health field. The lack of objective, replicable information about treatment and service systems outcome contributes to this perception, and also to the discrimination against persons with mental illness.

The process of developing appropriate outcome measures will not be a simple one. Because so many consumers of mental health services receive 'service packages', there is a need to develop comprehensive, multi-dimensional outcome models. To be useful in the context of public policy, the process of developing outcome measures should include:

- identification of specific outcomes of importance to various constituency groups – consumers, family members, clinical and administrative staff, provider organisations and systems managers;
- development of consensus around the *minimum* set necessary to meet needs;
- mechanisms for putting an outcomes-based monitoring system into place, including bolstering of evaluation capacity at the State, the local government, and the provider levels; and
- linkage of the public and private sectors' interests.

Finally, results must be presented to policy-makers and the public in a *distilled* manner, so that the complexity of the data does not obscure the core results and what they mean for policy. The research and service communities should capitalise on the current interest in competition and customer satisfaction in order to enlist consumer and provider participation in research and advocacy for cogent outcome measures.

The complexity of organising systems of care

The task of informing public policy and decision-making must take into consideration the complexity of funding streams and systems of care, the coexistence of multiple systems of care, and the dynamics of interaction of various governmental entities. Koyanagi & Goldman (1991) have provided an excellent analysis of Federal involvement in US mental health policy during the 1980s, and a synopsis of the primary funding streams and Federal programmes which provide for the needs of individuals with severe mental illnesses within the public system of care.

Federal funding provides partial support for the public system of mental health care, which is funded primarily at the State level. There is also the private system of care, funded primarily by insurance reimbursements but also with some funding by reimbursements from public funds. The coexistence of these two systems, and the lack of parity of insurance benefits for individuals with mental illnesses with benefits for other illnesses, results in continual migration of severely mentally ill individuals from the private system to the public system. There are usually low lifetime benefit limitations on insurance coverage for mental illnesses (typically enough to support two or three relatively brief hospitalisations or a few years of outpatient care). When these limits are reached, individuals must rely on the public sector for their care.

As described succinctly by Koyanagi & Goldman (1991), in 1978 the President's Commission on Mental Health, established by President Jimmy Carter, reviewed mental health needs and prepared recommendations for Federal action. Among other things, the Commission recommended legislation in the form of a comprehensive Mental Health Systems Act. The Commission also launched a process to develop a national plan for caring for severely mentally ill individuals; the plan was to focus on the primary Federal funding streams for mental health services. The Commission's legislative recommendations resulted in passage of the Mental Health Systems Act in October 1980 – just prior to the election of President Ronald Reagan. As a result of this change in political leadership, the Mental Health Systems Act was repealed the very next year, and its provisions never were put into effect.

Changes in policy during the 1980s led to a decline in Federal support for programmes specifically for mentally ill individuals; nearly all existing categorical programmes were combined in a block grant to States for mental health and substance abuse treatment. The block grant considerably reduced the total specific funding available for mental health services. In the period from 1983 to 1990, block grant funds dropped from 11% to 6% of community programme expenditures (Center for Mental Health Services and National Institute of Mental Health, 1992). During the same period, Federal support for low income housing also was sharply reduced.

Despite these setbacks, progress did occur during the 1980s, by expanding eligibility for individuals with severe mental illnesses for 'mainstream' Federal programmes for support of individuals with disabilities. These include:

- the *Social Security Disability* Insurance programme, for workers and their dependents who become disabled;
- the *Supplemental Security Income* programme, for individuals who are aged, blind or disabled and who have limited financial resources and limited or no income;
- *Medicaid*, a jointly funded Federal–State programme to pay medical expenses for certain low-income individuals; and
- *Medicare*, a health insurance programme provided to persons who are aged or disabled.

Through small gradual changes in these mainstream financing programmes, many of the Carter Commission's recommendations were implemented, providing access to some additional resources for persons with a mental illness. Koyanagi & Goldman (1991) attribute these events to a redirection of energy on the part of advocates and others towards effecting seemingly minor changes in existing health funding programmes, which have substantially increased the eligibility of individuals with severe mental illnesses for these types of public assistance. Of great significance was the fact that the perceived threat of policy change and cutbacks in the early 1980s brought together groups within the mental health community and the disability community that had not previously worked in concert. More recent evidence of the effectiveness of these coalitions was the passage in 1990 of the Americans with Disabilities Act, which explicitly includes individuals with mental disabilities.

Intergovernmental dynamics

Because in most countries mental health services are supported by multiple levels of government, intergovernmental relationships and responsibilities are of great importance to policymakers. In the United States, the level of Federal involvement – in terms of policy, legislation and funding – has varied. During the 1980s, the balance underwent a definite shift away from Federal involvement towards re-emphasising the role of the States. In many States there is now a trend towards increased control and authority at local levels.

The current Federal role is embodied in legislation, enacted in 1986, which mandated that States develop and implement plans for organised community-based systems of care for adults with severe mental illness and children with serious emotional disturbance. Plans under Public Law 99-660 were to include access to mental health services; reductions in the rate of hospitalisation of individuals with severe mental illness; provision of case management services; outreach for homeless persons with mental illness; and linkages to housing and other supportive services necessary for individuals with severe mental illness to live in their communities.

The legislation mandated creation of a planning council in each State to include individuals with mental illnesses and their families; providers; and individuals with related responsibilities within State government such as education, criminal justice, welfare, health and housing. The product was to be a State plan addressing a number of specific requirements, aiming toward the establishment of an organised, comprehensive community-based system of care. The legislation contained a penalty provision that if States failed to comply, they could be assessed a penalty of up to 10% of their Block Grant funds. Initially, some funds were provided to States to carry out this planning process, but specific funding for planning was phased out.

Compliance with the specifics of this law has been a major challenge for States. There is general agreement that, by providing the vehicle for all interested parties to work together towards the improvement of services for individuals with mental illnesses, the State planning law has been effective in encouraging improvements in systems of care.

The positive aspect of these laws is that existing Federal funding is leveraged to produce systems change. A negative aspect is the continuing pressure on States to carry out this and other 'unfunded Federal mandates' in an economic climate of declining resources at all levels. Ross & Mazade (1991) cite this as a significant problem in Federal–State relations. States believe that although reductions in Federal funding have led to a reduced Federal role, the burden of Federal reporting requirements and services standards that are a condition for receiving Federal funds has increased substantially. The challenge of working within the myriad funding streams – all of which have separate requirements, eligibility criteria and application processes – siphons energy and resources at the State level which might otherwise be directed towards coordination and integration of services.

States have struggled to find the resources to effect changes that, in the long run, have the potential to provide much more effective care at lower cost. In keeping with the emphasis on influencing mainstream health and social support programmes to the benefit of persons with mental illness, a major issue at the State level in recent years has been an effort on the part of a number of States to ensure that they use Medicaid to the full extent permitted by Federal law. States which have been successful in accomplishing this have greatly enhanced the funding available for treating individuals with severe mental illnesses. An increasing number of States have implemented new ways of drawing upon this funding source.

A number of States are using combinations of Federal and State funds to pay for mental health services. One of these is Ohio, which implemented the Ohio Mental Health Act in 1988, the purpose of which was to create an integrated system of care that gives local communities more control over how mental health dollars are spent. The Act assigns responsibility for local services to local Boards, reaffirms the importance of inpatient care as part of a full range of mental health services, and redefines the State's role in operating both hospital and community-based programmes.

The process of change in Ohio has been well documented, as a result of a policy commitment to research and evaluation as well as a legislative mandate establishing an independent study committee to review changes.

The Ohio study committee has recently completed an assessment of the implementation of the legislation (Study Committee on Mental Health Services, 1993). The Committee reported five key findings:

1 Substantial progress has been made in implementing the Mental Health Act since its passage in 1988. State hospitals have been downsized and local Boards have assumed responsibility for providing community-based services to people who previously received care in State hospitals. Funds have shifted from State hospitals to community settings at a rate slower than authorised by the Act.

2 More persons are receiving community services than in 1988 – particularly those identified as priority populations in the Act: adults with a serious mental illness and children and adolescents with serious emotional disturbances. However, people who did not meet these definitions experienced a *decline* in the availability of services over the 5-year period.

3 Funding shortages have prevented some communities from developing improved community support systems – and have slowed efforts to enhance communities' capacity to meet mental health needs. Capacity building funds were not allocated in amounts anticipated as needed; the mental health system's share of State General Revenue funds has declined.

4 Development of essential community support services, including employment services, vocational rehabilitation and housing assistance, has not kept pace with growing demands for services and/or the movement of people from State hospital inpatient care to community-based programmes. Waiting lists for housing and other community services are getting longer as the demand for community services continues to grow.

5 Local Boards and providers have not universally implemented approaches and technologies to outreach, diagnosis, treatment and programme development. For example: African-Americans are disproportionately served in hospital settings and their access to community-based services is more limited than for other populations; the lack of appropriate, effective services for people with mental illness compounded with substance abuse problems is one of the most pressing clinical problems experienced by the system; and the development of mental health services for children/youth and their families continues to lag behind those developed for adults.

The Study Committee articulated about 30 recommendations, including the establishment of an improved evaluation process that attempts to measure the impact of service delivery on consumers' quality of life; support of service system evaluation and research, particularly outcome research; expansion of dissemination of findings from research projects; facilitation of local evaluation efforts; funding of innovative programmes and plans for evaluating programme outcomes and disseminating findings; and other recommendations which provide the type of information decision-makers will need in order to track the progress of implementation of the law and take corrective action as needed.

Ohio's considerable progress to reform the mental health system has been enhanced by the State's emphasis on services research, evaluation, and the improvement of data systems within the State. Such information gives the various constituencies which have participated in the process uniform information on which to base decisions and recommendations. Without sound information, it is difficult to bring together the divergent points of view of advocates and other constituents to obtain a consensus which gives policy-makers and politicians the ability to effect change.

The State of New York provides another example of a long-range, comprehensive planning process for mental health services which is much broader than that mandated by Federal planning laws. New York's most recent published plan (Office of Mental Health, 1993) articulates the State perspective on challenges for the 1990s; provides an overview of the State mental health system; sets out programmes, special populations and research plans; sets out plans for capital and facility planning; and describes the planning process.

The document mentions statutory changes within the State which are expected to affect the financing of the State public mental health system, including a continuing process of shifting the locus of services and funding from State inpatient care to a comprehensive, community-based system of care. An accompanying shift to local government of an increasingly greater part of programme planning and implementation responsibility is anticipated. New Medicaid programme options are envisioned within the State's Medicaid managed care legislation.

The New York plan articulates a number of principles that the plan is intended to ensure, and in so doing illustrates the interests of the policy and advocacy communities. These principles are:

- that the participation of current and former recipients of services and their families in decision-making at all levels is expanded;
- that significantly greater resources (capital and programme) are allocated to serving persons who are homeless and diagnosed with serious mental illness;
- that existing incentives that encourage children, especially those

with serious emotional disturbances, to be sent away from their homes are replaced with local arrangements for appropriate care;
- that new job opportunities and training are available for State workers displaced by State hospital closures and downsizing;
- that incentives exist for community providers to serve patients who are at 'high risk' of engaging in violent behaviour and often fall through the 'cracks' in the system;
- that incentives encourage excess general hospital inpatient capacity (where it exists) to convert to outpatient and community services for recipients of mental health services; and
- that the administration of mental health services in New York City is streamlined by merging City and State administrative functions.

As is clear from the complexity of this agenda at the State level, the information needed to inform such a process is immense, and New York State has long been a leader in the development of research and evaluation data to support policy development and programme monitoring.

Researchers and the policy process

In the face of varying and shifting intergovernmental arrangements, multiple funding streams, and separate but overlapping systems of care for individuals with mental illnesses, how can the research and evaluation communities participate in the introduction and support of new services for persons with mental illness?

Data that are to the point, and presented in a clear, concise manner, are just the beginning. In his analysis of the administrative barriers to effective systems change in mental health, Yellowlees (1990) observes that apathy and passive resistance are key obstacles, and that new transitional funding for the process of change must be found since 'old' services need to be kept operating until newer systems are in place. Yellowlees likens achieving change to a battle: 'The battle to be fought, therefore, is primarily one "for hearts and minds" – including the paramount need to generate effective political will – so that willing co-operation may replace negative apathy and that money which has to be found – is found.' The solid knowledge and credibility of the research and evaluation communities are essential assets for 'the battle'.

It is possible to answer key questions that can inform and impel policy-makers to adopt policies and to advance legislation that will effect systems change and improvement. Hoult (1990) describes how a research project led to the development of new community-based services for persons with mental illness in the Australian State of New South Wales. Mental health services are funded primarily by the State government, with services organised through 11 regional health areas. Hoult's research, undertaken with both Commonwealth and State funding, began in 1979, and was published in 1983. The culmination of his initial studies coincided with establishment of a New South Wales Public Inquiry into Services for the Psychiatrically Ill and Developmentally Disabled, known as the Richmond Inquiry. His presentations to the Inquiry and continuing involvement in the implementation of the Richmond Report provide an excellent case history. As clinical and evaluation experts, Hoult and his colleagues observed at first hand interactions with multiple levels of government (State Treasury, Health and Housing officials, Commonwealth officials, administrators in New South Wales' health regions), and with a diverse array of interest groups (unions representing doctors, nurses and other health workers, the media, clinicians, and advocacy groups).

In summing up his experiences, Hoult points to the importance of a number of factors, among them persistence in the face of frustration, delay and opposition; exploiting opportunities to develop and exert leadership roles; maintaining credibility via continuing evaluation as new projects were implemented; maintaining support at various organisational levels; and advocacy. (Interestingly, advocates for the developmentally disabled played a much stronger role than did advocates for the persons with mental illness.) Clear, unambiguous communication of results was key, as was personal contact with policy officials. As Hoult notes, 'submissions and proposals which are left to find their own way in the world solely on their merits do not go far. Success depends on persistent but appropriate lobbying of the bureaucrat who has the power to make the decision'.

Advocacy and the political process

Hollingsworth (1992) examined the care of chronically mentally ill persons in the United States, Germany and the United Kingdom, in the context of the structure of each country's general medical care system. The status of community services – 'frail and inadequate' in all three countries – was found to be related less to the organisation of health care than to the national priority given to mental health services. Her conclusion points to the importance of the advocacy and policy processes.

The improvement of systems of care for individuals with mental illnesses can come about when there is adequate information to reach sound recommendations that can be put forward and implemented by policy-makers. But moving from idea to implementation requires a consensus among concerned parties, and their ability to draw in funding support. The role of advocacy groups at the local, State and Federal levels is key.

The principal advocacy groups within the mental health community are those which represent consumers, family members, and associations which represent the mental health professional, provider and administrative communities. As noted above, the perceived threats to care for individuals with mental illnesses in the early 1980s led to greater cooperation and collaboration among those groups and also cooperation with other constituencies representing individuals with other types of disabilities.

Surles (1994) describes the 'turbulent environment' of mental health administration in the context of developments in the last two decades. In describing changes in eight areas, he characterises the current level of political support as 'only marginal' in the face of increasingly limited resources for health and social services. He also notes the importance of family and mental health consumer organisations as participants in the policy development process. Organisations representing family members emerged as a powerful force in the early 1980s. Equally significant in the past few years has been the increasing voice that consumers of mental health services have demanded – and won – in determining services and systems of care.

Consumers can be the voice for others with emotional disorders who may not be able adequately to express their feelings. Consumers promote the concepts of recovery and wellness, in which they have the most fundamental stake. On a daily basis, they live with the successes and failures of the mental health system. Family members, too, have 'been through it all'. They know the inadequacy of insurance coverage for mental illnesses. They have witnessed their relatives with mental illnesses being imprisoned in jails that have no linkages with local mental health systems. They know what it is like to be denied information about their adult child's condition and treatment alternatives, despite the fact that they are the primary caregiver for that individual.

When one talks with consumers – individually and with representatives of organisations of consumers – one hears a lot about the person-specific outcomes and the system characteristics they want to see:

- a reduction in financial and system-imposed barriers to care;
- participation in treatment decisions, and in system decisions and policy development;
- jobs; training programmes that include less repetitive tasks and less sheltered environments; job exchanges promoting real work opportunities – both short and long term; and support for continuing education programmes;
- the opportunity to have friends and companionship;
- practical, understandable, research-based information;
- support for consumer teams to educate mental health professionals in consumer needs perspectives;
- a mental health system that offers hope, and promotes the concept of recovery;
- respect, dignity, and the right to choose.

Mental health consumers really do not want much that is different from general health consumers. Stressing this commonality of interests between health and mental health consumers may help the general public and policy-makers to appreciate the mental health field.

The evaluation research community is in a unique position to contribute to policy development, and in implementation of policy on programmes to meet the needs of persons with mental illness. But fulfilling the promise of that position requires attention to the interests and needs of policy-makers and their constituents. Many evaluation scientists have recognised the benefits – to their work and to the utilisation of their work – of active dialogue with the full range of constituent and advocacy groups, but this dialogue needs to expand.

References

Center for Mental Health Services and National Institute of Mental Health (1992). *Mental Health, United States, 1992.*

Hollingsworth, E.J. (1992). Falling through the cracks: care of the chronically mental ill in the United States, Germany, and the United Kingdom. *Journal of Health Politics, Policy, and Law*, **17**, 899–928.

Hoult, J. (1990). Dissemination in New South Wales of the Madison Model. *In Mental Health Care Delivery: Innovations, Impediments and Implementation*, ed. I.M. Marks. Cambridge: Cambridge University Press.

Koyanagi, C. & Goldman, H. (1991). *Inching Forward*. Alexandria, Virginia: National Mental Health Association.

Office of Mental Health (1993). *Statewide Comprehensive Plan for Mental Health Services 1994–1998*. Albany: State of New York.

Ross, E.C. & Mazade, N. (1991). Doing more with less: mental health responses to Federal mental health policies. *Administration and Policy in Mental Health*, **18**, 461–7.

Shore, M. & Cohen, M. (1992). Grant watch: observations from the program on chronic mental illness. *Health Affairs*, **11**, 227.

Study Committee on Mental Health Services (1993). The Results of Reform: Assessing Implementation of the Mental Health Act of 1988. Final Report.

Surles, R. (1993). Significant changes in mental health: 1972–1992. *Administration and Policy in Mental Health*, **21**, 123–8.

Yellowlees, H. (1990). Administrative barriers to implementation and diffusion of innovative approaches to mental health care in the United Kingdom. In *Mental Health Care Delivery: Innovations, Impediments and Implementation*. Ed. I.M. Marks. Cambridge: Cambridge University Press.

PART II

COMPREHENSIVE SERVICE
EVALUATION PROJECTS

5

The Copenhagen Community Psychiatric Project (CCPP)

HELLE CHARLOTTE KNUDSEN, ALLAN KRASNIK, MERETE NORDENTOFT, BIRGIT JESSEN-PETERSEN AND HENRIK SÆLAN

Introduction

In a typical study evaluating the changes produced in a community by the introduction of community psychiatric services, an assessment of the utilisation of psychiatric care is made *before* the introduction of these new services and utilisation is then *assessed* after the services have been in place for some period of time. The impact of the community mental health centres (CMHCs) is measured by the pre–post changes observed and may be attributed to the effects of the introduction of the new services (Wing & Hailey, 1972; Häfner & Klug, 1982; Stefansson & Cullberg, 1986; Rudas, 1990; Tansella *et al.*, 1991; Søgaard, 1993). Few studies of service-level outcome have employed a control district (Haroutun & Babigian, 1977; Valbak *et al.*, 1992). Only, however, if changes observed in the intervention districts are not noted in the control districts can we be justified in attributing the changes in utilisation of services to the introduction of the new services.

Most research evaluating the effects of the institution of community psychiatric services describes changes in inpatient, outpatient and CMHC utilisation. The introduction of a CMHC may, however, affect other parts and functions of the community such as the social welfare system, privately practising psychiatrists and general practitioners. Indeed this is often an aim of these centres. Thus, potentially important effects of the new CMHC may be overlooked if the assessment of the effects is not comprehensive.

This chapter presents data which speak to the issue of control districts and comprehensiveness of design by describing an evaluation project conducted in Copenhagen: The Copenhagen Community Psychiatric Project (CCPP). The remainder of this chapter will include a description of the Danish mental health care system and the background of the evaluation project, details of the methodology of the project, results of the changes in utilisation which followed the introduction of the CMHC and data relating to our attempt to increase the comprehensiveness of an assessment of change. In appropriate analyses the importance of control groups will be highlighted.

Background

The Danish social welfare system ensures basic economic support for all residents of Denmark. Health services (including psychiatric services) are a part of a national health system. Privately practising psychiatrists are paid by the public health authorities for a limited number of visits for each patient referred by general practitioners to the psychiatrist (Knudsen et al., 1992b).

Mental health services in the city of Copenhagen are organised with acute wards in general hospitals of inner-city Copenhagen and a major mental hospital outside the city.

In 1969, the Municipality of Copenhagen (about half a million people) was divided into four catchment areas, one for each of the city's general hospitals. In December 1987 (Københavns Hospital-sdirektorat, 1987) the City Council legislated a system for the development of community psychiatry. Two experimental CMHCs were opened on 1 April 1989. The focus of the CMHCs is the assumption of total responsibility for the mental well-being of the population of their catchment area (about 30 000 people). The specific goals of the CMHCs in Copenhagen are to:

- provide psychiatric treatment locally for patients;
- provide preventive interventions (at the primary, secondary and tertiary levels) for at-risk district residents and through changes in district structures and functions;
- coordinate the work of the health services, the social welfare system and other services involved in the care of the mentally ill;
- provide multidisciplinary cooperation to encourage continuity of care.

The City Council also took the extraordinary decision of mandating independent research evaluative procedures to help guide the future development of CMHCs (Københavns Kommune, 1987). This action of the City Council was the impetus for the initiation of this evaluation research project.

Research methods

Research design

An experimental CMHC was established in an intervention district (ID) within the catchment areas of each of two of the general hospitals of the city of Copenhagen. From each of the catchment areas of these two general hospitals, control districts (CDs) were selected. It was agreed that no mental health or social welfare system interventions would be instituted in these two CDs during the course of the evaluation study.

We attempted to match CDs and IDs for size of population, age distribution, type of housing and number of social welfare clients (Statistisk Kontor, København, 1988). The most important criterion for definition of a CD, however, was that it was in the same general hospital catchment area as the ID.

Intervention and control districts

ID-1 and CD-1 are similar in terms of the background population's distribution of age, sex, unemployment rate, and family structure (Fig. 5.1). ID-1, however, is better off with respect to educational level, average income, number of residents on disability pension and social welfare support.

ID-2 and CD-2 are similar in their background population's age and sex distributions (Fig. 5.1); they differ with respect to educational level, level of unemployment, disability pensions, social welfare support and family structure. With respect to all of these differences, ID-2 is relatively disadvantaged.

The two IDs differs markedly from each other, ID-1 being the most prosperous district of Copenhagen and ID-2 being the socially most deprived district of Copenhagen.

The community mental health centres

The CMHCs are *additional* psychiatric services for the populations of their districts. They are under the administrative control of the

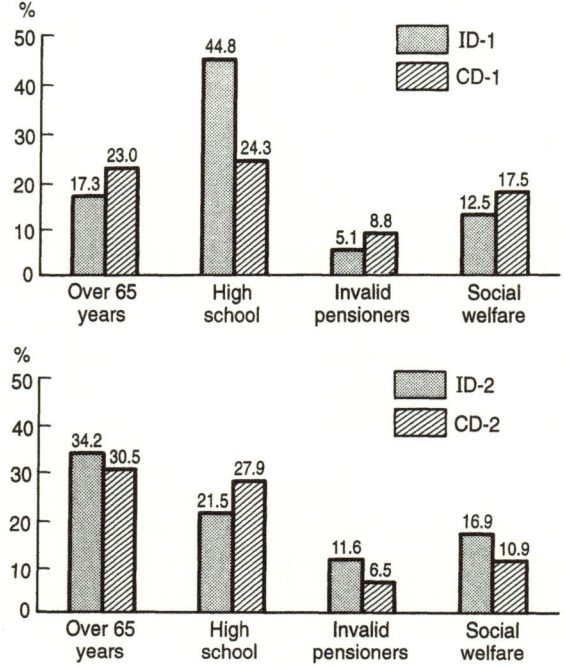

Fig. 5.1. Socio-demographic characteristics of the background population aged 18 years or more in the intervention districts (ID-1, ID-2) and control districts (CD-1, CD-2). (Reproduced by permission of W. an der Heiden.)

psychiatric departments of the general hospitals of their catchment area. In terms of day-to-day operation, however, the CMHCs are autonomous. Each CMHC is staffed by 21 full-time employees: three psychiatrists, two psychologists, four nurses, three social workers, two auxiliary nurses, two full-time and one half-time occupational therapists, one half-time physiotherapist, two secretaries, one cleaner and one research assistant. The CMHCs have an outpatient clinic with an emergency room and a day-care unit. Patients are either self-referred or referred by general practitioners, the social welfare office, the mental hospital or the psychiatric departments of the general hospitals. The IDs and CDs *must compete* for hospital beds with the other districts in the catchment areas of their general hospitals. (In 1989 the total number of psychiatric beds for the Copenhagen population was 991, equal to 2.2 beds per 1000 population.)

Overview of the research plan

The research attempted to measure aspects of the impact of the CMHCs on service provision and the population's utilisation of services using a *pre-intervention assessment* and a *2 years post-intervention* assessment. The research consisted of both cross-sectional and longitudinal studies (Schene *et al.*, 1992).

The cross-sectional studies were conducted with hospital inpatient, and CMHC and hospital outpatient and day patient units (Knudsen *et al.*, 1992a; Knudsen, 1994), psychiatrists in private practice (Knudsen *et al.*, 1992b), and general practitioners (Krasnik *et al.*, 1992). We also examined the effect of these new CMHCs on the handling of psychiatric patients by social welfare system representatives (Knudsen *et al.*, 1992a).

Because an important aim of the new CMHCs was improvement of the provision of care to the chronic psychiatric patient a special longitudinal study was made of chronic patients and their relatives (Knudsen, 1994). Another part of the evaluation study involved a sociologist who conducted a qualitative assessment of formal and informal social network structures in the local communities and of collaboration within and between agencies (Knudsen *et al.*, 1992a).

Definition of the samples in the cross-sectional studies

Psychiatric patients were included in the cross-sectional studies if they met the following criteria: 18 years or older and resident in one of the IDs or CDs on 1 January 1989 or 1 January 1991, respectively.

The pre-intervention patient sample

The hospital *inpatient and day-patient samples* consisted of those registered on the second Wednesday of January 1989 as patients in either of the two Copenhagen general hospitals or the mental hospital outside the City (day- or 24-hour patients). The *outpatient sample* consisted of those registered in the outpatient psychiatric clinics of one of the three hospitals on 2 January 1989 and who attended an appointment at the outpatient clinic between 2 January and 31 March 1989.

We surveyed the *private psychiatrists* in full-time practice in Copenhagen and identified the residents of the IDs and CDs who were registered as their patients on 5 April 1989 (point-prevalence sample).

In the practices of *general practitioners* we studied residents of the two IDs and two CDs who attended the practice between 7 and 17 November 1989.

In *social welfare services* individuals living in one of the two IDs and who were receiving social welfare support in the form of: (1) general social welfare, (2) sick pay or (3) disability pension were identified. From those receiving general social welfare or sick pay a random sample was drawn; clients with psychiatric problems were identified and the social interventions were registered as they appeared in the social records. From those receiving disability pension for psychiatric reasons a random sample was drawn; needs for intervention and for treatment were registered as they appeared in the social records.

The post-intervention sample

The post-intervention assessment took place in 1991, in the same months as in 1989, after the CMHCs had been operative for almost 2 years. The rules for selection of subjects for all groups were the same as for the pre-intervention assessment. In 1991, the CMHC day- and outpatients were sampled in the same manner as the hospital day- and outpatients.

Definition of the sample in the longitudinal study

From hospital records psychiatric patients living in one of the IDs or CDs and who fulfilled one of the following criteria were identified (Kastrup, 1987a, b):

Long-stay patients: Admitted as an in- or day-patient for at least the preceding year.

Outpatients: Having had continuous contact with the psychiatric hospital system as an outpatient for the preceding $2\frac{1}{2}$ years, with breaks of no more than 3 months (except for stays as an in- or day-patient).

Revolving-door patients: Having had at least four separate in- or day-patient episodes in the preceding $2\frac{1}{2}$ years, without continuous outpatient contact in the intervening periods.

One-hundred and seventy-one patients fulfilling these criteria were included in the study. Each of these patients was also asked for permission to interview a close relative.

Pre- and post-intervention assessments

Cross-sectional study

The methods and content of the 1989 and 1991 assessments were identical. In accordance with the criteria described, in the case of the in- and day-patients we counted the number of patients in treatment and the length of their stay. For outpatients we counted the number of patients in treatment. For the psychiatrists in private practice we counted the number of patients in treatment. For general practitioners in the IDs and CDs, we recorded the number of patients who the general practitioners judged to have psychiatric problems according to a specified list. In the social welfare offices we counted, in accordance with the criteria descibed above, the number of clients suffering from psychiatric problems.

Longitudinal study

For the chronic patients we recorded the number of days of hospitalisation for the period of the preceding 1 year, and for the second year after the introduction of the CMHCs.

For all classes of patients we noted their age, sex, level of education, marital status and economic status. For patients in the health care system we also recorded age at first psychiatric treatment episode, lifetime duration of hospital stay and psychiatric diagnoses. In this report we present a portion of the findings of the total study.

Results

Cross-sectional studies

Psychiatric hospital-based services

As has been reported in other studies (Haroutun & Babigian, 1977; Häfner & Klug, 1982; Stefansson & Cullberg, 1986) the proportion of the population in psychiatric treatment (as in-, day- or outpatient) increased markedly and significantly in both the IDs after the introduction of the CMHCs. In fact the proportion almost doubled (ID-1: 1989, 5.1/1000; 1991, 8.8/1000 population. ID-2: 1989, 6.0/1000 population; 1991, 12.0/1000 population). The proportion of the population in treatment in the CDs did not change. As we have indicated, the CDs belonged to the same hospital catchment area as the corresponding IDs. The lack of change in CDs assured us that the changes in the IDs were not likely to be due to some unknown alteration of the admission policy of the catchment area hospital or any other unregistered and uncontrollable changes in the catchment area. The odds ratio comparing the IDs' and CDs' utilisation of services in 1989 was compared with the odds ratio for 1991 by logistic regression. The increases in the odds ratios in the IDs in comparison with their CDs were highly significant.

The pattern of results in ID-1 and CD-1 was very similar to the results in ID-2 and CD-2. It is important to point out that these results represent independent replications of the findings.

Inspection of the figures reveals that the bulk of the increase in total utilisation of psychiatric services seen in the preceding analyses is due specifically to the increased level of utilisation of the outpatient services. The pattern of results for day-patients is very similar to that for the outpatients. At the same time, however, there was no significant change in the proportion of the population who were hospital inpatients in each of the two IDs relative to their CD.

In ID-2 the proportion of the population in inpatient treatment increased by 90% (ID-2: 1989, 1.0/1000 population; 1991, 1.9/1000 population). This increase within ID-2 was highly statistically significant. There was, however, also an increase in utilisation of inpatient services in CD-2 and the changes between ID-2 and CD-2 were not statistically significant. The fact that the 90% change in ID-2 was not significantly different from the changes in the CD points up the importance of including CDs in this type of research. As noted, the CD made it possible for us to assess the effect of unknown and otherwise uncontrolled intervening factors. In this case we suspect that the increase in the utilisation of inpatient services in these two districts is in part due to a decrease in the size of the catchment area of the general hospital resulting in an increase in the number of psychiatric beds available to both ID-2 and CD-2.

It has been an aim of the CMHCs to shorten hospital stays of psychiatric patients. We examined changes in duration of hospital stay for short- and medium-term admissions (1 year or less) before and after the introduction of the CMHC. The introduction of CMHCs in the two IDs was not associated with a decrease in median length of inpatient hospitalisation in either of the IDs (Knudsen, 1994).

Other services caring for mentally ill

Häfner & an der Heiden (1989) have indicated the importance of the inclusion of primary health care and specialist services in the evaluation of changes in the mental health care system. In this study we have attempted to include private psychiatric specialist services, general practitioners and services associated with the social welfare system in our assessment.

Privately practising psychiatrists

We examined the changes in the pattern of population's attendance in the practices of private psychiatrists. There were 17 psychiatrists in full-time private practice in Copenhagen; of these, 12 agreed to take part in this study.

We first studied the characteristics of the patients of these psychiatrists. As might be expected, private psychiatrists care for less severely ill patients; there are 3 times as many women as men in the care of the private psychiatrists. As we have shown in a previous paper, the socio-demographic characteristics of the patients of the private psychiatrists are comparable to those of the background population and superior to those of the hospital patients (Knudsen *et al.*, 1992b).

The introduction of the CMHCs was associated with a reduction in the number of patients being cared for by the privately practising psychiatrists. In ID-1 the difference almost reached statistically significance; in ID-2 this decrease was significant. Note that in both CDs the number of patients in private practice increased. There was not a differential effect for any diagnosis or social characteristic.

General practitioners

We attempted to assess the effect of the CMHCs on the practices of the general practitioners in the IDs (Krasnik *et al.*, 1992; Knudsen *et al.*, 1992a) compared with the general practitioners in the CDs. We noted no changes in the number of patients with mental health problems seen by general practitioners after the introduction of the CMHCs. We noted a significant tendency for the general practitioners in one ID to decrease the referral rate (to somatic specialties) of the neurotic patients in their care. This was also the district with the closest working relationship between the general practitioners and the CMHC (as recorded by the staff sociologist). It is possible that the collaboration between CMHC and general practitioners and the training afforded to the general practitioners in this district made them better able to treat neurotic patients in their practice.

Social welfare system

One of the goals of the establishment of the CMHCs was cooperation and coordination with the social welfare system in order to improve the level of psychiatric treatment of the social welfare clients in the IDs.

Fifteen per cent of the clients receiving general social welfare were noted to merit a diagnosis of a psychiatric/psychological illness; 69% of these clients did not receive appropiate treatment. Twenty-one per cent of the clients on sickleave pay, and 39% of clients receiving disability pension had a psychiatric diagnosis as their first or second diagnosis. In both IDs the proportion of social welfare clients with psychiatric problems who were in psychiatric treatment after the introduction of the CMHCs increased significantly (Knudsen *et al.*, 1992a).

A questionnaire answered by social workers and a sociologist documented a major increase in consultations and meetings between the social welfare workers and the CMHC during the 2 years following the introduction of the centres. These finding suggest that the consultation with the CMHC made the social workers more aware of clients with psychiatric problems and resulted in an increased rate of treatment contacts among patients.

Longitudinal study

Long-term mentally ill patients

As mentioned above, a special study was made of a group of chronic psychiatric patients (long-stay patients, outpatients and revolving-door patients). Among other questions we were interested in possible changes in their utilisation of hospital inpatient services after the introduction of CMHCs. For the entire group of 81 chronic patients (in both ID-1 and ID-2) there was no significant change in utilisation of hospital inpatient services. We examined the subgroup of 21 chronic patients who attended the day-care unit at the CMHC in their district at least once a week at some time during the 2-year follow-up period. For each of these patients a comparable control patient was selected, living in one of the control districts and matched for sex, age, main diagnostic category, inclusion criteria and Global Assessment Scale score (Nordentoft, 1994; Knudsen *et al.*, 1992a). For the 21 chronic patients attending the CMHCs their mean length of total inpatient hospital stay in 1 year decreased by 75.2 days; the matched controls' mean length of total inpatient hospital stay in 1 year decreased by only 6.5 days. This difference was significant (Nordentoft, 1994).

Discussion

Summary of results

The introduction of the CMHCs was associated with the following changes in patients' utilisation of services and in provision of care:

1 There was a doubling of the proportion of the population utilising psychiatric services.
2 This doubling was based on an increase in the proportion of the population utilising outpatient services as well as day-patient services.
3 There was no change in the population's utilisation of inpatient services or in the length of inpatient stays for short- or medium-stay patients.
4 A selected group of severely mentally ill patients attending the CMHCs reduced significantly their number of days spent in psychiatric wards.
5 The number of patients in the IDs in treatment with private psychiatrists decreased significantly.
6 There was no marked effect on the handling of psychiatric patients by general practitioners.
7 There was a significant increase in the proportion of social welfare clients with psychiatric disorders who were receiving treatment.

Disadvantages of the study

1 The follow-up assessment was made after the CMHCs had been in operation for 2 years. It is possible that we have missed the long-term effects which might only be evident after the initial 2-year period.
2 We utilised a cross-sectional design for a large part of the research

we have reported. This design is limited in that it does not follow the fate of individual patients who are affected by system changes. This method does, however, permit the monitoring of changes in the utilisation of mental health care at the aggregate level.

3 The cross-sectional design samples subjects in a point-prevalence frame. The method has disadvantages relative to a period-prevalence sampling frame. The point-prevalence method yields fewer subjects and may be influenced by transitory local conditions existing on the day of sampling. This method also oversamples chronic patients.

4 The interpretation of the research results would have been facilitated by an assessment of the need for care (Wing *et al.*, 1992) of the background population of the districts. This would have enabled us to estimate the extent to which the CMHCs reached the goal of meeting these needs, as well as enhancing our understanding of our findings.

5 An assessment of the health economic implications of the interventions would have been useful in estimating the cost-effectiveness of these changes. For example it would have been of interest to calculate the relative costs and benefits of the privately practising psychiatrists' and the CMHCs' outpatient services. It is possible that what might be interpreted as a transfer of patients from private psychiatrists to the hospital-based outpatient services (including the CMHCs) represents a reduction in cost-effectiveness.

Advantages of the design

Research at the programme level of service outcome includes random assignment of subjects to intervention and control groups. In the area of service utilisation research, however, the use of CDs is not common. Rossi & Freeman (1989) and Häfner & an der Heiden (1989) have supported the importance of control groups in service utilisation studies.

In this chapter the usefulness of CDs in the interpretation of the results has been emphasised. At several points in the findings there have been instances in which the changes in the IDs were not significantly different from changes in the CDs. These changes were very probably valid for the entire catchment area and were not a function of the introduction of the CMHC. Finding significant differences in service utilisation within an ID before and after the introduction of a new CMHC may simply reflect larger trends in the society.

It may be useful to highlight the fact that the study had the advantage of observing effects in two IDs and their two CDs. This gave us the opportunity to test for independent replications of our findings within the context of the single study. We give extra credence to significant findings which were observed in both IDs.

The follow-up study of the chronically mentally ill patients gave us a wider context in which to interpret our results. The chronically mentally ill patients decreased their utilisation of inpatient services significantly while the background population's utilisation of inpatient services did not change after the introduction of CMHCs. The CMHCs reduced the chronically mentally ill patients' inpatient stays and at the same time reached out to groups of patients not in contact with the services at the time when the intervention began. As noted above it is the aim of the CMHCs to assume the 'total responsibility for the mental well-being of the population of the catchment area'. Part of this aim involves the coordination of the work of the health services and the social welfare system. These aims emphasise the necessity of a comprehensive assessment of potential changes in services other than those directly associated with the hospital system. Effects of the introduction of a CMHC may spill over into the practices of general practitioners, as well as psychiatrists in private practice. In this study we have noted that the introduction of the CMHC was associated with a reduction in the number of patients being seen by the private psychiatrists. As we have also observed in this study, an increased awareness of the problems of the mentally ill by workers in the social welfare system might benefit the psychiatric patient. In this analysis we benefited from the work of a sociologist who observed and described the relations between the CMHCs, the social welfare workers and other organisations and services involved in the care of the mentally ill patients.

We attempted, in this study, to increase the comprehensiveness of our assessments compared with most research in this area. These efforts are described in order to open the discussion of these issues in research.

References

Häfner, H. & an der Heiden, W. (1989). The evaluation of mental health care systems. *British Journal of Psychiatry*, **155**, 12–17.

Häfner, H. & Klug, J. (1982). The impact of an expanding community mental health service on patterns of bed usage: evaluation of a four-year period of implementation. *Psychological Medicine*, **12**, 177–90.

Haroutun, M. & Babigian, M.D. (1977). The impact of community mental health centers on the utilization of services. *Archives of General Psychiatry*, **34**, 385–94.

Kastrup, M. (1987a). Predicting profile of the long-stay population: a nation-wide cohort of first time admitted patients. *Acta Psychiatrica Scandinavica*, **76**, 71–9.

Kastrup, M. (1987b). Who became revolving door patients? Findings from a national cohort of first time admitted psychiatric patients. *Acta Psychiatrica Scandinavica*, **76**, 80–8.

Knudsen, H.C. (1994). *Kontakt- og ydelsesmønster i et regionalt sundhedsvæsen før og efter reorganiseringen af den psykiatriske service.* Copenhagen: Afdelingen for Social Medicin, Københavns Universitet. (Pattern of utilisation and provision of care in a local health service before and after the reorganization of the psychiatric services.) PhD dissertation.

Knudsen, H.C., Jessen-Petersen, B., Klitgaard, V., Krasnik, A., Nordentoft, M. & Sælan, H. (1992a). *Distriktspsykiatri i København. En evaluering af de første to år.* Copenhagen: Københavns Sundhedsvæsen. (Community Mental Health Centers in Copenhagen. An evaluation of the first two years.)

Knudsen, H.C., Krasnik, A., Jessen-Petersen, B., Nordentoft, M. & Sælan, H. (1992b). Patients in the care of private psychiatric practitioners: comparison with public hospital patients and the background districts' population. *Social Psychiatry and Psychiatric Epidemiology*, **27**, 156–60.

Københavns Hospitalsdirektorat (1987). *Forslag til psykiatriplan for Københavns Kommune 1988–2000.* Copenhagen: Københavns Hospitalsdirektorat. (Suggestions for development of the psychiatric services in Copenhagen 1988–2000.)

Københavns Kommune (1987). *Borgerrepræsentationens forhandlinger. No.. 29, 10 December 1987.*

Krasnik, A., Knudsen, H.C., Jessen-Petersen, B., Nordentoft, M. & Sælan, H. (1992). The role of general practice in community mental health: a survey in four districts of Copenhagen. *Nordic Journal of Psychiatry*, **46**, 223–7.

Nielsen, J., Nielsen, J.A., Kastrup, M. & Strömgren, E. (eds.) (1981). *The Samsø Project: a Community Psychiatric Project in a Geographically Delimited Population.* Aarhus: Acta Jutlandica LV, Medicine Series 23.

Nordentoft, M. (1994). *Hjemløshed, social integration og livskvalitet hos psykiatriske patienter i København.* Copenhagen, Århus, Odense: FADL. (Homelessness, social integration and quality of life among mentally ill patients.) PhD dissertation.

Rossi, P.H. & Freeman, H.E. (1989). *Evaluation: A Systematic Approach.* Newbury Park: Sage Publications.

Rudas, S. (1990). On measuring the changes in psychiatric care systems: results in an urban area (Vienna). *Psychiatric Bulletin*, **14**, 262–6.

Schene, A.H., Henderson, J.H., Knudsen, H.C., Rijkschroeff, R. & Thornicroft, G. (1992). The evaluation of mental health care transformation in the cities of Europe. *International Journal of Social Psychiatry*, **38**, 40–9.

Statistisk Kontor, København (1988). *The Social Districts of Copenhagen, Figures no. 4*. Copenhagen: The Municipality of Copenhagen.

Søgaard, H.J. (1993). *Rapport over evaluering af den distriktspsykiatriske ordning i Viborg Amtskommune. Sammenfattende rapport 1990–1992*. Århus: Psykiatrisk Hospital Århus. (Report on the evaluation of the district psychiatric organisation in the county of Viborg. The summarising report.)

Stefansson, C.-G. & Cullberg, J. (1986). Introducing community mental health services: the effect of a suburban patient population. *Acta Psychiatrica Scandinavica*, **74**, 368–78.

Tansella, M., Balestrieri, M. & Micciolo, R. (1991). Trends in the provision of psychiatric care 1979–1988. *Psychological Medicine*, Supplementum **19**, 5–16.

Valbak, K., Sørensen, L.V. & Lindhardt, A. (1992). Evaluation of community psychiatry: a cross-sectional study. *Acta Psychiatrica Scandinavica*, **85**, 183–8.

Wing, J. & Hailey, M. (1972). *Evaluating a Community Psychiatric Service: The Camberwell Register 1964–71*. London: Oxford University Press.

Wing, J., Brewin, C.R. & Thornicroft, G. (1992). Defining mental health needs. In *Measuring Mental Health Needs*, ed. G. Thornicroft, C.R. Brewin & J. Wing, pp. 1–17. London: Gaskell.

6

The Mannheim Project

HEINZ HÄFNER AND WOLFRAM AN DER HEIDEN

Introduction

After World War II psychiatry in Germany carried a terrible burden. From 1933 onwards the ideology of national socialism had disastrous consequences for the mentally ill. The eugenic laws demanded the compulsory sterilisation of every individual suffering from functional psychoses, familial epilepsy and familial retardation. The inhumanity culminated in the programme of euthanasia. Between 80 000 and 100 000 mentally ill people were killed. Some of the leading German psychiatrists had been actively involved in this programme.

Understandably, psychiatrists and psychiatric institutions thereafter met with a fundamental distrust. It took a long time until the problems of mental health care could again be brought before the public. Therefore, until 1970, German psychiatry was comparatively little influenced by the community psychiatry movement initiated in the United States, Britain and other European countries. As a consequence, the maximum of occupation of psychiatric beds, indicating the culmination of custodial care, was reached in Germany approximately 15 years later than in Great Britain or the United States.

Mental health care in Germany in the early 1960s was characterised by a sharp demarcation between inpatient and outpatient care. Ninety-seven per cent of all psychiatric beds were in mostly remote, large public hospitals, four of them with more than 4000 beds. The majority were in an obsolete state. The average length of stay was 215 days, 26% of the patients staying in hospital for more than 10 years. Only 3% of the psychiatric beds were located in units of general hospitals with a bed ratio of 1:12.6 and an average length of stay as short as 35 days. Outpatient psychiatric care rested almost completely with psychiatrists and psychotherapists in private practice. Among their clientele patients with severe mental disorders and socially disabled chronically mentally ill individuals in particular, as well as psychogeriatric patients, were considerably underrepresented. Complementary services, such as day hospitals, supervised homes and apartments, and sheltered workshops, were lacking almost completely, and there was no prospect of a change in this system, especially in the rehabilitation of dischargeable long-stay patients.

Provision of care for mentally ill old people was extremely deficient. In the mostly isolated mental hospitals somatic care to modern standards was impossible. For the same reason and due to the large catchment areas of the rural mental hospitals psychiatric emergency care and crisis intervention were hardly available. Almost all general hospitals lacked a psychiatric liaison service, which resulted in the neglect of psychiatric care for the physically ill, in particular of suicide attempters.

The recommendations of the Expert Commission on Psychiatry, 1972–1975

This being the situation we proposed to the then Federal Minister for Health, E. Schwarzhaupt, in 1965 that a commission of experts be set up to analyse the state of mental health care in the Federal Republic of Germany, a model institute for research in social psychiatry be founded and 2-year training courses in community psychiatry be offered to nurses working in the profession. The proposals were favourably received and, with regard to the setting up of an expert commission, adopted by the Parliament. The Commission presented its report in 1975. The report formulated five principles to reform mental health care:

1 For every person in need of psychiatric care the best possible treatment in terms of effectiveness and cost must be available without undue financial and geographical barriers.
2 Physically and mentally ill individuals must be granted an equal status from a legal, social and financial point of view.
3 Psychiatric care must be integrated into the system of general health care as far as possible.
4 Inpatient psychiatric care must be organised in the form of

community-based services. The intention should be to remove the mentally ill from contact with family, society and work place for no longer than is necessary and to make their rehabilitation easier.

5 For the socially disabled chronically ill a network of complementary services should be built up.

In the years following the recommendations were gradually realised in both the provision of mental health care and legislation, though not completely. The well-developed social system in Germany, which guarantees full payment of all forms of treatment and social care for anyone in need, favoured the development of community mental health services.

Preparations for the establishment of community mental health services in Mannheim

In 1963 we introduced an advanced training course in community psychiatry with the aim of obtaining well-trained and experienced nurses capable of running complementary services or working in other domains of community psychiatry. In the meantime the advanced training courses in psychiatry have been officially recognised, and similar institutions have been established in 43 locations in Germany (including former East Germany).

Behind the concept of founding a model institute for mental health care and research lay the notion that to establish modern mental health care in Germany it would be necessary, for one thing, to demonstrate how good community mental health services worked and, for another, to re-build the almost totally collapsed research capacity of German psychiatry. In this context priority was given to those research fields that were particularly underdeveloped or especially important for the establishment of modern community care, such as psychogeriatrics, child- and adolescent psychiatry, psychiatric epidemiology and services research.

Opening of the Central Institute of Mental Health in Mannheim in 1975

In 1975, before the recommendations of the Expert Commission for Psychiatry were published, the Central Institute of Mental Health

(CIMH) opened in Mannheim. It was founded by the Federal government, the State government of Baden-Württemberg, and the Volkswagen Foundation. As a research institution it has been rated by the Scientific Council of the Federal Republic as an institute of national interest and supra-regional importance. As a provider of mental health care it serves the 305 000 inhabitants of the city of Mannheim. At present the CIMH, located in an inner city district, has a department of psychiatry with 106 beds, ten of which are in an intensive care unit with competence in internal medicine and psychiatry. There is a psychogeriatric day hospital with 10 places within the Institute and another day hospital with 20 places for chronic schizophrenics situated within walking distance of the Institute in a well-preserved inner city residential area.

Besides the psychiatric department there is a child and adolescent department with 48 beds and a department of psychotherapy and psychosomatic medicine also with 48 beds. There are eight further departments engaged primarily in research and five working groups. In the field of teaching the CIMH is responsible for the subjects of psychiatry, child psychiatry, psychosomatics and forensic psychiatry at the University of Heidelberg and clinical psychology at the University of Mannheim.

In the planning phase of the Institute, Mannheim (a mainly industrial city of about 305 000 inhabitants at the confluence of the rivers Rhine and Neckar in the mid-western part of Germany) had no psychiatric hospital of its own. The mentally ill in need of inpatient treatment were referred to a large public hospital situated about 50 kilometres outside Mannheim. In 1969 a second medical school of the University of Heidelberg opened in Mannheim, and the large municipal hospital – without a psychiatric department of its own – became a teaching hospital. In the wake of these developments the CIMH had an opportunity to take charge of teaching the disciplines represented at the Institute and to establish a psychiatric liaison service.

Four CIMH psychiatrists are currently available at the municipal hospital during office hours. Outside office hours one psychiatrist is in charge of an emergency service. Although there are nearly twice as many places for chronic mental patients available in complementary facilities as there are beds at the CIMH, CIMH's bed capacity does not satisfy the needs of the Mannheim population and the 170 000 inhabitants of the adjacent city of Ludwigshafen, which is separated from Mannheim only by the river Rhine. To alleviate the situation until an adequate bed capacity is reached, a division of work has been agreed with the Wiesloch public hospital some 50 kilometres from Mannheim. The CIMH is resposible for acute and severe cases and provides and coordinates complementary care for chronic mental patients with social disabilities in complementary services. The Wiesloch public hospital offers a special programme for the long-term treatment or detoxication of patients with substance abuse and alcohol-related disorders. In addition, it is responsible for the small proportion of chronic patients in need of 24-hour nursing and medical care over long periods of time (more than 1 year) due to severity of illness or highly disordered behaviour.

The CIMH was established to provide care according to the principles of modern psychiatric prevention, treatment and rehabilitation (WHO, 1980). One of the main objectives was the gradual realisation of a community-based system of rehabilitation and long-term care for psychiatric patients with social disabilities. This and interdisciplinary research in all branches of psychiatry, clinical psychology, social epidemiology, biological psychiatry and molecular biology, are the two main aspects of the CIMH's work.

The implementation of a comprehensive community mental health service in Mannheim

The development of a community psychiatric service in Mannheim was under way long before the opening of the CIMH. In 1958 the Municipal Council established the first sheltered workshop for psychiatric patients. In 1967 an outpatient service for psychiatric and psychogeriatric patients and children and adolescents was introduced at the general hospital and the first supervised home for psychiatric patients went into operation. In 1969 the CIMH Department for Community Psychiatry started its work with the aim of creating a network of community mental health services in Mannheim and coordinating their activities. From 1972 until moving into its present building in 1975 a psychiatric unit with three wards and 55 beds was run in the premises of the University Hospital as a forerunner of the CIMH.

In cooperation with the City of Mannheim, welfare organisations, university hospitals and medical agencies, sheltered workshops, supervised psychiatric homes, group homes and apartments were created.

The Mannheim psychiatric case register

At an early stage it was deemed necessary to build up a psychiatric information system that would enable the evaluation of the effectiveness and costs of the new system of care and continued monitoring of the use made of it or of its components and that would also provide appropriate indicators for accomplishing this task. The psychiatric case register, funded by the German Research Association (Deutsche Forschungsgemeinschaft), went into operation in 1973. Incompatible with the new data protection laws, it was forced to close in 1981.

The Institute is situated in a socially heterogeneous inner city area characterised by a high percentage of immigrants, bars and night clubs, but also numerous well-preserved middle-class houses. The high utilisation of the outpatient departments and the emergency and crisis intervention service at the CIMH indicates that the Institute has been accepted by those needing such services. Over time it has acquired a favourable image with the local population, partly as a result not only of its permanent public relations work but also of the growing number of patients treated there.

The network of complementary services

In 1993 there were 216 places in supervised homes for the socially disabled mentally ill available in Mannheim. Besides sheltered workshops for the mentally retarded and physically disabled, which are not under the supervision of the CIMH, there are two further sheltered workshops for psychiatric patients counselled by the CIMH Department for Community Psychiatry. The Department cooperates with numerous voluntary workers especially in promoting the social integration of and organising leisure activities for the socially disabled mentally ill. Since its foundation, the Department has helped to set up nine patients' clubs for the mentally ill. Some of these clubs now operate on their own and as self-help institutions are no longer in need of counselling by specialists.

In the field of child and adolescent psychiatry there are two kindergartens for children with behavioural disorders counselled by child psychiatrists, two supervised homes for children and adolescents with mental or behavioural disorders as well as special groups in sheltered workshops for psychotic adolescents. In addition, the Department for Child and Adolescent Psychiatry operates an extensive network of child-psychiatric counselling in social services. For instance, a child and adolescent psychiatric consultant works full time at the city's child guidance centre.

The complementary services are funded by the City of Mannheim and the large welfare organisations – the Protestant and the Catholic Church and a social welfare organisation. Thanks to its training capacity the CIMH has provided a considerable proportion of the staff for these services. Until recently all the community psychiatric services in Mannheim were planned and partly also commissioned and run by the CIMH Department for Community Psychiatry on its own responsibility; only after attaining a stable level of functioning could they start working on their own. The Department for Community Psychiatry was thus responsible for the needs-led planning and coordination of the total network of community mental health care. In 1989 the CIMH handed the task of coordinating the planning of, division of work between and cooperation among the various services over to the Deputy Mayor for Health and Social Affairs of the City of Mannheim, who has set up a Social Psychiatric Advisory Board at the Municipal Council to assist him in this task. On this board the CIMH acts as an expert.

The task of case management, that is, the coordination of the care provided by the various agents and facilities, rests with a social psychiatric service, which was founded in 1989 and is run by the CIMH. The six social workers of this service come from the welfare organisations, which are also responsible for the main facilities.

In the past few years increasing unemployment has dramatically reduced the chances of occupational rehabilitation of the mentally ill, especially of those suffering from chronic schizophrenia or alcoholism. In 1983 the CIMH therefore called into being a special service for occupational rehabilitation, 'the Mannheim Project of Starthilfe' (help for starting). In collaboration with more than 100 Mannheim-based enterprises and shops it offers to the mentally ill who have lost their jobs supervised on-the-job training for up to 3 months. In 1992, there were 58 former patients who underwent such a training, 18 of whom managed to obtain a regular job thereafter (Waschkowski, 1993).

The centrepiece of the CIMH's mental health work in the community and of the extramural services is the Department for Community Psychiatry. This is unique in Germany. The Department continues to advise all the community mental health services operating in Mannheim. Since the closure of the case register a continuing evaluation of the community mental health services has become increasingly difficult.

Evaluative research

With respect to the implementation of a community mental health care system in Mannheim the CIMH has taken over the task of evaluating psychiatric services, their effectiveness and efficiency at different levels of care. In the 1970s the evaluation was mainly carried out with the help of the cumulative psychiatric case register, the first and, up to now, the only one in the Federal Republic of Germany. With the case register an instrument was established that is one of the most important of evaluative research.

With the implementation of a strong network of complementary services a change seemed to occur in the function of the psychiatric hospital, even for those diagnostic groups with a high proportion of chronic courses or persisting social disabilities. Even when needing long-term residential care, patients have a much better chance of finding accommodation and adequate support in terms of treatment, housing and social activities within their community.

The transition from long-term hospital to complementary care

In 1975 Mannheim had one home for 19 psychiatric patients. In 1993 there were five sheltered homes with a total of 151 places, mainly for chronic psychiatrically ill persons. These services were supplemented by a total of 65 places in nine sheltered group homes. Consequently, the number of Mannheim inhabitants with a diagnosis of schizophrenia in psychiatric hospitals in the Mannheim area decreased consistently from 155 to 110 at a yearly census day between 1973 and 1980,* whereas the number of patients of the same diagnostic group in psychiatric homes nearly doubled to 100 in the same period (Häfner & an der Heiden, 1984).

* Data are available only until 1980, because the cumulative psychiatric case register was closed down in 1981.

Among the total number of schizophrenic long-stay patients (i.e. those with a stay of more than 1 year) the proportion of those cared for in psychiatric homes increased from 32% on a census day in 1973 to 60% in 1980. Seventy-five per cent of the patients who became new long-stay patients in 1980 were admitted to psychiatric homes, and only 25% began a stay of 1 year or more in a mental hospital.

What is effective in comprehensive community care?

Looking at individual patterns of utilisation, as we did on the basis of a cohort study of 145 schizophrenic patients over 18 months, it is possible to investigate the effects of particular components of care. While controlling for chronicity, psychopathological status and type of accommodation (living alone/in family/in sheltered accommodations) we were able to demonstrate that outpatient medical care had a significant influence on reducing re-admissions to hospital (an der Heiden *et al.*, 1989): the greater the number of contacts with an outpatient psychiatric facility, the greater the probability of staying out of hospital.

If the direct costs of community mental health care for our patient cohort are compared with the costs of continuous psychiatric inpatient treatment over the same period, community mental health care amount only to 43% of the costs of hospital care (Häfner & an der Heiden, 1991).

So, at least with respect to direct costs, complementary care seems more economical than long-term hospitalisation. This is true despite the fact that very often patients contact several facilities at the same time – in our cohort, up to five within a 2-week interval. Most instances of multiple utilisation consist of visits to a physician combined with stays in sheltered homes and attendance at a sheltered workshop and a patients' club.

Emergency care and crisis intervention

When the proportion of schizophrenic patients in complementary services is so high that even patients with considerable behavioural

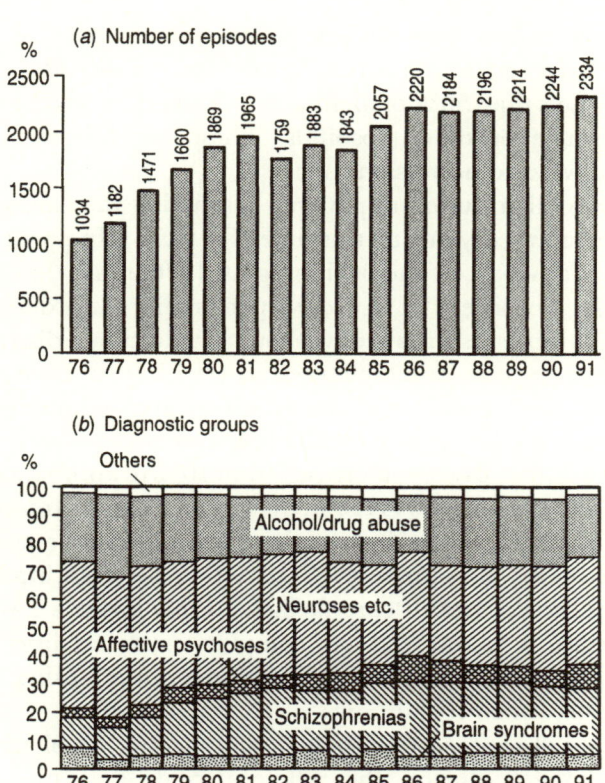

Fig. 6.1. Utilisation of the psychiatric emergency service in Mannheim, 1976–1991. (Data from CIMH, Mannheim.)

disorders or frequent relapses are cared for outside hospital, an emergency service is required to offer home staff counselling and outpatient intervention or hospital admission when crises occur. A 24-hour psychiatric emergency service constitutes an essential part of a comprehensive community-oriented care system. It provides care for mentally ill and disabled persons who can only stay outside hospital when sufficient psychiatric care is provided. To function effectively one emergency service in Mannheim is attached to the emergency unit of the general hospital where many patients get referred to because of attempted suicide or intoxication. Another emergency service is attached to the CIMH.

Between 1976 and 1991 the utilisation of the crisis intervention and emergency service more than doubled (Fig. 6.1a). A detailed analysis based on case register data by Häfner *et al.* (1986) for the years up to

1980 showed that a little over 50% of the emergency cases came on their own initiative or on the initiative of relatives directly to the service facility. Less than 50% of them were admitted by psychiatrists in private practice or other hospitals. These are the two most important pathways to admission.

The diagnostic distribution of patients contacting the emergency service changed markedly during this time (Fig. 6.1b). In particular, two changes are obvious. At the beginning, in 1976, more than 50% of all diagnoses consisted of neurosis, personality disorders and temporary psychiatric disturbances without an additional diagnosis. This diagnostic group was still the largest in 1991 but its share of the whole spectrum of diagnoses had decreased to approximately one third. In contrast, the proportion of schizophrenic patients and those with schizophrenia-like diseases increased from 10% to approximately 25% – in spite of a roughly 100% rise in the total number of treatment episodes – almost parallel to the increase in patients in complementary residential care. This may prove the interaction between inpatient and outpatient mental health care facilities: Only when a 24-hour emergency service is guaranteed can complementary facilities care also for those chronic patients who are in danger of relapsing, even under modern treatment conditions.

The frequency of contacts due to drug and alcohol problems was relatively unchanged during the whole period, and made up approximately one quarter of the patients. For most of these people an emergency service is necessary because of severe intoxication or complications such as delirium and attacks. The smaller proportion of patients suffering from dementia and organic psychoses or patients with other diagnoses showed no significant changes. Affective psychoses recorded a small increase.

Services research in child psychiatry

Besides the examples shown, single components of the health care system and services for special patient groups have been the subject of scientific investigations. Studies on the utilisation of the Child Psychiatric Clinic and the evaluation of the underlying causes for referral and utilisation showed that external events, such as entering school, are of greater importance in leading to a first consultation than the severity of illness or a disrupted family life (Corboz *et al.*,

1983; Remschmidt & Schmidt, 1983). A comparative study of the effectiveness of various treatment modalities – home treatment, combined inpatient and outpatient treatment – for a wide range of psychiatric disorders in childhood and in adolescence was also conducted (Remschmidt & Schmidt, 1985).

Mental health of immigrant workers

Several studies have been carried out on psychiatric morbidity among immigrant workers and the psychiatric care provided for them (Häfner *et al.*, 1977; Häfner, 1980; Weyerer & Häfner, 1992). In 1980 in Mannheim the proportion of immigrant workers was about 14% – almost twice as high as the figure for the whole country. A cohort study comprising 200 Turkish workers from Central Anatolia (Häfner *et al.*, 1977) revealed that, immediately after their arrival in West Germany, about 25% of the population showed some kind of psychopathological characteristics, mainly depressive symptoms. Eighteen months later, some 33% suffered from predominantly minor psychiatric disorders, in most cases unspecified psychosomatic symptoms. As a substantial proportion of the cases had already manifested mental disorders or neurotic symptoms over an extended period prior to emigration it can be concluded that with respect to the risk of falling ill emigration as such seems less important than certain personality traits.

An analysis of case register data for the period 1974–77 showed markedly lower rates of psychiatric illness in the most important groups of immigrant worker – Turks, Italians and Yugoslavs – as compared with the German population. This was especially true for those diagnostic groups with a chronic course, such as schizophrenia, chronic brain diseases and alcohol-related disorders. The lower rates are mainly due to the characteristic age structure of the immigrant population, which has an overrepresentation of the younger age groups. For Turks the rates remained significantly different even when controlling for age. Although a field study on two samples of 13- and 14-year-old Turkish and Italian children (Poustka, 1984) revealed a higher rate of psychiatric disorders compared with the rates in the adult population of immigrant workers, the prevalence rates of 18% and 22% proved to be slightly lower than those for German children of the same age group. In contrast, among 'other foreigners', including refugees from Eastern European countries, the prevalence of neuroses and depressive disorders in some age groups exceeds that for the German population. The differing morbidity figures were explained in terms of different selection mechanisms in the countries of origin acting to different extents on male emigrants, their wives and children.

Psychogeriatrics

Special attention was paid to studies on the treatment of psychiatrically ill older people. Cooper & Sosna (1983) found that among the elderly in nursing homes and to a lesser extent in residential homes the proportion exhibiting mental disorders and especially dementia was markedly higher than among those living in private accommodation.

The general practitioner is by far the most important provider of medical care. The study proved a high utilisation rate (90% per year) of the elderly in general practices and also an astonishingly high sensitivity of diagnosing dementia by medical doctors. But there is still insufficient utilisation of mental health services by the mentally ill elderly population. Another study was aimed at the reduction of health risks among the elderly through intensified support given by social workers after discharge from hospital (Cooper, 1987; Bickel et al., 1993).

Now, 20 years after the completion of the CMIH, the structure of the mental health care system in Mannheim has been completed in many respects. But there is still a process of accumulating needs for complementary care by the socially disabled chronically ill, together with the unforeseeable emergence of new and special needs such as AIDS cases, new immigrant populations and asylum seekers. The implementation of new facilities at different levels of care will be a continuing subject for evaluation.

References

Bickel, H., Cooper, B. & Wancata, J. (1993). Psychische Erkrankungen von älteren Allgemeinkrankenhauspatienten: Häufigkeit und Langzeitprognose. Nervenarzt, 64, 53–61.
Cooper, B. (1987). Psychiatric disorders among elderly patients admitted to

hospital medical wards. *Journal of the Royal Society of Medicine,* **80,** 13–16.
Cooper, B. & Sosna, U. (1983). Psychische Erkrankungen in der Alten-bevölkerung: eine epidemiologische Feldstudie. *Nervenarzt,* **54,** 239–49.
Corboz, R., Schmidt, M.H., Remschmidt, H., Schieber, P. & Göbel, D. (1983). Multiaxiale Klassifikation in Berlin, Mannheim und Zürich. Gemeinsamkeiten und Differenzen der Inanspruchnahmepopulationen dreier Kliniken: Artefakt und Realität. In *Multiaxiale Diagnostik und Jugendpsychiatrie,* ed. H. Remschmidt & M.H. Schmidt. Bern: Huber.
Häfner, H. (1980). Psychiatrische Morbidität von Gastarbeitern in Mannheim: epidemiologische Analyse einer Inanspruchnahmepopulation. *Nervenarzt,* **51,** 672–83.
Häfner, H. & an der Heiden, W. (1984). Evaluation von Veränderungen in einem psychiatrischen Versorgungssystem. In *Psychotherapie: Makro-/ Mikroperspektiven,* ed. U. Baumann, pp. 52–72. Göttingen:, Hogrefe.
Häfner, H. & an der Heiden, W. (1991). Evaluating effectiveness and cost of community care for schizophrenic patients. *Schizophrenia Bulletin,* **17,** 441–51.
Häfner, H., Moschel, G. & Özek, M. (1977). Psychische Störungen bei türkischen Gastarbeitern: eine prospektiv-epidemiologische Studie zur Untersuchung der Reaktion auf Einwanderung und partielle Anpassung. *Nervenarzt,* **48,** 268–75.
Häfner, H., Rössler, W. & Haas, S. (1986). Psychiatrische Notfallversorgung und Krisenintervention: Konzepte, Erfahrungen, Ergebnisse. *Psychiatrische Praxis,* **13,** 203–12.
an der Heiden, W., Krumm, B. & Häfner, H. (1989). *Die Wirksamkeit ambulanter psychiatrischer Versorgung: Ein Modell zur Evaluation extramuraler Dienste.* Berlin: Springer.
Poustka, F. (1984). *Psychische Störungen bei Kindern und Jugendlichen ausländischer Arbeitnehmer. Eine epidemiologische Untersuchung.* Stuttgart: Enke.
Remschmidt, H. & Schmidt, M.H. (1983). *Multiaxiale Diagnostik in der Kinder- und Jugendpsychiatrie. Ergebnisse empirischer Untersuchungen.* Bern: Huber.
Remschmidt, H. & Schmidt, M.H. (1985). *Evaluation in der Kinder- und Jugendpsychiatrie.* Stuttgart: Thieme.
Waschkowski, H. (1993). Mannheimer Starthilfe-Projekt. Jahresbericht 1992 (unpublished).
Weyerer, S. & Häfner, H. (1992). The high incidence of psychiatrically treated disorders in the inner city of Mannheim: susceptibility of German and foreign residents. *Social Psychiatry and Psychiatric Epidemiology,* **27,** 142–6.
WHO (1980). *Advisory Committee on Medical Research, Report to the Director-General on its twenty-second session,* held at WHO headquarters, Geneva, 13–16 October 1980, ACMR22/80.

7

Psychiatric evaluation as a process of quality assurance

CLAES-GÖRAN STEFANSSON

The Nacka Project revisited

Ten years after the introduction of the Community Health Services system in the United States, a study by the National Board of Health and Welfare in Sweden recommended that adult psychiatric services should be reconstructed so as to provide more open forms of care managed by multiprofessional teams and based on a total care responsibility for a defined catchment area. One of the first clinics in Sweden to be organised according to these principles was located in a Stockholm suburb. The Nacka Project (NP), as it was called, was to be run as a pilot scheme for 2 years (1975–76) whilst undergoing continual evaluation.

The aim of the present study is to describe how the evaluation of this organisational change was carried out, as well as some of the effects of the change. A further aim is to give an account of how continual evaluation in close association with clinical practice can be used to monitor and guide the enterprise towards targeted goals and/or improved efficiency. Discussions about the quality of care often start with Donabedian's concepts – structure, process and effect quality – from the patient's perspective (Donabedian, 1966). The present study adopts instead a perspective by which the care organisation in its entirety, as well as its relationship to the catchment area population, is focused upon. It is an attempt which can be characterised as population-focused quality assurance.

Study area and method

The study population consisted of all persons aged 18 years and above in two outer suburbs of Stockholm who had sought psychiatric care in the catchment area at any time during 1972–3 (the old organisation) and 1975–6 (the new organisation, i.e. the NP). Data from these patients was included in a psychiatric case register for these periods. A new patient register was set up during the period 1981–5, containing the same type of information for the area. Patient and treatment characteristics could thus be compared over three periods of time, thereby reflecting organisational changes.

In 1975, the inhabitants of the catchment area numbered 71 400, of whom 51 300 were aged 18 and above. Ten per cent of the population lived in rural, sparsely populated areas. Twenty-five per cent were under 17 years and 10% were 65 years and older. The proportion of immigrants was 12%, but in certain densely populated sub-areas could exceed 25%. The study area had, and still has, a mixture of social classes and various types of housing. There are more affluent neighbourhoods of owner-occupied houses and other areas with blocks of rented flats. Many people commute to work in central Stockholm.

From 1972 to 1975, the adult population increased by 8% and in the years up to 1985 by another 12.5%. The age group 35–45 years increased in comparison with the younger section of the population. A certain shift towards higher social classes has taken place due to the building of private housing developments.

The content of the case register

Table 7.1 shows the main features and content of the psychiatric case register in operation during the period 1981–5. The content of the register is the same as that which was set up for the evaluation of the NP in 1975–6. The administration of data collection is, however, somewhat different, involving a follow-up procedure whereby every patient was checked three times in the course of a year.

On the first visit, some administrative information was recorded in the register. The second check-up took place about 1 month later. Social and demographic information was then recorded, together

Table 7.1. *The Nacka Project's psychiatric case register: data collecting stages and contents*

Data collected at first visit	Data collected after 1 month					Data collected after 1 year
	Social and demographic data	Current diagnosis[a]	Supplementary diagnosis	Social and psychological functioning	Significant distress 1 year before first visit	
Patient identification	Previous psychiatric contact (out patient and/or inpatient	Presenile or senile dementia	Alcohol abuse: light or occasional	Good functioning, no disturbances	Relationship disturbances	**Main outpatient treatment**
Reception unit		Schizophrenia	Alcohol abuse: severe	Fairly good functioning, some disturbances with respect to social relations, work or leisure time	Divorce/ separation	Diagnostic judgement only
Date		Psychosis from brain injury or intoxication	Drug abuse		Somatic disease (*patient/ significant other*)	Supportive treatment
Emergency visit or not	Age	Other acute psychosis	Narcotic abuse		Long-term psychiatric illness	Psychotherapy (*individual, family- or group settings*)
	Sex		Mental retardation			Non-verbal therapy
Referring institution	Civil status	Paranoid state	Psychosomatic disease	Poor functioning with respect to some of the factors above	Disease of significant other	
Therapist(s) responsible for treatment	Nationality	Uni- or bipolar depression	Somatic disease			**Medication**
	Children (at home)	Brain injury dysfunction (*not psychotic*)	Attempted suicide		Child-care arrangements	Sedative/ hypnotics
	Cohabitation form					Antidepressant
	Dwelling type					Antipsychotic: depot

and sub-area

Occupation or non-occupation status

Social class

Borderline syndrome

Neurosis

No personality disorder

None of above alternatives

Diagnosis missing

Poor functioning with respect to all factors

Reproduction

Education

Ageing

Work situation (*unemployment*)

Work situation (*relationships, stress, etc.*)

Habitation isolation

Economy

Authority intervention

Other reasons (*what?*)

Antipsychotic: other

Lithionite

Anti-alcoholic

Care utilisation (*Nos. during 1 year*)

Outpatient visits

Outpatient emergency visits

Admission to psychiatric hospital

Compulsory admissions

Inpatient days

Revised diagnosis

Terminated/referred

[a] Reduced ICD-8 diagnosis.

with psychiatric data including diagnoses. All diagnoses were made under the supervision of the head psychiatrist. At this stage, the register was computerised. After 1 year, the remaining data was recorded and merged with the 1-month data. A 1-year cohort with a 1-year follow-up was thus established. A check was made as to whether the treatment had been terminated during the year. If not, the patient's file was transferred to the next year's cohort and the procedure for that particular patient started all over again from the 1-month stage. These variables were used when comparing the NP (1975–6) organisation with the old one (1972–3) as well as the NP organisation with the same organisation after 10 years (1984–5). A 2-year period of prevalence was chosen in order to include cases within small diagnostic categories.

The effects of changing from hospital-based to outpatient-based community mental health services

The establishment of the NP entailed a radical growth in psychiatric outpatient resources. Three outpatient teams were set up close to the large population centres they were to serve. Each team consisted of slightly more than ten therapists: 2.5 psychiatrists, two psychologists, two medical social workers, two psychiatric nurses as well as two auxiliary nurses. The team bases were situated in ordinary residential areas close to population centres. A broad spectrum of treatment was available with the possibility of both medical-psychiatric and psychotherapeutic help. Apart from direct treatment, supervision and consultation was to be made available to other care professionals. Primary preventive inputs aimed at various groups in the area were also developed. The outpatient teams, however, lacked inpatient care facilities, i.e. beds. Admissions took place at a mental hospital situated approximately 20 kilometres from the catchment area. Outpatient services for the area had previously consisted of 1.5 psychiatrists and a social worker. Patients were even then given inpatient care about 25 kilometres away from the area although on modern psychiatric wards at a general hospital.

The new organisation resulted in major changes in the composition of the patient population and care consumption (Stefansson &

Cullberg, 1986). The total number of patients increased by 30% allowing for the increase in the total population. A completely new patient group which had not been previously treated by the psychiatric services now sought care. This was the case for patients with acute crisis reactions (Table 7.2: PII–PI). This group comprised mainly younger individuals who had never before sought psychiatric care. They tended to come from lower social classes with a prevalence of substance abuse problems often in combination with suicide attempts.

Outpatient visits increased threefold. Inpatient care decreased with regard to both the number of persons admitted and the number of days in hospital. Contrary to expectation, the number of individuals admitted to compulsory inpatient care increased however.

Feedback of the evaluation's outcome into clinical praxis in order to improve the quality of care

The evaluation of the effects of the introduction of a new outpatient-oriented psychiatric care organisation showed that most of the appointed goals had been achieved. Accessibility for those amongst the population with mental disorders had increased. They were offered a variety of outpatient services replacing earlier inpatient care. New groups of the population with mental disorders sought care at an earlier stage without other patients, especially those suffering from psychotic problems, seeking care at other institutions. Outpatient care increased and inpatient care decreased. The continual evaluation showed, however, that there were many aspects of the new care organisation which indicated inadequate quality of care and which needed to be singled out and investigated.

This was the case with, for example, the new patient group, i.e. patients with acute crisis reactions, which had increased by a large measure. It was established that these patients had suffered from mental disorders and at the same time had had obvious social problems. This combination of psychiatric and social problems was so widespread within this patient group that it warranted its own description under the concept of 'anomic syndrome' (Cullberg, 1993).

The psychiatric services were confronted here with a group of patients who, according to experience, could be regarded as being at

Table 7.2. *The NP (period II) compared with the old organisation (period I) and with the same organisation after 10 years (period III): total patients, patients by diagnosis (ICD-8) and care utilisation per 100 000 inhabitants (⩾ 18 years)[a]*

	Period I, 1972–3 (PI)	Period II, 1975–6 (PII)	Period III, 1984–5 (PIII)	Relative differences	
				PII–PI	PIII–PII
Total patients	4 309	5 620	3 534	+30	−40
Patients without previous psychiatric contacts	2 194	3 327	1 521	+52	−54
Diagnoses					
Main diagnosis					
Schizophrenia	196	218	225	+11	+3
Other functional psychosis	181	183	180	+1	−2
Affective disorder	99	115	171	+16	+49
Senile dementia	72	94	33	+31	−65
Brain injury syndrome	59	70	16	+19	−77
Toxic psychosis	93	51	17	−45	−67
Neurosis including personality disorders[b]	2 716	2 613	1 906	−4	−27
Acute crisis reaction[c]	530	1 773	455	+236	−74
Other or no diagnosis	363	503	351	+39	−30
Supplementary diagnoses					
Alcohol abuse	610	991	586	+62	−41
Other addiction	169	211	164	+25	−22
Somatic illness	392	669	474	+71	−29
Suicide attempt	276	310	187	+12	−40
Care utilisation					
Total outpatient visits	14 669	39 437	46 390	+169	+18
Outpatient visits by psychotic patients	2 604	5 520	10 366	+112	+88
Admited patients	1 171	774	709	−44	−8
Compulsorily admitted patients	211	257	275	+22	+7
Hospital days	65 200	46 930	54 100	−28	+15

[a]Inhabitants (⩾ 18 years): 47.358 (1972–3), 51.294 (1975–6) and 57.752 (1984–5)
[b]ICD-8: 300–302, 305, 306
[c]ICD-8: 307

the start of a progressive development of symptoms. If these patients' problems were tackled in the right way then considerable secondary preventive gains might be expected, both for society and for the individual patient. The question remained, however, especially when considering what priority should be given to various patient groups in terms of resources, as to whether this specialist psychiatric care was the most appropriate for their needs.

This was also true in the case of the treatment spectrum available within the psychiatric services to special groups of patients. The number of patients with alcohol problems within the new organisation increased considerably. It could at the same time be established that those suffering from more serious alcohol related conditions, e.g. alcoholtoxic psychoses in need of acute detoxification, had to be treated outside the catchment area. Hence the services were found to be inadequate for alcohol abusers.

Another group of patients which in the first analysis appeared to receive quite unsystematic treatment comprised those with long-term psychoses. Their situation also evoked discussion as to how to improve services. This question became more acute in that the larger mental hospitals (two larger institutions each with approximately 2000 beds as well as a smaller one were in operation at that time in Stockholm) were successively closed down.

The compulsory admission rate increased for patients with long-term psychosis and, above all, for patients with neurotic or borderline syndromes among whom many were suicidal. One reason was the change of hospital setting from modern wards at a general hospital to wards at an older mental hospital. The former had a closed ward for intake. The patients could be persuaded to accept medication, to stay over night for observation, etc. This 'soft violence' avoided in many cases the need to use compulsory measures. Another reason was the staff's commitment to fulfil the aims of the organisation, of which one was to give priority to offering treatment outside the hospital for as long as possible. Sometimes the patients were kept in such a treatment too long and a compulsory admission had to be accomplished as a last resort. Could the organisation be changed in order to achieve improvements in these areas of concern?

The following section gives examples of how these issues were thought through, responded to and fed back to the care organisation. In this way, a basis for change was provided which aimed to raise the quality of the contact between the psychiatric services and the

population. The first issue concerned itself with which approach the
psychiatric services should adopt towards the large group of patients
presenting symptoms of psychosocial disorders ('anomic syndrome' as
it is called) and, who it was shown, came chiefly from particular
housing areas.

Home environment and psychiatric care

Epidemiological studies have shown that the prevalence of mental
disorders varies geographically according to the character of various
housing areas (Faris & Dunham, 1967). Likewise there is a connection
between prevalence and home environment (Dalgard, 1980). Choice
of housing area and type of housing are, along with profession, those
components which most reflect the individual's freedom of choice in
society, opportunities and therefore status. Financial resources often
have a bearing on this type of freedom of action. The areas with a high
prevalence of mental disorders and major consumption of the
psychiatric services are those which are above all characterised by
inhabitants with limited financial resources. People with mental
disorders, especially those of a long-term nature, generally have
limited financial resources and congregate to a large extent in these
areas.

A cartographic method known as MAPS (Stefansson, 1984) was
developed which linked the psychiatric patient register with a
database containing social and demographic data for 72 smaller
homogeneous sub-areas. Age-standardised treatment rates were
calculated for these various areas. Many areas showed a significantly
high prevalence of psychiatric disorder. Analysis showed that the
differences among areas could above all be associated with an area's
social structure and its age. Important factors regarding the area's
social structure which showed a high correlation with the seeking of
psychiatric care were: number of households moving in and out of the
area; the proportion of foreign nationals; percentage of single-parent
families; low income and crowded housing conditions. Areas with
high scores in these variables were given the operational definition
'low-status areas' and those with low scores, 'high-status areas'. By
also making a division according to age (areas which were younger
than 5 years and those which were older than 10 years), approximately
half of the catchment area's 72 sub-areas could be grouped into four

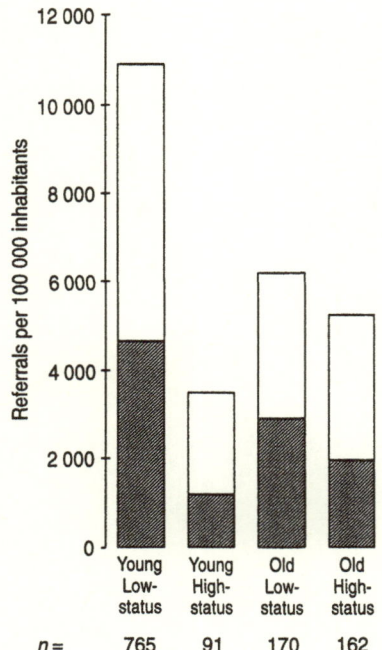

Fig. 7.1. Referrals to psychiatry per 100 000 inhabitants from various residential areas (age-standardised). Open columns, patients without previous psychiatric contact; hatched columns, patients with previous psychiatric contact. For definitions see the text.

contrasting areas. Fig. 7.1 shows the rates of treatment prevalence for these areas.

Low-status areas showed much higher levels of care consumption than high-status areas. This was especially true of the young low-status areas. A study of various diagnostic categories showed that the latter areas above all were overrepresented – approximately 6 times more than any other housing area – regarding the number of patients attempting suicide (Fig. 7.2). An inventory of the patients' problems in the case register also showed that these mental disorders were to a significant degree associated with social problems.

This information led to the following question: To what degree will the new psychiatric service organisation function as a social service institution where social problems dominate amongst the patients although in combination with mental disorders? In the earlier description of the new patient groups which sought care from the NP, it was established that this type of psychosocial problem was

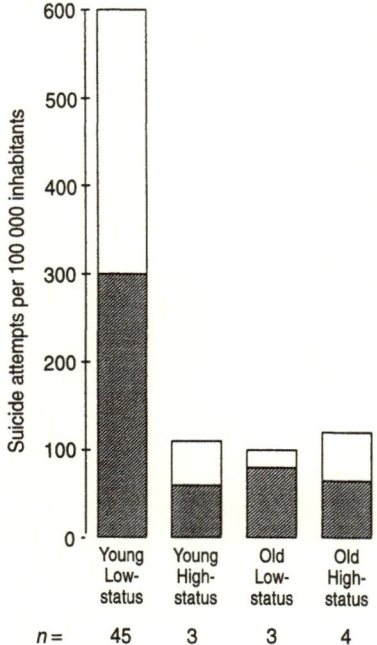

Fig. 7.2. Suicide attempts amongst psychiatric patients per 100 000 inhabitants from various residential areas (age-standardised). Open columns, patients without previous psychiatric contact; hatched columns, patients with previous psychiatric contact. For details see the text.

prevalent amongst crisis patients without earlier contact with the psychiatric services. A study where a psychiatric assessment was made of 30 randomly chosen medical records of patients with this diagnosis ($n = 679$) showed that one third could be considered to have problems of a type which could be addressed more adequately by a care service other than the psychiatric service. In many cases family counselling would have been the appropriate treatment alternative, preferably with the cooperation of the psychiatric services. In the remaining cases, psychiatric care was deemed to be suitable. The study was carried out, however, using data from medical journals, i.e. when the patient had already been assessed and afforded psychiatric care. How would a psychiatric assessment of the problem facing these patients in these housing areas look if it were carried out before they sought psychiatric care?

Table 7.3. *Measures taken by psychiatric field staff concerning 41 persons from so-called low-status areas attending psychiatric care for the first time*

Measures	Nos.	%
Referred to psychiatry	11	27
Offered psychiatric care or self-support group but moved out of the area	2	5
Referred to self-support group outside psychiatric care organisation	17	41
Referred to other care organisation	6	15
Psychiatric assessment in home only (*no further measures*)	5	12
Total	41	100

Adaptation of the organisation to meet the needs of low-status housing areas

A 'sub-office' to the main outpatient team was set up in a part of a housing area with approximately 1300 inhabitants of 18 years and above and with the highest frequency of individuals seeking psychiatric outpatient care. Each new visit to the psychiatric services, i.e. self-referrals or when the patient was referred, from the area was passed to this unit. Two of the staff, which consisted of a psychiatrist, a psychologist and an auxiliary nurse, then made two home visits in order to make a diagnostic assessment. The aim was to try to identify those patients with genuine psychiatric problems and refer them to psychiatric care. Patients with non-psychiatric problems were to be referred to other agencies or helped by other means without them being taken care of by the psychiatric services. It was considered that psychiatric assessments in the home environment would provide a better opportunity for carrying out this screening (Levander, 1987). When this operation had been running for some time it was evaluated (Table 7.3).

Forty-one new referrals from the housing area in question were examined. The problems of 25% of the area's patients who had referred themselves to the psychiatric services were assessed to be of a nature which required psychiatric care. In 75% of the cases the assessment was that the psychiatric problems were secondary. These patients would all have been accepted as psychiatric cases by the care organisation. In most of these cases it was a question of psychological reactions to social problems in combination with the lack of a functioning social support structure (family, etc.). Over half of the latter cases were referred to self-help groups such as women's groups or immigrant associations which were organised in the housing area by unit personnel. One conclusion was that home assessments, or above all those made outside the psychiatric surgery, contributed considerably to an increased understanding of the importance of social aspects with regard to the development of psychiatric problems. Home assessments were later incorporated into the daily work of other psychiatric outpatient units within the organisation.

'Patients with psychotic problems are psychiatry's main area of responsibility' (Nacka Project's Clinic Director)

One of the organisation's goals was to develop an outpatient service for patients who had been hospitalised for long periods. In most cases, these were patients with psychotic problems, especially schizophrenics. An earlier survey of these patients' out- and inpatient care consumption as well as treatment offered by the old and new organisation showed small changes. The utilisation of inpatient care decreased for these patients whereas compulsory admissions increased, contrary to intentions. There was certainly more contact with outpatient services but the treatment offered was scanty. In most cases, treatment consisted of supportive contacts often in combination with the dispensation of neuroleptic medication.

Organisational adaptation to meet the needs of patients with long-term psychosis

Stein & Test (1980) and other researchers have pointed out that the development of resources necessary to cope with long-term psychotic patients must be comprehensive in order to lead to a reduction of inpatient care as well as an integration of the patient into society with, it is hoped, an improved quality of life as a result.

In order to offer such an alternative to patients within the NP who were suffering from psychotic problems, a start was made in the early

1980s to reorganise outpatient services. One of the three general psychiatric outpatient teams was made into a psychosis unit. The unit comprised three sub-sections operating from the same building: a treatment section where psychiatric/medical and therapeutic treatment of a systematised nature was offered; a housing section where patients were able to practise living on their own but under the auspices of the psychiatric unit; and a psychosocial section where the chief contributions centred around building up and maintaining a functioning social network for the patients. The various housing and work-experience schemes as well as independent work cooperatives were expanded in stages.

To solve the shortcomings concerning the elevated rate of compulsory admissions, it was decided to establish resources for hospital treatment in the catchment area. Two wards (32 beds altogether) were opened at a somatic hospital close to the psychiatric outpatient units.

Easily available hospital beds as well as a varied outpatient programme for patients with long-term, mainly psychotic, problems were thus created. Group projects and training in living alone, in combination with work rehabilitation, could be developed. New therapeutic approaches which had already been tested and systematised within general psychiatric outpatient services, e.g. so-called ego-strengthening psychotherapy, could be further developed.

The importance of social conditions for problems and symptoms was also afforded greater priority in treatment. A method called social linking was developed. Social linking aimed actively to coordinate all social help inputs in order to create a tailor-made support structure for each patient. This method can be regarded as a parallel development to that which internationally came to be known as case management.

The effects of changing from general community mental health services to sub-specialised psychiatric care

The new organisation afforded an improved outpatient service to patients suffering from psychotic problems without any major increase in personnel. A comparison was once again made of the patient populations and care consumption in the catchment area with the help of the patient register (Table 7.2: PIII–PII) (Stefansson *et al.*, 1990). This time it was the NP which was the old organisation whilst the changed organisation of 1984–5 was the new one.

This comparison showed that the new organisation now treated approximately a thousand fewer patients than previously from the same area, which meant a reduction in the patient population by 40%. An increase might have been expected in that the general population had grown by 12.5% during the periods under comparison. The rate of diagnosis of functional or other psychoses as well as affective disorders increased as a result of the focus on patients with illnesses of long duration. All other diagnostic groups showed a decrease. Outpatient contacts for these patients increased considerably, especially for the psychotic patients. More admissions to hospital were recorded along with a larger amount of time spent as inpatients. This occurred without any appreciable increase in the number of patients receiving hospital care. There were thus more admissions but for shorter periods, i.e. that which is usually termed a revolving-door pattern. The number of compulsory psychiatric admissions increased.

The change in the pattern of inpatient care was mainly due to the fact that the post-reorganisation psychiatric care services now served a group of patients who had previously received long-term care outside the catchment area but who had needed and still needed much inpatient treatment. Inpatient care had also become more accessible.

Those patient groups which disappeared from the care services were for the most part those which had previously increased so considerably with the advent of the NP (period II). This development was not compatible with the original goals of the reorganisation. The possibilities for certain groups amongst the population to come into contact with the psychiatric services had diminished considerably. This led once more to the changes which had been made in the care service organisation being called into question.

One question again concerned the long-term psychotic patients. It was indeed the case that they had received improved outpatient care, but that which was provided on an inpatient basis was of a traditional nature and barely adequate for these patients. They still had a high proportion of involuntary care too. At this time it was decided to establish a completely new outpatient unit for these patients that would combine the firm and protective structure of the hospital with extensive outpatient activities. It was a matter of creating, as Wing & Furlong (1986) termed it, 'a haven for the disabled'.

For those who had become psychotic for the first time it was also considered essential to develop new forms of care less stigmatising than hospitalisation in an emergency ward. Such care would be tailored to help them or patients with psychotic problems whose symptoms had increased or who otherwise were experiencing a crisis to handle this crisis better. Help would also be available for patients' relatives. Despite financial setbacks, such a treatment unit which should fulfil these intentions was started in 1993.

Another question concerned those patients who suddenly disappeared from the outpatient clinics. The designated goals and the principle of total responsibility for the total population's mental health stimulated an initiative to find out where these individuals now sought care.

In search of the vanished patients

Psychiatric epidemiology tells us that the prevalence of mental disorders amongst the total population, i.e. that proportion which gets a psychiatric diagnosis, is in the region of 15% (Hagnell *et al.*, 1994). We also know from earlier studies that the population with mental disorders seeks care from their general practitioner or from somatic emergency units. The question which emerged at this point was the extent to which the patient groups which had previously sought psychiatric care and which had now disappeared turned to the somatic care services and, in particular, to general practitioners.

The first thing that was established was that the primary care capacity had radically increased during the same period that the psychiatric services heavily invested resources in patients with chronic illnesses. Fig. 7.3 shows how the number of new visits/referrals to general practitioners and psychiatric services respectively changed during the 1970s and 1980s.

It was decided to chart the extent to which persons with mental disorders had contact with primary care services in the catchment area. The investigation was carried out within the framework of an inter-Nordic multi-centre study the aim of which was to investigate the 'pathways to psychiatric care' as referred to in Goldberg & Huxley's (1980) earlier studies. In November 1990, 374 consecutive adult patients (18 years and above) in two primary health-care areas within the catchment area answered a self-assessment questionnaire

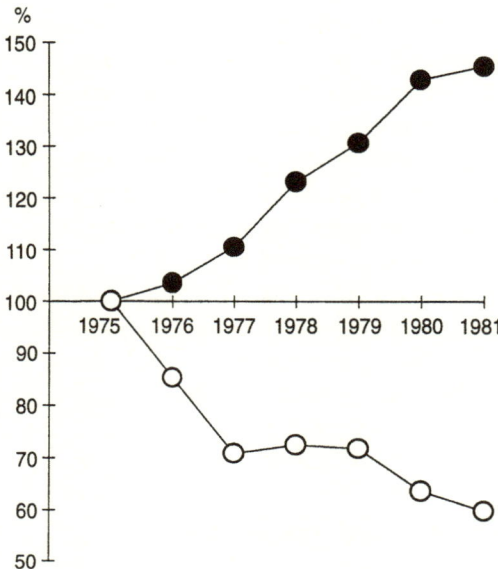

Fig. 7.3. Development of new visits 1975–1981 to general practitioner surgeries (filled circles; n = 29 000 in 1981) and psychiatric outpatient clinics (open circles; n = 680 in 1981).

(HSCL-25). They were also diagnosed by a general practitioner according to ICD-9. A random sample of the patients were interviewed using the Present State Examination. This study has been presented elsewhere (Nettelbladt *et al.*, 1993; Stefansson & Svensson, 1994).

The data were specially processed in order to ascertain to what extent the type of patient who had earlier sought care from the psychiatric services was now a patient in the primary care sector. The occurrence of the combination of mental illness and social problems, as well as the extent to which they occurred in the previously researched housing areas, were studied in particular. According to HSCL-25, the percentage of patients suffering from mental illness was calculated to be 19.6% (cut-off point 1.75). Table 7.4 shows the annual prevalence of those who claimed to have had social problems and to what extent they came from various housing areas divided up according to types used in an earlier study.

The primary care population was from a smaller part of the catchment area, which is why only two of the earlier area types are

Table 7.4. *Different categories of patients attending a general practitioner per 100 inhabitants from 'high-status' and 'low-status' housing areas*

Patient categories	Type of housing area	
	'High-status'	'Low-status'
Total patients	29	54
Self-reported mental illness (HSCL-25)	5	10
Self-reported social problems	7	10
Mental illness and social problems	3	4

represented. We can see, however, that the number of adult patients during 1 year from the 'low-status area' was almost double that from the 'high-status area', as was the proportion of patients with a mental illness according to HSCL-25. We can also note that primary care services were visited by a large part of the population during the course of a year. Approximately half of the population from these areas seeks such care during a year and a high percentage of these people are suffering from mental illness.

A 1-year follow-up found that one fifth of patients with mental illness sought psychiatric care. There is much to indicate that many of the patients who sought help from the NP and whose number later diminished with the reorganisation of psychiatric services now sought help within primary care.

This type of care is expanding more and more in Sweden. The goal is one general practitioner per 2000 inhabitants. There is a risk that part of the population suffering from mental illness but without a psychosis will receive less qualified help, adversely affecting the course of the illness. Psychiatry's new organisatory task is to find ways of once again increasing the possibilities for these population groups to obtain professional help, this time perhaps in conjunction with primary care.

The evaluation of the psychiatric care organisation in the catchment area will continue. Today the implementation of a market system and market thinking in care is fashionable. Further investigations will reveal how this system affects the treatment and quality of life of psychiatric patients, especially the long-term ill. It is also of importance to follow up the availability and care quality of the psychiatric services for that section of the total population suffering from mental illness. The present study is intended to give some clues as to how to proceed in that direction.

Conclusions

There were two things above all which characterised the evaluation studies carried out at the NP and which are also present in other internationally published evaluation projects. The first was the close link with clinical reality. The negative and of course the positive effects of the organisational changes could be swiftly uncovered. Various organisatory experiments could be made which could then perhaps, after a new evaluation, be implemented within the organisation. An important factor was also that the clinic management was interested in changing the organisation on the basis of the results provided by the evaluation. The NP clinic director was moreover part-time head of the unit which carried out the evaluation and which also consisted of 2.5 personnel. This meant that the evaluation could be carried out whilst maintaining an open dialogue with the clinic's personnel. From a larger perspective, it can be seen that this evaluation process went through a number of delimited phases.

Initially, a number of goals had been set up within the NP. For example, the new organisation aimed to reach new groups of patients at an early stage without dropping other patients in need of psychiatric care. Another goal was to increase outpatient services whilst decreasing inpatient services. These objectives came to be widely adopted as goals or standards within psychiatric care. It was not generally the case that such more or less operational goals were set up for clinical work, at least not during the 1970s. Such an approach was unnecessary as clinics were financed by annual budgets and the content and volume of their work were considered to reflect the needs of the population.

After the organisational changes had been made or after a certain time had elapsed, a broad description was made of the activities of the whole clinic. This description was population-focused due to the fact that a general goal was that the clinic should be responsible for all psychiatric services for the whole adult population in the catchment area. This description showed population groups, social and demographic, which were over- or underrepresented regarding care as well as utilisation of care

The next phase involved more in-depth studies of specific problem areas. Such studies, which sometimes took the form of research projects, often entailed the involvement of the staff. The latter were given the opportunity of leaving their ordinary clinic duties for a limited time in order to carry out studies under the supervision of qualified researchers from the Research and Evaluation Unit.

The organisatory changes were effected in the following phases. Psychiatric care was altered in various ways so as to improve those aspects which had been shown to function badly. An evaluation capability in the form of follow-up instruments, etc., was built into these development projects. After a time, a broad description was again made of the clinic's spectrum of care available to the population. The evaluation process could then begin again. This process, with its oscillation between goal-related description, deeper analysis and organisational changes, can in many ways be regarded as that which is aimed at today, i.e. quality assurance.

The second important prerequisite and condition necessary for this process to be feasible was that documentation should be collected in a systematic way. In this case, a psychiatric patient register was created along the lines of the model used in Camberwell (Wing & Hailey, 1972). Internationally, a 20-year period (1965–85) saw the establishment of many psychiatric patient registers. They have provided valuable knowledge as to how psychiatric care functions in relation to the population of the catchment area (ten Horn *et al.*, 1986; Wing, 1989). We have also seen most registers disappear, falling victim to either legislation or lack of funding. Registers have often been created for specific evaluation projects (as with the NP) and discontinued when the study was concluded. Many attempts have been made to put such registers on a permanent footing so as to be able continually to evaluate and monitor the quality of psychiatric care.

A trial was made with 25 participating clinics in Sweden during the 1980s. Only a few clinics have at the time of writing been able to maintain a register and this has often been due to the efforts of one or more persons committed to the idea. At a conference where experience from this project was discussed, several reasons were put forward to explain why it was so difficult to maintain patient registers of this type. One argument was that a psychiatric patient register was experienced as alien to the everyday work of the clinic. To describe the personal relationship to the patient in statistical terms was felt to be an objectification of this relationship. It was also considered that the patient's right to secrecy would be in jeopardy. This was despite the fact that the registers were usually kept under the supervision of a government body, the Data Inspection Authority, and that it could be demonstrated that a computerised register was considerably less vulnerable to intrusion than traditional medical records. Manual routines were often employed in the collection of data. It was considered that filling in forms other than the usual ones was burdensome and time-consuming. The most important reason, however, was that registers were not integrated into the everyday work of the clinic. Large sections of the staff were excluded from the evaluation process and the annual budget was granted regardless of the clinic's performance.

The situation is slightly different today. In the first place, demands have been made on the care services' management to regularly account for and monitor the quality of care. Secondly, in Sweden as in other countries, there is a demand that the financing of care should no longer be based purely on a budget but should also be performance-related. These two demands give very strong incentives for organising a regular and systematic collection of clinic data. Thirdly, and perhaps most important, is that computer technology has advanced so that there is today an increasing use of computerised medical record systems. Such a system which unites several aspects – quality control, clinical follow-up of treatment inputs for individual patients as well as descriptions of the care organisation and its relation to the population in the catchment area – may become the clinically integrated evaluation system which has up until now been missing.

References

Cullberg, J. (1993). *Dynamic Psychiatry*, 4th edn. Stockholm: Natur och Kultur. (In Swedish.)

Dalgard, O.S. (1980). Mental health, neighbourhood and related social variables in Oslo. In *Epidemiological Research as Basis for the Organization of Extramural Psychiatry*, ed. Strömgren, Dupont & Nielson. *Acta Psychiatrica Scandinavica Supplementum*, **285**, 298–304.

Donabedian, A. (1966). Evaluating the quality of medical care. *Millbank Memorial Foundation Quarterly*, **44**, 166–206.

Faris, R.E.I. & Dunham, H.W. (1967). *Mental Disorders in Urban Areas*. Chicago: University of Chicago Press.

Goldberg, D.P. & Huxley, P. (1980). *Mental Illness in the Community: The Pathway to Psychiatric Care*. New York: Tavistock.

Hagnell, O., Öjesjö, L., Otterbeck, L. & Rorsman, B. (1994). Prevalence of mental disorders, personality traits and mental complaints in the Lundby Study: a point prevalence study of the 1957 Lundby Cohort of

2612 inhabitants of a geographically defined area who were reexamined in 1972 regardless of domicile. *Scandinavian Journal of Social Medicine, Supplement,* **50**, 1–77.

Levander, S. (1987). Community work as part of the psychiatric services of Nacka. *Acta Psychiatrica Scandinavica Supplementum,* **337**, 23–9.

Nettelbladt, P., Hansson, L., Stefansson, C.-G., Borgquist, L. & Nordström, G. (1993). Test characteristics of the Hopkins Symptom Check List-25 (HSCL-25) in Sweden, using Present State Examination (PSE-9) as a caseness criterion. *Social Psychiatry and Psychiatric Epidemiology,* **28**, 130–3.

Stefansson, C.-G. (1984). Map analyses of psychiatric services: the application of a computerized psychiatric case register to geographical analysis. *Acta Psychiatrica Scandinavica,* **70**, 515–22.

Stefansson, C.-G. & Cullberg, J. (1986). Introducing community mental health services: the effects on a suburban patient population. *Acta Psychiatrica Scandinavica,* **74**, 368–78.

Stefansson, C.-G. & Svensson, C. (1994). Identified and unidentified mental illness in primary health care: social characteristics, medical measures and total care utilization during one year. *Scandinavian Journal of Primary Health Care,* **12**, 24–31.

Stefansson, C.-G., Cullberg, J. & Steinholtz-Ekecrantz, L. (1990). From community mental health services to specialized psychiatry: the effects of a change in policy on patient accessibility and care utilization. *Acta Psychiatrica Scandinavica,* **82**, 157–64.

Stein, L.I. & Test, M.A. (1980). Alternative to mental hospital treatment. *Archives of General Psychiatry,* **37**, 392–7.

ten Horn, G.H.M.M., Giel, R., Gulbinat, W.H. & Henderson, J.H. (1986). *Psychiatric Case Register in Public Health. A Worldwide Inventory 1960–1985.* Amsterdam: Elsevier

Wing, J.K. (1989). *Health Services Planning and Research: Contributions from Psychiatric Case Register.* London: Royal College of Psychiatrists/ GASKELL.

Wing, J.K. & Furlong, R. (1986). A haven for the severely disabled within the context of a comprehensive psychiatric community service. *British Journal of Psychiatry,* **149**, 449–57.

Wing, J.K. & Hailey, A.M. (1972). *Evaluating a Community Psychiatric Service: The Camberwell Register 1964–71.* Oxford: Oxford University Press.

PART III

METHODS: MEASUREMENTS, STRATEGIES AND NEW APPROACHES

8

Strategies of measurement and analyses

WILLIAM W. EATON

Introduction

'Strategy' means 'the science or art of military command as applied to the overall planning and conduct of large-scale combat operations'. The definition orients us to useful aspects of our war on mental illness, and in particular the evaluation of success in that effort. It suggests the value of overall planning in the face of a variety of alternatives. Inclusion of the idea of 'combat' emphasises the need for continuing energy and vigilance. The definition allows for the rationality of science or the intuition of art to be used in the work. In this chapter the notion of strategy is applied to the issue of measurement in the evaluation of community psychiatric services. It is important to note that 'services' is in the plural form. This form appropriately indicates that evaluation of an individual treatment service is not the focus – rather the focus is on evaluation of the *service system*. The focus is appropriate because the psychiatric service system is so fragmented that evaluation of a single service unit is rarely likely to be very useful. Much of the discussion will concern choices to be made, and alternatives to be avoided, given the strategic focus.

Strategies of measurement include three separate issues. First, there is a need to decide what content should be measured. Second, we must choose how to measure the chosen content. Third, there must be a technology to evaluate the success or failure of the measurement process itself. After a presentation of these three issues, there is a discussion of several strategic choices that must be made in designing measurement and analysis systems.

The content of measurement in the evaluation of mental health services

Measures can be applied at levels smaller than or greater than the individual human being. For evaluation of mental health services, the content of measurement can be divided roughly into outcomes at the level of the individual, and at the level of the service system. For the task of system evaluation, service outcomes are more important than individual outcomes. Also, other chapters of this book will focus in appropriate depth on individual outcomes. But it is useful to review both domains in order to guide and justify the strategic choices.

Individual outcomes

In the domain of individual outcomes, the major content of measurement includes measures of distress, psychopathology, diagnosis, functioning and quality of life. *Distress* is the feeling of discomfort which is aroused in stressful situations, when the perceived demands of the environment are greater than the potential responses of the individual (Mechanic, 1968). I do not distinguish the concept of distress from the concept of demoralisation (Frank, 1974): both are indicated by feelings of discomfort and a desire to change the situation on the part of the individual. Usually stressful situations are departures from the normal state of affairs, and distress tends to be transient. There are a variety of good indicators of distress, some as short as just a handful of questions (Cohen *et al.*, 1983). The best measure of distress is the initial version of the General Health Questionnaire (Goldberg, 1972). An entire generation of research in psychiatric epidemiology was dominated by measures of distress, and sociologists, and others, continue to be very interested in its causes and consequences (Aneshensal *et al.*, 1991).

Measures of *psychopathology* concern mental disturbances that reflect an aberrant causal process. There are thousands of relevant measures, depending on the nature of the psychopathology. For purposes of evaluation, a high priority is placed on feasibility of measurement, with scales such as the Center for Epidemiologic Studies Depression (CESD) Scale (Radloff & Locke, 1986). These measures blend imperceptibly into diagnostically oriented measures of psychopathology, such as the Diagnostic Interview Schedule (DIS:

Robins *et al.*, 1985) the CIDI (Robins *et al.*, 1988) or the SCAN.

Functioning is the success with which the individual meets the tasks of living. These tasks vary from those required for survival, such as eating and obtaining shelter, and clothing oneself, to those which make life more interesting and pleasant, such as social and recreational activities. But the notion of functioning connotes that they are tasks and that success can be evaluated. There are several measures concerning functioning, including the Global Assessment Scale (GAS), the Katz Adjustment Scales (Katz & Lyerly, 1963) and a set of scales which arose from studies of functioning in elderly populations, the Activities of Daily Living (ADL: Lawton & Brody, 1969).

Quality of life is the degree of enjoyment, and breadth of meaning, an individual takes from everyday living. Good quality of life is expected to be absent from persons in distress, and those not functioning well, but the concepts are different, even if empirically related. Scales of the quality of life have been developed for the general population (Mor & Guadagnoli, 1988) and adapted for the seriously mentally ill (Lehman, 1983).

For the evaluation of mental health services, measures of functioning are the strategic choice. Distress is too widely present in the general population to be useful in evaluating mental health services. Measures of psychopathology and diagnosis are useful for evaluating individual treatment effectiveness but not as important for the service system in general, because many disorders do not change sufficiently that improvements in the service system can be noticed. Measures of quality of life are important as outcomes but may reflect many other social processes, and are not as high a priority within the context of limited resources. Measures of functioning fluctuate widely, have important individual and social costs attached to them, and are amenable to a wide variety of interventions.

Service outcomes

An obvious and important measure of service outcome is the *volume of service*. Units of service are customarily defined and counted as part of the accounting and fiscal mechanism of treatment units – days of hospitalisation, and outpatient visits, for example. Volume of service can also be obtained in population-based surveys (Shapiro *et al.*, 1985), but care must be taken to define the unit of service, and the facility, precisely, before asking about the number of visits or days.

Volume of service is a dynamic indicator, in that the time interval for the volume must be specified.

Rate of rehospitalisation is a widely used measure of service outcome. Hospitalisation is costly and often involves a social crisis, so a low rate of rehospitalisation is good. Rehospitalisation varies widely between treatment systems (Eaton *et al.*, 1992) and between treatment modalities (Hogarty *et al.*, 1974). Therefore, the effects of changes in the service system are probably noticeable.

Continuity of treatment refers to the degree to which the service system links episodes of treatment in a seamless whole (Bass & Windle, 1972). The linkage tends to be more difficult when the intensity of the treatment episodes varies, as occurs, for example, between hospitalisation and maintenance outpatient treatment. The problem is exacerbated by the nature of the onset of recurrent clinical episodes, which shift the appropriate intensity of treatment in unexpected ways. The percentage of unfulfilled dispositions is one (inverse) indicator of continuity of treatment, and others are available (Bass & Windle, 1972).

Client satisfaction is another measure of service outcome. It is obtained through surveys of client populations (Larsen *et al.*, 1979).

In the context of this era of community care, measures of continuity of treatment are the strategic choice. Volume of service is too crude a measure, and may well reflect inappropriate use of services, due either to clients or to treatment providers. Rehospitalisation is more important for disorders in which hospitalisation usually occurs, such as schizophrenia; but much less important for disorders usually treated in an outpatient setting, such as the depressive and anxiety disorders. Client satisfaction is less useful because, in some situations such as involuntary hospitalisation, clients might not be expected to be 'satisfied' with the services received, and in other situations high levels of satisfaction might not reflect good treatment. The concept of continuity of care applies to the entire treatment system, which is appropriate. It measures one of the most important predictors of clinical success which is dependent on the service system itself.

Modalities of measurement

The modality of measurement refers to the process by which measurement occurs. Modality is closely associated both with the cost of measurement and with its accuracy. Therefore, choice of modality is a highly strategic issue.

The *clinical modality* arises out of medical practice. Its basic quality is that the clinician decides upon the presence or absence of phenomena to be measured. In the context of psychiatry, where interview material is most important, other distinctive aspects of the clinical modality are use of cross-examination, and rating of behaviours and signs in the absence of a complaint.

The *survey modality* also relies on the interview, but the burden of determining the presence or absence of the measured phenomena rests with the respondent, client or patient. The survey approach works best when the structure of questions is fixed and they are asked in verbatim form by the interviewer.

Paper and pencil modality is related to the survey modality in its reliance on the respondent, but no interviewer is involved. The respondent reads the question and fills out an answer sheet. Psychological testing is most often conducted in this format. This format is not useful for illiterate persons or those whose consciousness is not clear.

Computer-assisted modality involves use of a computer to assist in either the clinical, survey or paper and pencil modality. Computer-assisted modality is relatively new, and has been used most extensively in conjunction with paper and pencil tests. Recently, computer-assisted forms of commonly used survey (Blouin, 1986) and clinical (Wing *et al.*, 1990) instruments have been made available in computer-assisted modality. In the near future, many psychophysiological, performance-oriented tests will be available in computer-assisted form.

The *record-based modality* involves use of records that are already available. Table 8.1 shows different types of record systems in use in psychiatry. The 'traditional medical record' has evolved out of standard clinical care, and is oriented towards treatment of a single patient. Billing patients for treatment received requires that each treatment event be counted and operated upon. Monitoring the service system involves counting the volume of care rendered in a way that allows comparison across types of treatments and facilities, i.e. a uniform reporting system. Evaluation of the service system requires that records in a uniform reporting system be linked, so that effects of changes in one part of the system are noticed in other parts. The point here is that evaluation of the service system, *as a system*, and not as individual treatment units, requires that records be linked. Finally,

Table 8.1. *Record systems in psychiatry*

Purpose	Record system
Clinical care	Traditional medical records
Billing	Event reporting system
Monitoring	Uniform event reporting system
Service system evaluation	Linked uniform reporting system
Epidemiological research	Comprehensive population-based register

for basic epidemiological research, the linked uniform reporting system must be based in a general population – this is the situation of the psychiatric case register.

The content of measurement, as discussed above, affects the modality of measurement somewhat. In theory, all areas of content could be addressed via all modalities, but some association between content area and modality exists. Standard records do not normally contain evidence about distress because it is so transient, for example. Diagnoses are often required in medical settings, so they are available from records: but diagnoses are generally not made from paper and pencil tests.

Assessment of measurement

A variety of procedures allow assessment of the success of measurement. The *sine qua non* of measurement is *reliability*, which is loosely defined as the consistency of measurement, and more precisely defined as either the correlation between equivalent measures or the ratio of true score variance to total variance (Bohrnstedt, 1983). Without measures of reliability, there is always the possibility that the fertile human mind can create concepts and engage in measurement operations which appear to generate a reality that is in fact non-existent: if reliability is low, there is no clear proof as to the existence of the phenomena under study. Table 8.2 displays various procedures for assessment of the success of measurement, with a metric for measuring that success, and a minimal or standard value using the given metric. For reliability, the kappa statistic is a commonly used metric (Cohen, 1960) and a suggested minimum value for it is 0.50. If a kappa value for a measured concept being analysed is below 0.50, it is hardly worth the effort to analyse the data.

Table 8.2. *Standard values in the assessment of measurement*

	Metric	Minimum or standard value
Reliability	Kappa	>0.50
Validity	Rho	>0.50
Cost	Dollars	$0.01–$1000 per measure
Response burden	Hours	1 minute–4 hours
Temporal comprehensiveness	% career events linked	Depends on severity/prognosis (schizophrenia: 5 years)
Geographical comprehensiveness	Square miles	Maximum of 1 day's drive
Facility comprehensiveness	% service events linked	Depends on severity/prognosis (schizophrenia: 90%)

Validity is the degree to which the target concept is actually measured by the instrument at hand. As is well known, measures can be reliable without being valid. An example is the measure of the presence of the divinity, which might be measured very reliably by pronouncing words, or by the presence of an icon. Many would challenge the idea that the presence of an icon is a valid indicator of the presence of the supreme being. Validity is assessed in a variety of procedures, all involving the notion of correlation or association (indicated by 'rho' in Table 8.2) with some true value. The minimum acceptable value for validity is also somewhere around 0.50.

The *cost of measurement* is an obvious measure of success. In this case, less is better! Cost can be measured in dollars, and the standard or minimum value can vary enormously. A paper and pencil test, administered in a structured setting, might cost only a few cents per subject to collect. A 10-minute telephone interview might cost $25 per subject. A full-fledged psychiatric epidemiological survey, with 2-hour household interview, might cost $500 per subject. If there is an examination by a psychiatrist, the per subject cost can easily rise to $1000. Finally, for epidemiological studies with full medical and biological assessments, as well as clinical and survey assessments, the cost can be thousands of dollars per subject.

Response burden is important in assessing measurement. Every measure entails some sort of demand from the respondent. The nature of the demand can vary in its intensity and duration. An example of variation in intensity is the comparison of demand created by measures taken through unobtrusive observation as compared with the demand required for a spinal tap. In the field of psychiatry, many measures undertaken involve only mental alertness by the respondent, and the most useful metric is response burden hours. Epidemiological research projects sponsored by the United States government are required to obtain approval for their total response burden hours, and each agency within the public health service has a response burden budget. In the situation of service outcomes, response burden can be estimated for the treatment unit which is providing the information, if that is the measurement situation. Service outcomes, in general, involve far fewer response burden hours than patient outcomes, because the service outcome data are often already collected, and have just to be organised.

There are a series of measurement qualities which have to do with the content area of continuity of treatment. These qualities involve the comprehensiveness of the measurement in various areas. Measuring continuity of treatment involves linkage of data of various types, to form a treatment career. Without the notion of the individual career of treatment, continuity has little meaning. The linkage will be successful only to the degree it involves all possible data points, i.e. its comprehensiveness. Comprehensiveness can be judged temporally, geographically, by service and by population. *Temporal comprehensiveness* is the length of time covered by the data linkage effort. The most complete measurement of continuity of treatment will include the entire treatment career, which can be many years long. Clinical episodes that are not recorded because they occur before or after the data collection has taken place may have an important effect on the measures of continuity. The standard value for temporal comprehensiveness will vary dependent on the severity of the disorder. For a relatively chronic disorder such as schizophrenia, it would not make much sense to measure continuity of treatment without at least a few years of measurement.

Geographical comprehensiveness is the area covered by the data linkage effort which is used to measure continuity of treatment. Several research efforts (Person, 1964; Mellsop, 1969) have shown that the distance from the residence to the service facility affects the probability that the individual will actually obtain services. Data linkage efforts which are geographically confined to a small area will miss service episodes from outside the area that would otherwise contribute to estimates of continuity. The metric is in square miles or kilometres. It would seem that one possible minimum standard would be the maximum distance which permits the individual to obtain outpatient treatment without staying overnight away from home, i.e. one-half day's drive (a circular area with a radius of about 150 miles (250 kilometres), with an area of approximately 70 000 square miles (200 000 square kilometres)).

Data linkage involves several types of service facility, ranging from hospitalisation in a chronic care mental hospital, to emergency room visits at an acute care general hospital, to brief outpatient visits from an outreach team. *Service comprehensiveness* is the degree to which all types of facilities are involved in measures of continuity of treatment. The costs of linkage rise as the number and breadth of facilities included in the linkage effort increase. Linkage systems typically attempt to link data from some circumscribed subset of all possible facilities. The metric is the percentage of the total number of service events which are linked by the measurement system. The minimum standard again depends on the severity and prognosis of the disorder, but is similar to consensually accepted standards for non-response bias in field surveys, i.e. about 70%. It is hard to imagine a measure of continuity of treatment being credible if it linked less than 70% of the total service events.

Some systems of data linkage apply to only some subset of the population. For example, Medicaid and Medicare data systems in the United States apply only to the elderly, the poor, and certain other subgroups. For data linkage to be successful in creating careers of treatment events, a large proportion of the general population must have unchanging eligibility to use the service system.

Strategic choices

To summarise the presentation so far, the strategic choice for measurement in mental health services evaluation is to measure continuity of treatment in the record-based modality, using a system of measurement which includes at least 70 000 square miles (200 000 square kilometres), extends for at least several years in time, covers 70% or more of the service events, and more than 70% of the population residing in the service region. These qualities are met in the situation of many psychiatric case registers. Therefore, a brief discussion of psychiatric case registers is warranted.

Psychiatric case registers

A psychiatric case register is a population-based system for collecting a minimum amount of data for each service event, and linking these data across time and facilities, to enable construction of a service career for each individual in the population. The notion of the population is included in the definition of the register, and the population referred to is all persons eligible for treatment, not simply those treated. In the days prior to deinstitutionalisation, the service system was so much simpler (the state hospital) that the service career could be credibly constructed and analysed usefully, without a great deal of effort at record linkage (since the pertinent records tended to be in one place). The service system now is more complicated. Evaluation of a *treatment* is still feasible without record linkage, but evaluation of *the mental health service system* will not be useful without record linkage. Therefore, psychiatric case registers (or, at least, linked uniform reporting systems with every quality discussed above, except possibly population comprehensiveness) should be in place where service systems are under evaluation.

There is a sizable literature on psychiatriac case registers (Baldwin, 1973; ten Horn *et al.*, 1986). The registers span the globe, and vary in size from populations of less than 50 000 to more than 5 000 000. Many were started in the early 1960s, at the beginning of the era of deinstitutionalisation, when some planners had correctly foreseen the need for record linkage to combat the disorganisation in treatment that would follow use of many facilities instead of one hospital (Kramer, 1967).

Most registers started with the aim of combining one or more of the functions listed in Table 8.1, but their success has been limited. Register data is not always useful for research, because the diagnostic and clinical measures are not good enough for research, and because the research has required comprehensiveness across facilities (for accurate prevalence data) or a duration of operation (for accurate incidence and longitudinal data) which was never achieved. Most registers were able to provide counts of service events, categorised by patient and facility characteristics, but these were not widely useful. Registers have never been very useful for clinical purposes because of the delay in processing records, which could be from several days to several months. Thus, the registers were expensive and did not live up to the initial hopes of mental health planners. Registers were also challenged by public advocacy groups concerned about the implications of record linkage, when the records are as sensitive as is the situation in psychiatry. In the United States, although there are now many linked uniform reporting systems, they generally have very poor population comprehensiveness, and many registers there have fizzled out. It is probably fair to say that almost all psychiatric case registers have had important challenges to their existence over the last several decades.

The original vision of the registers leaped ahead of available technology. Even now, registers suffer from rapid changes in computer technology. Over the last 5 years important developments have taken place, however, which have strong implications for the clinical use of the linked record systems. I believe these uses will be so positively evaluated as to lead to a resurgence of interest in psychiatric case registers generally. Managers of mental health service systems, and psychiatric researchers, have always been interested in organised and linked record systems; but in the near future they will have strong allies among clinicians who see the systems as vital to good clinical care.

Statistical analysis for evaluation

Many strategic choices must be made in the realm of data analysis for evaluation of mental health service systems. Data analytic methods for evaluation are developing very rapidly. Evaluation has such a strong implication of process that only techniques for analysis of longitudinal data are discussed here. These procedures for the analysis of longitudinal data can be characterised as to whether the outcome of interest is described as continuous or discrete; and likewise as to whether the passage of time is demarcated in relatively large, discrete clumps or continuously in small or even infinitesimal bits. To apply the methods requires a theory, model, or at least a question being asked of the longitudinal data. Therefore, we have to organise the multitudinous questions asked about the longitudinal nature of psychopathology into a coherent form. The basic organisation involves two distinct types of questions about the ebb and flow of psychopathology. One question concerns timing: How fast or slow does the psychopathology change? As an aside, it may be of interest to note that some of the words we have for psychopathology (e.g. 'lunacy') imply this interest in timing. A second question focuses on aetiology: What causes the psychopathology to change? As an aside, it is of interest to note that early uses of some of our words for psychopathology imply this interest in cause (e.g. the 'insane root' in *Macbeth*).

These two questions help to subdivide the types of statistical analyses undertaken on longitudinal data. Table 8.3 reflects this subdivision as to purpose. The discussion here provides only a brief orientation to the general area, with references to textbooks and articles for more detail. Cell A, discrete time and dichotomous outcome, reveals simple analyses of *incidence* and *outcome* when the goal concerns timing; and *logistic regression* when the goal is aetiological. Statistical procedures for these types of analyses are described in Kleinbaum *et al.* (1982). Cell B, continuous time and dichotomous outcome, now splits into *survival curves* on the one hand; and *proportional hazards regression* on the other (both subsumed under 'survival analysis' and described in Lawless, 1982). Cell C, with continuous levels of psychopathology and discrete time, breaks into uncomplicated models of ebb and flow such as *change scores* (e.g. as discussed in Kessler & Greenberg, 1981) versus the more complex *structural equation models* (as described in Bollen, 1989). Finally, cell D, continuous time and continuous measures of psychopathology, reveals two sets of analyses: *growth models* (e.g., Rogosa *et al.*, 1982), where the interest is strictly temporal; and *random effects models*, where the interest is in causes (Ware, 1985).

The dual dichotomies simplify too much, unfortunately. Outcomes can be categorical but not dichotomous. Also, there can be mixtures of continuous and discrete variables in one model. The description of time as discrete or continuous is arbitrary – rather it is relatively chunky or relatively smooth. The fifth cell, at the bottom of the table, reflects these complexities. For categorical variables, including dichotomous and polytomous variables, where the interest is in timing, the *discrete-time* and *continuous time Markov models* (e.g. Feller & Higgins, 1968) are appropriate, if clumsy. For mixtures of variables, the change in metric has not allowed development of techniques which allow simultaneous study of timing, as far as I know. For mixtures of variables where the interest is more in causes, there is a technique I will call *latent probit regression*, where time is measured in larger chunks (Muthen, 1984); and a type of time series that has not yet received an easy label or glib acronym that is called *discrete/continuous time series* (Zeger & Liang, 1991), for want of something more facile.

Table 8.3. *Potential analytical strategies*

	Time	
Psychopathology	Discrete	Continuous
Discrete	*Temporal description*: Incidence, outcome	*Temporal description*: Survival curves
	Search for causes: Logistic regression	*Search for causes*: Proportional hazards regression
Continuous	*Temporal description*: Change scores	*Temporal description*: Growth models
	Search for causes: Structural equations	*Search for causes*: Random effects models
Mixed	Markov models Latent probit regressions Discrete/continuous time series	

The statistical procedures discussed above have generally grown out of observational, as opposed to experimental, paradigms. But they are completely amenable to studying the effect of a randomly assigned treatment. They also handle the more frequent situation which arises in evaluating mental health service systems: that of a quasi-experimental design (Cook & Campbell, 1979).

Record-based visual aids for treatment history

One example of a clinical use of linked data systems is the graphical presentation of treatment history. Using new developments in computer screen graphics allows Adolph Meyer's (1919) concept of the life chart to be adapted to presentation of treatment history in the context of integrated information systems. The goal is to encourage the treating psychiatrist to learn the treatment history for each patient, and to assist the psychiatrist in doing so. Fig. 8.1 is an example. The horizontal dimension represents time, passing from left to right. Three characteristics of the treatment history are presented: the treatment agency, including the intensity of treatment; the diagnosis, including co-morbidity and hierarchy; the medication prescribed, including dosage. In anticipated usage, the visual presentation of treatment history will take advantage of colours on a colour monitor (for categorical qualities such as agency, diagnosis, and type of medication), and width for qualities with intensity such as intensity of treatment, number of diagnoses, and dosage). Here the reader will

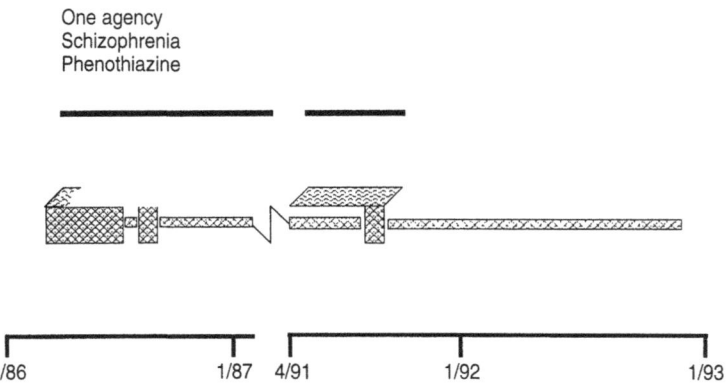

Fig. 8.1. Visual aid to treatment history: patient A.

have to imagine the effects of gradations of colour, since the figure is in black and white.

In Fig. 8.1, patient A has an episode of schizophrenia in hospital X, which has the colour light green (diagonal cross-hatching) assigned to it. The episode involves inpatient care (wide band) for several months along the time axis. It is followed by outpatient care through the same agency; the outpatient level of intensity is denoted by the lesser width of the horizontal light green (diagonal cross-hatched) line. Shortly thereafter another, shorter hospitalisation occurs, which is followed by outpatient follow-up care. During this treatment episode the patient is diagnosed as having schizophrenia, denoted by the light mauve rectangle (wavy lines inside) on the front-to-back dimension. Phenothiazine is prescribed at a recommended level (thick dark line at top). In February 1987 the patient disappears from the record system, to reappear at the outpatient clinic nearly 4 years later, in April 1991. The diagnosis of schizophrenia is given and the same medication is prescribed. Another hospital episode occurs in the middle of 1991, followed by outpatient care until 1993.

Fig. 8.2 shows the more complex situation of patient B. Two treatment agencies are involved, and an additional diagnosis of depression is made – perhaps this explains the reluctance to release the individual until the depression subsides. At any rate, the additional antidepressant medication is included in the appropriate area of the chart (square cross-hatching). As with patient A, the system loses track of the patient in 1987 until 1991, but for this patient there is an emergency room visit, precipitated by an attempted

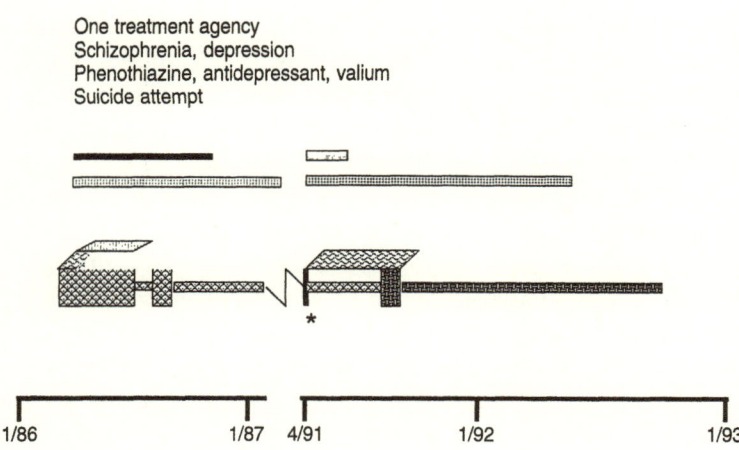

One treatment agency
Schizophrenia, depression
Phenothiazine, antidepressant, valium
Suicide attempt

1/86   1/87 4/91   1/92   1/93

Fig. 8.2. Visual aid to treatment history: patient B.

suicide. Again, the width indicates overnight stay, and light green (diagonal cross-hatching) indicates hospital X; but here the light green is surrounded by red to indicate the emergency room visit (colour red not shown in black and white reproduction). The asterisk denotes a danger. At the emergency room, and for several days thereafter, valium was prescribed (light orange rectangle – dots inside).

It is possible to imagine, and display in colour, much more complicated situations. For example, there could be three separate psychiatric agencies (hospitals X, Y and Z, denoted by light green, light blue, and violet, respectively), and a primary care physician (light grey). The primary care physician becomes involved first, leading to a hospital stay eventually, where three diagnoses are received, and noted hierarchically (schizophrenia, depression, phobia). In the hospital, the dosage is increased in several stages, and then reduced after discharge to the outpatient care. An inpatient stay at hospital Y follows, and this hospital agrees with the diagnosis, but prefers another form of phenothiazine. The patient is discharged to a day treatment centre for several months, and then to outpatient treatment. In 1987 the patient is lost to the system, until a visit to the emergency room of hospital Y due to a suicide attempt. The patient is released to outpatient care, and eventually to the care of the family physician, which is followed by an inpatient episode at hospital Z. This hospital thinks the patient is bipolar (dark blue in diagnosis area), and tries lithium (blue in medication area). The patient is released to outpatient care, and eventually lost again to the system, until June of 1992, when he ends up at hospital Y again. He is discharged to day treatment, then outpatient visits, and finally to the primary care physician. During treatment for an infection, the primary care physician enters a notation that the patient is allergic to penicillin. Another short but uneventful emergency room stay occurs, and then outpatient treatment until the present.

This manner of visual presentation could take of the advantage of the zoom facility now available in many graphical programs. For example, zooming on the asterisks might inform as to the details of the emergency; zooming on the agency might give the name and telephone number of the treating clinician. Automatic rescaling should be possible also, so that a single visual presentation could include a psychiatric career of 2 years', or 20 years', duration. Finally, there is room for a few details about the patient, such as name, age, sex, and identifying number.

All the information needed for these visual aids is present in the medical record now. In many linked uniform reporting systems, the data are available in magnetic form. What is required is computer programs to organise the data visually.

Empirically based discharge planning

Another example of clinical use of linked record systems is locally based empirical discharge planning. It is pretty hard to predict future need for services for an individual patient, especially at their first episode. The diagnosis, and the type of onset, will help to some extent, but there is not much else to go on. However, as time passes the prediction may improve because more information about the history of that particular individual's need for treatment becomes available. Some of this information can be built into statistical algorithms. For example, the probability of being hospitalised might be a function of diagnosis, type of onset, number of hospitalisations to date and time since latest contact with a mental health professional. Fig. 8.3 shows the rate of retention ('survival') in the community in four service systems in Denmark, Maryland, Salford (England) and Victoria (Australia), respectively. The curves have similar shapes but differ in level, indicating that the rate of rehospitalisation varies markedly between service systems. The shape is approximated in parametric form such as the Weibull (Fig. 8.4), a probability distribution related

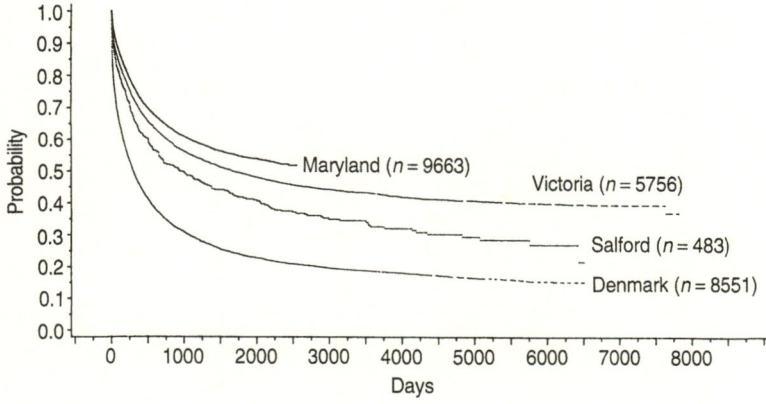

Fig. 8.3. Schizophrenia: probability of remaining in the community after the first discharge.

to the exponential (Lawless, 1982) which is widely used in various analyses of duration (Eaton & Whitmore, 1977). The Weibull parameterises the probability of rehospitalisation as a function which changes with time in a linear fashion. For many duration distributions the change is a linear decline – that is, the longer an individual goes without having the rehospitalisation, the less likely it is that the rehospitalisation will occur. It seems likely that locally based algorithms would be more accurate than algorithms merging service data from widely dispersed populations. Therefore, each system should have a unique algorithm for projecting the need for services after discharge. The statistical form of the algorithm – for example, parametric survival curve such as the Weibull, gamma or mixed exponential – could be generic to many systems, with the variables used for prediction being unique to each local system.

An algorithm for an individual patient might be helpful in planning such things as the frequency of future contacts. An alarm system could be built into the algorithm, to alert clinicians to the possibility of dangers, or costly hospitalisations. As with the visual aid presented above, many data useful for this sort of prediction are already available in the medical record, and in many places, in magnetic form. They just need to be organised and used.

These data-based tools would help psychiatrists treat the individual patient, by providing information efficiently, and identifying areas of doubt or danger. They would inform the psychiatrist about the current structure of the treatment system. These systems would

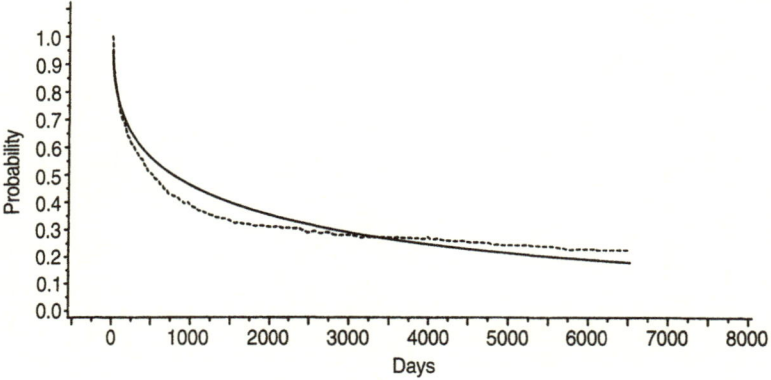

Fig. 8.4. Comparison between the Kaplan–Meier curve (broken line) and the Weibull model (continuous line) for the first episode in Denmark (see Fig. 8.3).

sensitise the psychiatrist to both errors in treatment of the patient, and weaknesses in the treatment system. Finally, use of these systems would tend to improve the quality of data. Clinical use of linked data record systems will benefit evaluation efforts, because linked data are of such good use for evaluation.

Priorities and costs

The high priority placed on comprehensive linked record systems is not meant to exclude other forms of measurement in the evaluation of community psychiatric service systems. What is recommended here is that evaluation efforts be built upon the foundation of registers. If we cannot tell where the client is, and who is treating him or her – in effect, if we cannot construct a relatively seamless treatment career – it is difficult or impossible to conduct evaluations of the service system. In the context of a service system with comprehensive record linkage, many important evaluations can be conducted that are more intensive. As indicated above, for outcomes at the level of the client, measures of functioning are recommended as most pertinent to evaluation efforts.

How much does record linkage cost? Is it worth the effort? It is not difficult to make estimates of costs, using data from existing registers. In the past, early cost estimates have often been optimistically low, because unanticipated resources were needed to upgrade normal records to a minimum standard to make them useful. Due to changes in computer technology, costs of this sort of activity are dropping each year. One would think that if a bank can follow a cheque around, and if express mail couriers can follow a package around, we should be able to keep track of our clients. Costs may depend heavily on seemingly small choices made – for example, how quickly records are linked. Real-time linkage is very expensive, but daily linkage may be almost as useful for our purposes, and much cheaper.

The costs of record linkage should be compared with the benefits. While it is possible, as noted above, to estimate costs very roughly, it is almost impossible to estimate benefits without a carefully controlled study. Benefits should appear in the form of fewer rehospitalisations and other social crises, lower levels of symptomatology and distress, better client functioning and higher quality of life for populations in communities with psychiatric services which are linked versus those which are not linked. Thus, the final recommendation is for evaluation studies of the costs and benefits of record linkage.

Summary

The strategic priority for evaluation of mental health services is measures of continuity of care in the record-based modality. A new consensus about minimum standards for quality of measurement for continuity of care must be created. Computerised record linkage systems provide the opportunity for this content and modality of measurement to flourish, if clinical uses for the data are developed and exploited.

References

Aneshensel, C.S., Rutter, C.M. & Lachenbruch, P.A. (1991). Social structure, stress, and mental health: completing conceptual and analytic models. *American Sociological Review*, **56**, 166–78.

Bachrach, L.L. (1981). Continuity of care for chronic mental patients: a conceptual analysis. *American Journal of Psychiatry*, **138**, 1449–56.

Bahn, A. K. (1962). Psychiatric case register conference 1962. *Public Health Reports*, **77**, 1071–6.

Bahn, A.K. (1966). Psychiatric case register conference 1965. *Public Health Reports*, **81**, 748–54.

Bahn, A.K., Gardner, E.A., Alltop, L., Knatterud, G.L. & Solomon, M. (1966). Admission and prevalence rates for psychiatric facilities in four register areas. *American Journal of Public Health*, **56**, 2033–51.

Baldwin, J.A. (1973). Linked record medical information systems. *Proceedings of the Royal Society of London, Series B*, **184**, 403–20.

Bass, R.D. & Windle, C. (1972). Continuity of care: an approach to measurement. *American Journal of Psychiatry*, **129**, 110–15.

Blouin, A.G. (1986). The computerized Diagnostic Interview Schedule. *DIS Newsletter*, **3**, 4–8.

Bohrnstedt, G.W. (1983). Measurement. In *Handbook of Survey Research*, ed. P.H. Rossi *et al.*, pp. 69–121. Orlando, FL: Academic Press.

Bollen, K.A. (1989). *Structural Equations with Latent Variables*. New York: Wiley.

Cohen, J. (1960). A coefficient of agreement for nominal scales. *Educational and Psychological Measurement*, **20**, 37–46.

Cohen, S., Kamarck, T. & Mermelstein, R. (1983). A global measure of perceived stress. *Journal of Health and Social Behavior*, **24**, 385–96.

Cook, T.D. & Campbell, D.T. (1979). *Quasi-experimentation: Design and Analysis Issues for Field Settings*. Boston. Houghton Mifflin.

Eaton, W.W. & Kessler, L.G. (1985). *Epidemiologic Field methods in Psychiatry: The NIMH Epidemiologic Catchment Area Program*. Orlando, FL: Academic Press.

Eaton, W.W. & Whitmore, G.A. (1977). Length of stay as a stochastic process: a general approach and application to hospitalization for schizophrenia. *Journal of Mathematical Sociology*, **5**, 273–92.

Eaton, W.W., Mortensen, P.B., Herrman, H., *et al.* (1992). Long-term course of hospitalization for schizophrenia. I. Risk for rehospitalization. *Schizophrenia Bulletin*, **18**, 217–28.

Feller, W. & Higgins, E. (1968). *An Introduction to Probability Theory and its Applications*, 3rd edn, vol. 1. Wiley Series in Probability and Mathematical Statistics. New York: Wiley.

Frank, J.D. (1974). *Persuasion and Healing: A Comparative Study of Psychotherapy*. New York: Schocken Books.

Goldberg, D. (1972). *The Detection of Psychiatric Illness by Questionnaire*. Maudsley Monographs 21. London: Oxford University Press.

Gulbinat, W., Dupont, A., Jablensky, A., Jensen, O.M., Marsella, A., Nakane, Y. & Sartorius, N. (1992). Cancer incidence of schizophrenic patients: results of record linkage studies in three countries. *British Journal of Psychiatry*, **161** (Supplement 18), 75–85.

Hogarty, G.E., Goldberg, S.C., Schooler, N.R. & Ulrich, R.F. (1974). Drug and sociotherapy in the aftercare of schizophrenic patients. *Archives of General Psychiatry*, **31**, 603–8.

ten Horn, T., Giel, R., Gulbinat, W.H. & Henderson, J.H. (eds.). (1986). *Psychiatric Case Registers in Public Health: A Worldwide Inventory 1960–1985*. New York: Elsevier.

Katz, M.M. & Lyerly, S.B. (1963). Methods for measuring adjustment and social behavior in the community. I. Rationale, description, discriminative validity and scale development. *Psychological Report*, **13**, 503–35.

Katz, S., Ford, A.B. & Moskowitz, R.W., *et al.* (1963). Studies of illness in the aged: the index of ADL. *JAMA*, **185**, 914–19.

Katz, S., Downs, T.D. & Cash, H.R., *et al.* (1970). Progress in development of the index of ADL. *Gerontologist*, Spring (part 1), 20–30.

Kessler, R.C. & Greenberg, XX. (1981). *Linear Panel Analysis: Models of Quantitative Change.* Quantitative Studies in Social Relations. New York: Academic Press.

Kleinbaum, D.G., Kupper, L.L. & Morgenstern, H. (1982). *Epidemiologic Research: Principles and Quantitative Methods.* Belmont, CA: Lifetime Learning Publications.

Kramer, M. (1967). *Epidemiology, Biostatistics, and Mental Health Planning.* Psychiatric Research Reports 22. Washington, DC: American Psychiatric Association.

Larsen, D.L., Attkisson, C.C., Hargreaves, W.A. & Nguyen, T.D. (1979). Assessment of client/patient satisfaction: development of a general scale. *Evaluation and Program Planning*, **2**, 197–207.

Lawless, J.F. (1982). *Statistical Models and Methods for Lifetime Data.* New York: Wiley.

Lawton, M.P. & Brody, E.M. (1969). Assessment of older people: self-maintaining and instrumental activities of daily living. *Gerontologist*, **9**, 179–86.

Lehman, A.F. (1983). The well-being of chronic mental patients: assessing their quality of life. *Archives of General Psychiatry*, **40**, 369–73.

May, P.R.A. (1975). Adopting new models for continuity of care: what are the needs? *Hospital and Community Psychiatry*, **26**, 599–601.

Mechanic, D. (1968). *Medical Sociology.* New York: The Free Press.

Mellsop, G.W. (1969). The effect of distance in determining hospital admission rates. *Medical Journal of Australia*, **2**, 814–17.

Mor, V. & Guadagnoli, E. (1988). Quality of life measurement: a psychometric Tower of Babel. *Journal of Clinical Epidemiology*, **41**, 1055–8.

Muthen, B.O. (1984). A general structural equation model with dichotomous, ordered categorical, and continuous latent variable indicators. *Psychometrika*, **49**, 115–32.

Nguyen, T.D., Attkisson, C.C. & Stegner, B.L. (1983). Assessment of patient satisfaction: development and refinement of a service evaluation questionnaire. *Evaluation and Program Planning*, **6**, 299–314.

Person, P.H. (1964). *The Relationship Between Selected Social and Demographic Characteristics and Hospitalized Mental Patients and the Outcome of Hospitalization.* Washington, DC: Government Printing Office.

Radloff, L.S. & Locke, B.Z. (1986). The community mental health assessment survey and the CES-D scale. In *Community Surveys of Psychiatric Disorders*, ed. M.M. Weissman *et al.*, pp. 177–90. New Brunswick, NJ: Rutgers University Press.

Rey, J.M., Gavin, W.S., Plapp, J.M., *et al.* (1988a). Validity of axis V of DSM-III and other measure of adaptive functioning. *Acta Psychiatrica Scandinavica*, **77**, 535–42.

Rey, J.M., Gavin, W.S., Plapp, J.M., *et al.* (1988b). DSM-III axis IV revisted. *American Journal of Psychiatry*, **145**, 286–91.

Robins, L.N., Helzer, J.E., Orvaschel, H., Anthony, J.C., *et al.* (1985). The diagnostic interview schedule. In *Epidemiologic Field Methods in Psychiatry*, ed. W.W. Eaton & L.G. Kessler, pp. 143–70. Orlando, FL: Academic Press.

Robins, L., Wing, J., Wittchen, H.U., *et al.* (1988). The composite international diagnostic interview. *Archives of General Psychiatry*, **45**, 1069–77.

Rogosa, D., Brandt, D. & Zimowski, M. (1982). Quantitative methods in psychology: a growth curve approach to the measurement of change. *Psychological Bulletin*, **92**, 726–48.

Shapiro, S., Tischler, G.L., Cottler, L., George, L.K., Amirkhan, J.H., Kessler, L.G. & Skinner, E.A. (1985). Health services research questions. In *Epidemiologic Field Methods in Psychiatry: The NIMH Epidemiologic Catchment Area Program*, ed. W.W. Eaton & L.G. Kessler, pp. 191–208. Orlando, FL: Academic Press.

Spitzer, W.O. (1987). Keynote address. State of science 1986: quality of life and functional status as target variables for research. *Journal of Chronic Disorders*, **40**, 465–71.

Turnage, J.J., Kennedy, R.S., Smith, M.G., Baltzley, D.R. & Lane, N.E. (1992). Development of microcomputer-based mental acuity tests. *Ergonomics*, **35**, 1271–95.

Ware, J.H. (1985). Linear models for the analysis of longitudinal studies. *American Statistician*, **39**, 95–101.

Weissman, M.M. & Bothwell, S. (1976). Assessment of social adjustment by patient self-report. *Archives of General Psychiatry*, **33**, 1111–5.

Weissman, M.M., Myers, J.K. & Ross, C.E. (1986). *Community Surveys of Psychiatric Disorders*. New Brunswick, NJ: Rutgers University Press.

Williams, J.B.W., Endicott, J. & Spitzer, R.L. (1986). Some biometrics contributions to assessment: PSS, CAPPS, SADS-L/RDS, and DSM III. In *Community Surveys of Psychiatric Disorders*, ed. M.M. Weissman *et al.*, pp. 377–402. New Brunswick, NJ: Rutgers University Press.

Wing, J.K. (1986). Describing and classifying psychiatric symptoms: the PSE-CATEGO System. In *Community Surveys of Psychiatric Disorders*, ed. M.M. Weissman *et al.*, pp. 429–48. New Brunswick, NJ: Rutgers University Press.

Wing, J.K., Babor, T., Brogha, T., Burke, J., Cooper, J.E., Giel, R., Jablenski, A., Regier, D. & Sartorius, N. (1990). SCAN. *Archives of General Psychiatry*, **47**, 589–93.

Zeger, S.L. & Liang, K.-Y. (1991). Feedback models for discrete and continuous time series. *Statistica Sinica*, **1**, 51–64.

9

Experimental and quasi-experimental design in evaluative research

WOLFRAM AN DER HEIDEN

Depending on the processes being assessed, the term 'evaluative research' is used for different approaches (Milne, 1987): 'effort evaluation' examines the relationship between the characteristics and activities of a programme or service (e.g. physician–patient ratio, utilisation of beds) and the money spent on it (e.g. for staff and equipment); 'process evaluation' is traditionally limited to a simple outline of services over time (number of patients, type and extent of services offered); 'efficiency evaluation' establishes the relationship between the cost of a service and the goal it aims to achieve; 'client satisfaction evaluation' examines the patients' acceptance of treatment measures. 'Outcome evaluation' is the core of evaluative research; here, the result of a measure is the focus of the study. This approach is chosen when the effectiveness of interventions or services is to be examined. Outcome evaluation relates most directly to the primary goal of treatment, 'which is to make the patient better' (Schwartz *et al.*, 1973).

In a mental health care system many events occur at the same time. So at first sight it seems rather arbitrary to assume that of all things happening one event 'treatment' is causally related to another event 'outcome', for example absence or presence of schizophrenic symptoms at a given point in time. Many factors besides treatment may influence psychopathological status. It is well known that the mere incidence or correlation of two events does not tell anything about which is the cause and which is the effect, whether two events are mutual interdependent or whether they are both dependent upon an unknown third variable (Simon, 1976). Chains of cause and effect are not observable in principle; it is also impossible to verify a causal relationship empirically. The testing of a causal hypothesis rather results by ruling out rival explanations for an effect (Kraak, 1966; Cook & Campbell, 1979).

According to Kenny (1979) three commonly accepted conditions must hold for a scientist to claim that the event X causes the event Y:

1 Temporal precedence of the cause: for X to cause Y, X must precede Y in time; such temporal precedence means a causal relationship is asymmetric.
2 Covariation: presence of a functional relationship between cause and effect. Implicit in this condition is the requirement that cause and effect are variables, that is, both take on two or more values.
3 Non-spuriousness: use of the 'control' concept to rule out alternative interpretations for a possible cause-and-effect connection.

The condition of non-spuriousness requires that extraneous factors that may exert an influence and obscure a 'true' causal relationship must be controlled. Cook & Campbell (1979; see also Campbell, 1957) discuss several threats to validity: 'History' is a threat when an observed effect might be due to an event that takes place in addition to the measure under observation. 'Maturation' is a threat which also takes place in addition to the measure one is interested in; in contrast to 'history' it is not a specific event but an effect which is systematic with the passage of time. A supposed amelioration in outcome might also be due to the number of times particular responses are measured and the increasing familiarity with tests ('testing'), or to a change in the measuring instruments ('instrumentation'). Other threats are known as 'statistical regression', 'selection' and 'mortality'.

In evaluative research the presence of some or most of the threats mentioned above is obvious. For example, it may be the case that after the implementation of a new extramural service there may be some new administrative regulations concerning admission to inpatient treatment ('history'). The outcome of schizophrenia may be influenced by therapeutic and rehabilitative measures but at the same time be the result of a chronic deterioration, reflecting the 'natural' course of a certain subtype of schizophrenia ('maturation'). Researchers become more experienced in rating behaviour or psychopathology ('instrumentation'), and so on.

In general the effects of such extraneous variables can be considered at two levels (Campbell, 1957): (a) as simple or main effects, where the effects occur independently of or in addition to the effects of the measure under study; (b) as interactions, where the effects appear in conjunction with the measure under study. Typically the main effects turn out to be relevant to internal validity, which means the validity that statements can be made about whether there is a causal relationship from one variable to another. On the other hand, interaction effects turn out to be relevant to external validity, that means to the extent to which conclusions can be drawn about the generalisability of a causal relationship across populations of persons, settings and times.

As mentioned above, the condition of non-spuriousness needs control. The control of most extraneous variables seems best accomplished within an experimental design. There are several features that seem indispensable for a true experimental design:

- random selection of samples from the same potential treatment population;
- random assignment of people to different treatment conditions (experimental and control group);
- manipulation and administration of treatment in a fully controlled situation.

Taking the simplest case the investigator will create an experimental and a control condition and afterwards observe the effects of the presumed experimental (independent) variable X on the presumed dependent variable Y (Campbell & Stanley, 1966; Edwards, 1970). Within this experimental framework Cook & Campbell (1979) separate three senses of the term 'control': (a) the ability to control the situation in which an experiment is being conducted; in the strictest sense control here means the experiment being conducted in total isolation to ensure the exclusion of extraneous sources of variance; (b) the ability to determine which units receive a particular treatment in a particular time; randomisation here plays the most important role; (c) the ability to identify and measure a particular threat to valid inference so that it can be used in data analysis to rule out the threat.

In the experimental 'Pretest–Posttest Control Group Design' the effects of the abovementioned threats seem so well controlled for that they are usually not made explicit. The control group design with random assignment to treatment groups is to ensure that the groups are comparable in terms of all relevant characteristics at the outset of the investigation. Known and unknown variables that are potential causes of an outcome variable are distributed at random to the experimental and control conditions and thus may not produce differential effects; probands differ systematically only by the variables controlled for in the design.

But even in the control group design not all of the abovementioned threats to validity are under control. For example, even a successfully implemented random assignment does not guarantee that the initial comparability between groups will be maintained over the course of the whole study, when the attrition from an experiment is systematically related to the experimental condition. This problem also sheds light on another crucial variable – especially in evaluative research – the time factor. From a methodological point of view status at outcome can best be ascribed to the effects of treatment when the time interval is short (Schwartz *et al.*, 1973). In psychiatric care delayed causation is often expected but the causal lag is not known. The longer the interval the higher the risk that additional events can take place ('history'), and therefore the less certain the causal relationship of treatment to outcome.

Although some modifications of the 'Pretest-Posttest Control Group Design' have been developed, e.g. the 'Solomon Four-Group Design', there are two classes of variables that may potentially restrict or confound the validity of research (see also Blalock, 1964):

- events that occur in the course of the experiment, that may be unknown or unmeasured, or that cannot adequately be assessed;
- events that are in some way systematically related to the independent variable; what appears to be a direct influence of the independent variable might in fact be covariation due to a third variable.

The control of these variables seem to be indispensable on theoretical grounds. In practice, however, it often cannot be achieved at all or at best only inadequately (Keenan, 1975; Schulberg & Bromet, 1981). Moreover, where control is possible, it is often at the price of reduced external validity (Campbell, 1957).

Although outcome evaluation in health service research is not limited to specified research methods (Attkisson *et al.*, 1978), the experimental design seems to be the method of choice when investigating treatment effects. It even seems so superior to other research strategies that some of the most frequently cited reviews on the evaluation of psychiatric services by Test & Stein (1978a) and May & Simpson (1980) included only studies described as 'prospective experiments' or 'controlled experimental design'.

At the level of single institutions or even whole systems of care, a chief characteristic of evaluation research is that it is carried out *in situ*. In field studies major features of 'true' experiments are not present: It is almost always impossible to find control conditions which are identical with experimental conditions; for methodological as well as ethical reasons the evaluation of psychiatric treatment does not allow the use of placebo control groups (Strayhorn, 1987). The same is true with respect to random assignment and physical isolation of respondents

Therefore, in most cases, one or more of the following prerequisites of 'non-spurious' experiments are violated in field settings (Kerlinger, 1973): manipulation of independent variables; random selection and randomisation of individuals between the experimental and the control groups. This design is referred to as 'pre-experimental' or 'quasi-experimental'. While Stouffer (1950) and Campbell (1957) first used the term 'quasi-experiments' for investigations that had most of the features of 'true experiments' but did not use random assignment for comparison purposes, the term was subsequently used in a much broader sense, even including correlational studies (Bortz, 1984).

Today there is agreement that quasi-experiments comprise a treatment, outcome measures, and different units to compare. However, instead of using random assignment the comparisons may depend on non-equivalent groups that differ from each other in many ways other than the presence of a treatment whose effects are being tested. Examples are the 'Posttest-Only Design with Nonequivalent Groups' and the 'Untreated Control Group Design with Pre- and Posttest' (Cook & Campbell, 1979). The former is characterised by the absence of a pretest, while in the latter there is a comparison between an experimental and a control group but no random assignment to one of the two groups.

The task of interpreting the results from quasi-experiments is basically one of separating the effects of a treatment from those due to the dissimilarity between the experimental and the control group; only the effects of the treatment are of research interest. To achieve this separation, the researcher has to explicate the specific threats to valid causal inference that random assignment rules out and then in some way deal with these threats.

Thus, also in studies with a quasi-experimental design the aim is to rule out rival explanations for given relationships in empirical data. However, as there are more threats to validity that are not controlled for by the design (history, maturation, regression, instrumentation, etc.) the internal validity of quasi-experimental trials is lower than that of experimental trials. In such cases, however, the lack of technical control provided by the design needs to be compensated by explicit measurement and data-analytic inclusion of additional variables as well as by specific assumptions concerning the effects of confounding variables (Kenny, 1975; Hodapp, 1984).

When randomisation techniques are not used, it becomes even more important to look at the characteristics of members of natural treatment groups. According to Schwartz *et al.* (1973) the exploration of the relationship of treatment to outcome in quasi-experimental situations requires the following:

1 definition of the group to be studied, which includes establishment of the diagnostic validity of the sample;
2 obtaining an assessment of patient condition prior to treatment;
3 documenting sociodemographic and symptom characteristics of patients belonging to various groups;
4 documenting characteristics of treatment; and
5 obtaining an assessment of patient condition at termination of treatment.

It should then be possible to control statistically for such characteristics in data analysis.

An observational study on the effectiveness of extramural psychiatric care: a model-based analysis of utilisation data

To analyse the efficacy of psychiatric outpatient care we studied utilisation of intra- and extramural services by a cohort of schizophrenic patients in Mannheim, Germany (for a more detailed description, see an der Heiden *et al.*, 1989). The cohort consisted of those inhabitants who were admitted to an inpatient facility serving the Mannheim area. One hundred and forty-eight patients were followed-up over a period of 18 months. Once in the sample, the patients were reassessed three times at equal intervals of 6 months. The interviews at cross-sections consisted of a semi-structured psychiatric interview, the Present State Examination (PSE; Wing *et al.*, 1974), an inquiry into

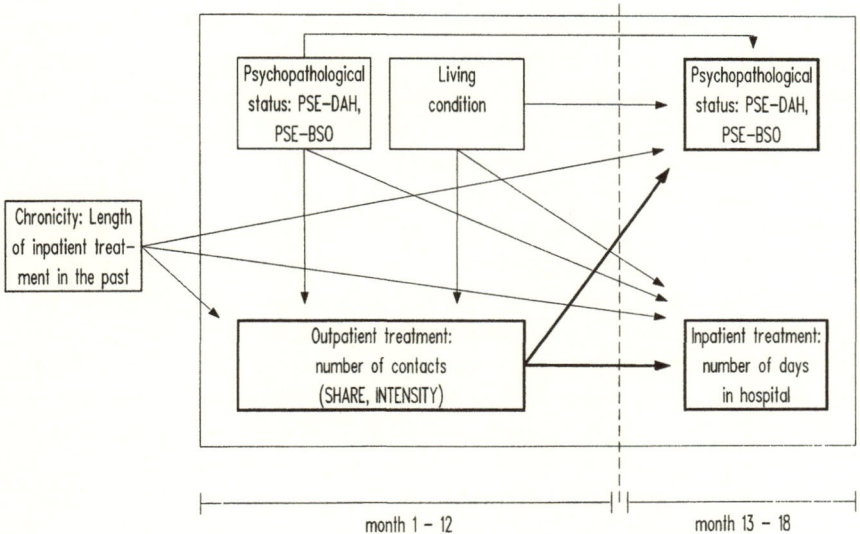

Fig. 9.1. Model of analysis.

socio-demographic variables and questions concerning type and duration of treatment before inclusion in the sample. Additionally, with the help of a special record system (an der Heiden & Klug, 1980), the demand for aftercare from different facilities was registered for the whole period of observation.

In clinical practice the decision for a certain quantity and/or intensity of medical care is not a random choice, but will be determined, at least partly, by attributes of the patient, such as psychopathological status (Franklin *et al.*, 1975; Mezzich *et al.*, 1984) living conditions (Test and Stein, 1978b; Vetter, 1985) and chronicity of illness (Rosenblatt & Mayer, 1974; Pokorny *et al.*, 1983). Not only the decision for an individual treatment plan but also the effects of the treatment may be influenced by these variables. These facts are evident in clinical practice but they may distort the interesting correlations when examining the effects of a certain treatment modality. As we were not able to eliminate these disturbing influences in a randomised control group design, we had to control them statistically within the model shown in Fig. 9.1.

The study aimed at analysing the effects of outpatient psychiatric care. One hundred and thirty-six out of 148 patients in our cohort were in contact with an outpatient psychiatric service and received drug treatment. So we used 'number of contacts' with an outpatient medical service as an operationalisation of our independent variable. We calculated two indices: 'percentage of outpatient care in total psychiatric care', and 'number of contacts with outpatient medical services during time outside hospital'.

Outcome evaluation implies measurement against an accepted criterion, so that it is possible to define the degree of the patient's improvement. In mental health services research there are few if any agreed standards and no accepted methods of measuring 'success' (Zusman & Reiff-Ross, 1969). Notwithstanding difficulties in operationalising 'response', 'recovery' or 'relapse' (Prien *et al.*, 1991), there is at least agreement that effectiveness cannot be measured by using a single outcome dimension. While in the past there seemed to be an overemphasis on symptom suppression (Collins *et al.*, 1991) or length of stay in hospital (Falloon *et al.*, 1983) as the only criteria of treatment effectiveness, other areas such as the quality of life and subjective experience of the patient have long been neglected. In schizophrenia research Strauss & Carpenter (1972, 1974) suggest a concept of outcome comprising four different semi-independent processes and areas: (a) social relationships, (b) work functioning, (c) psychopathological symptoms and (d) number and duration of hospitalisations. While adjustment in mental status seems only weakly correlated with social adjustment, and a patient's status at the end of a treatment episode bears little relationship to the rate of rehospitalisation or to consumer satisfaction (Strauss & Carpenter, 1981), one has to bear in mind that the multiplicity and complexity of the targets of success that characterise rehabilitation or treatment measures are hardly covered by just a couple of restricted criteria such as (in)ability to work or psychopathology. Since treatment outcome is multifaceted and multidetermined, multiple assessments must continue as vital procedures (Schwartz *et al.*, 1975).

As we expected that an effective outpatient treatment should have an effect on both the clinical status of the patient and his tenure in the community, we chose 'psychopathological status' (PSE subscores 'delusional and hallucinatory syndromes'/DAH and 'behaviour, speech and other syndromes'/BSO) and 'inpatient treatment' (number of days in hospital) as outcome measures.

The direction of causality depends on the knowledge of a time sequence (Kenny, 1979). Therefore the whole period of observation was divided into two periods of 12 months and 6 months respectively.

The control of the variables influencing the impact of outpatient care is based on the following considerations: For each combination of 'psychopathological status', 'length of illness' and 'living condition' of a patient in the first 12 months an 'average' intensity of treatment may be expected. This holds also true for months 13 to 18. The hypothesis is that a deviation from this average treatment in the first period with respect to the intensity of outpatient care will lead to a decrease or increase in inpatient treatment in the second period and also to a change in psychopathological status.

We calculated the average values of the 'treatment' and 'psychopathology' variables in the two periods by regression with the supposed confounding variables as predictor variables. In order to investigate the unbiased impact of outpatient care, we eliminated the influence of 'psychopathology', 'length of illness' and 'living condition' from the independent and dependent variables by subtracting the expected average values from the observed values. The resulting residuals were now used in all further computations. Fig. 9.2 displays the correlation coefficients between two indices of extramural care and the outcome criteria with the effects of the confounding variables removed. The coefficients represent the extent and direction of the influence exercised by outpatient psychiatric care in the first year of observation on inpatient treatment and psychopathological symptoms in the second interval.

The result reveals that the higher the share of outpatient medical treatment in total care, the less intramural care results in the follow-up period. This effect is also true for the standardised amount of outpatient contacts during the time outside hospital, say 'intensity of care'. This means that outpatient psychiatric treatment will reduce the necessity for inpatient treatment.

The correlations between the indices of outpatient care and the two subscores DAH and BSO of the PSE are low, yet they are all significantly negative. This means that contacts with outpatient psychiatric agencies will reduce symptomatology in the last 6 months.

Concluding remarks

The strongest approach to learning about the real effects of treatment is the controlled experiment. Random assignment of patients to different experimental and control conditions will rule out most

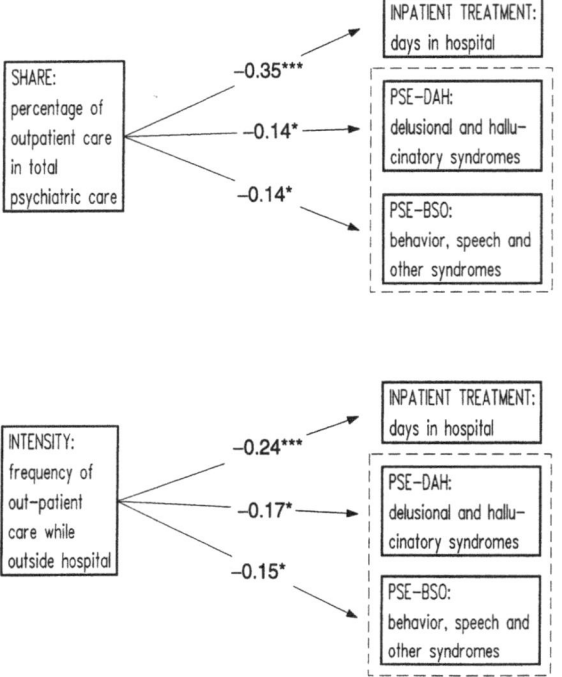

*Fig. 9.2. Impact of outpatient psychiatric care on length of stay in hospital and symptomatology. The figures are Pearson correlations after removing the effects of 'symptomatology', 'past inpatient treatment' and 'living conditions'. *p < 0.05; **p < 0.01; ***p < 0.001,*

alternative interpretations for a given correlation between treatment and outcome, thus increasing internal validity. However, the practice of mental health care normally does not allow random allocation, mainly because of ethical reasons. Also, researchers may be more interested in the generalisability of their results to complex field settings (external validity), which is often restricted in experimental situations.

Faced with the technical problems of internal and external validity, researchers in the field of evaluative research often tend to stress the need for external validity at the cost of reduced internal validity. Internal and external validity are indeed not independent of each other. Many of those measures that are suited to ruling out threats to internal validity, such as insulating patients from outside influences, will create artificial conditions that have nothing in common with 'real life'. Yet it is important to realise that – with respect to the quality of inferences about whether a causal relationship can be postulated from one variable to another – there is a priority for internal validity in both basic and applied research. Strict control of extraneous variables will allow for causal statements, at least for the particular conditions under observation. Jeopardising internal validity for the sake of increasing external validity usually entails a minimum gain for a considerable loss (Cook & Campbell, 1979).

Causal inference is much more problematic in field than in laboratory settings; using natural groups of patients, where allocation is not under the investigator's control, may confuse the results. All those confounding factors that in an experiment are controlled for automatically, must be made explicit in quasi-experimental settings. The next step is for the rearcher to separate the effect of the treatment from the effect of non-equivalence of the different units of observation. There are a number of statistical methods to handle this problem, such as analysis of (co)variance, path analysis, time series analysis and survival analysis. But even the most sophisticated methodology cannot compensate for an inadequate model of possible confounding variables. Unfortunately, in evaluative research the knowledge concerning those variables, besides treatment, that might have an influence on the outcome is rather limited (Nuehring *et al.*, 1980). Outcome evaluation in psychiatry is still in its infancy.

References

Attkisson, C.C., Hargreaves, W.A., Horowitz, M.J. & Sorensen, J.E. (1978). *Evaluation of Human Service Program*. New York: Academic Press.
Blalock, H.M. (1964). *Causal Inferences in Nonexperimental Research*. Chapel Hill: University of North Carolina Press.
Bortz, J. (1984). *Lehrbuch der empirischen Forschung*. Berlin: Springer.
Campbell, D.T. (1957). Factors relevant to the validity of experiments in social settings. *Psychological Bulletin*, **54**, 297–312.
Campbell, D.T. & Stanley, J.C. (1966). *Experimental and Quasi-experimental Designs for Research*. Chicago: Rand McNally.
Collins, E.J., Hogan, T.P. & Desai, H. (1991). Measurement of therapeutic response in schizophrenia: a critical survey. *Schizophrenia Research*, **5**, 249–53.
Cook, T.D. & Campbell, D.T. (1979). *Quasi-experimentation: Design and Analysis Issues for Field Settings*. Boston: Houghton Mifflin.
Edwards, A.L. (1970). *Experimental Design in Psychological Research*. New

York: Holt, Rinehart and Winston.

Falloon, I.R.H., Marshal, G.N., Boyd, J.L., Razani, J. & Wood-Siverio, C. (1983). Relapse in schizophrenia: a review of the concept and its definitions. *Psychological Medicine*, **13**, 469–77.

Franklin, J.L., Kittredge, L.D. & Thrasher, J.H. (1975). A survey of factors related to mental hospital readmissions. *Hospital and Community Psychiatry*, **26**, 749–51.

an der Heiden, W. & Klug, J. (1980). An integrated record system for the observation of the demand for medical and social aftercare as a basis for organising extramural services. *Acta Psychiatrica Scandinavica Supplementum* **285**, 54–9.

an der Heiden, W., Krumm, B. & Häfner, H. (1989). *Die Wirksamkeit ambulanter psychiatrischer Versorgung: Ein Modell zur Evaluation extramuraler Dienste*. Berlin: Springer.

Hodapp, V. (1984). *Analyse linearer Kausalmodelle*. Bern: Huber.

Keenan, B. (1975). Designing mental health studies: the pragmatics of nonexperimental design. *Hospital and Community Psychiatry*, **26**, 739–40.

Kenny, D.A. (1975). A quasi-experimental approach to assessing treatment effects in the nonequivalent control group design. *Psychological Bulletin*, **82**, 345–62.

Kenny, D.A. (1979). *Correlation and Causality*. New York: Wiley.

Kerlinger, F.N. (1973). *Foundations of Behavioral Research*. New York: Holt, Rinehart and Winston.

Kraak, B. (1966). Zum Problem der Kausalität in der Psychologie. *Psychologische Beiträge*, **9**, 413–32.

May, P.R.A. & Simpson, G.M. (1980). Schizophrenia: evaluation of treatment methods. In *Comprehensive Textbook of Psychiatry*, 3rd edn, vol. II, ed. H.I. Kaplan, A.M. Freedman & B.J. Sadock. Baltimore: Williams and Wilkins.

Mezzich, J.E. & Coffman, G.A. (1985). Factors influencing length of hospital stay. *Hospital and Community Psychiatry*, **36**, 1162–70.

Mezzich, J.E., Evanczuk, K.J., Mathias, R.J. & Coffman, G.A. (1984). Symptoms and hospitalization decisions. *American Journal of Psychiatry*, **141**, 764–9.

Milne, D. (1987). *Evaluating Mental Health Practice: Methods and Applications*. London: Croom Helm.

Nuehring, E.M., Thayer, J.H. & Ladner, R.A. (1980). On the factors predicting rehospitalisation among two state mental hospital patient populations. *Administration in Mental Health*, **7**, 247–70.

Pokorny, A.D., Kaplan, H.I. & Lorimor, R.J. (1983). Effects of diagnosis and treatment history on relapse of psychiatric patients. *American Journal of Psychiatry*, **140**, 1598–601.

Prien, R.F, Carpenter, L.L. & Kupfer, D.J. (1991). The definition and operational criteria for treatment outcome of major depressive disorder. *Archives of General Psychiatry*, **48**, 796–800.

Rosenblatt, A. & Mayer, J.E. (1974). The recidivism of mental patients: a review of past studies. *American Journal of Orthopsychiatry*, **44**, 697–706.

Schulberg, H.C. & Bromet, E. (1981). Strategies for evaluating the outcome of community services for the chronically mentally ill. *American Journal of Psychiatry*, **138**, 930–5.

Schwartz, C.C., Myers, J.K. & Astrachan, B.M. (1973). The outcome study in psychiatric evaluation research: issues and methods. *Archives of General Psychiatry*, **29**, 98–102.

Schwartz, C.C., Myers, J.K. & Astrachan, B.M. (1975). Concordance of multiple assessments of the outcome of schizophrenia: on defining the dependent variable in outcome studies. *Archives of General Psychiatry*, **32**, 1221–7.

Simon, H.A. (1976). Spurious correlations: a causal interpretation. In *Causal Models in the Social Sciences*, 4th edn, ed. H.M. Blalock, pp. 5–17. Chicago: Aldine.

Stouffer, S.A. (1950). Some observations on study design. *American Journal of Sociology*, **55**, 355–61.

Strauss, J.S. & Carpenter, W.T. (1972). The prediction of outcome in schizophrenia. I. Characteristics of outcome. *Archives of General Psychiatry*, **27**, 739–46.

Strauss, J.S. & Carpenter, W.T. (1974). The prediction of outcome in schizophrenia. II. Relationship between predictor and outcome. *Archives of General Psychiatry*, **31**, 37–42.

Strauss, J.S. & Carpenter, W.T. (1981). *Schizophrenia*. New York: Plenum Press.

Strayhorn, J.M. (1987). Control groups for psychosocial intervention outcome studies. *American Journal of Psychiatry*, **144**, 275–82.

Test, M.A. & Stein, L.I. (1978a). Community treatment of the chronic patient: research overview. *Schizophrenia Bulletin*, **4**, 350–64.

Test, M.A. & Stein, L.I. (1978b). The clinical rationale for community treatment: a review of the literature. In *Alternatives to Mental Hospital Treatment*, ed. L.I. Stein & M.A. Test, pp. 3–22. New York: Plenum Press.

Vetter, P. (1985). Die Rehabilitation psychisch Behinderter in Wohngemeinschaften und ihr Einfluss auf die Hospitalisierungsdauer. *Nervenarzt*, **56**, 359–64.

Wing, J.K., Cooper, J.E. & Sartorius, N. (1974). *Measurement and Classification of Psychiatric Symptoms*. London: Cambridge University Press.

Zusman, J. & Reiff-Ross, E.R. (1969). Evaluation of the quality of mental health services. *Archives of General Psychiatry*, **20**, 352–7.

10

An informal introduction to graphical modelling

SVEND KREINER

Introduction

The purpose of this chapter is to give a short introduction to graphical models, a new class of multivariate statistical models characterised by a so-called independence graph representing relationships among variables. Fig. 10.1 shows an independence graph depicting the associations between variables from a comparative study of the social situation of two different cohorts of 70-year-olds in Denmark. Six variables are included in the model – Dwelling, Work, Marriage, Education, Gender and Cohort Year – some of which are connected by undirected edges while others are connected by arrows.

This section gives a very brief introduction to independence graphs and graphical models and reviews some of the advantages of graphical models. The following section will discuss the methodological prerequisites from the social sciences and epidemiology that graphical modelling is related to. The discussion in this section eventually focuses on *conditional independence*, the fundamental notion on which graphical models are founded. It will also lead to a principle of *complete elaboration* and a precise definition of the concept of association on which the graphical models are implicitly based. The third section presents the formal definition of graphical models and a few key results from the theory. Finally, we return to the graphical model shown in Fig. 10.1 and discuss some of what this model may tell us about how the data should be analysed.

The independence graph (Fig. 10.1) is one part of the end result of the analysis of the six-dimensional contingency table by graphical models. It is at one and the same time a visual representation of a

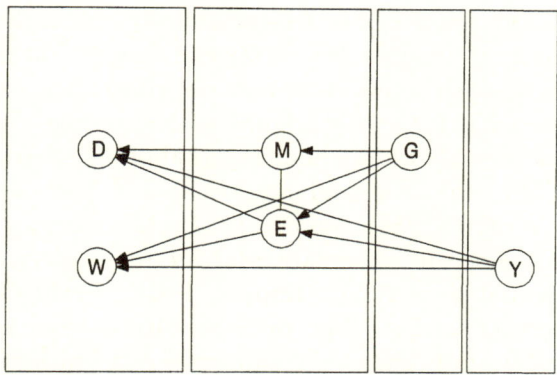

Fig. 10.1. Independence graph showing the relationships between variables from a study of the social situation of two cohorts of 70-year-olds in Denmark. D, dwelling; W, work; M, married; E, education; G, gender; Y, year.

special log-linear model for the table and a mathematical model in its own right.

The edges and arrows of independence graphs represent direct relationships, that is relationships between pairs of variables where correlations can not be explained by controlling with respect to the remaining variables included in the table. The directions of arrows indicate asymmetrical relationships corresponding to causal or temporal structure. The asymmetrical relationships define a so-called block recursive structure in which all asymmetrical relationships point in one direction only, distinguishing for each pairwise relationship between antecedent, intervening and consequent variables.

Graphical models originated in a series of research reports and research papers in the late 1970s and the early 1980s, most notably in the seminal paper by Darroch, *et al.* (1980). They have since spread into several areas of research due to the very general nature and high degree of applicability of these models. Some recent examples of the use of graphical models may be found in Schultz-Larsen *et al.* (1993) and Lidegaard (1993). The central premise behind the graphical models is that any kind of relationship should be analysed as a conditional relationship: that a relationship between two variables exists if and only if the association does not disappear completely, when one controls for the effect of antecedent and/or intervening variables. This is in no way a new idea, nor are graphical models the only models that make use of it. In statistics the idea is shared with other multivariate techniques such as standard regression techniques and log-linear analysis of multidimensional contingency tables. In the social sciences it is, for instance, found as the central component of the paradigms of elaboration and explanation (Lazarsfeld 1955; Rosenberg 1968) and in causal modelling and path analysis as developed by Wright (1934), Simon (1957) and Blalock (1964). In philosophy of science it is fundamental for the understanding of causality in probabilistic terms (Suppes, 1984). It should also be noted that the epidemiological concern with controlling for confounding and effect modification aims for conditional relationships between exposure and outcome in order to obtain undistorted estimates of the effect of risk factors.

One of the main advantages of graphical modelling compared with established methodological paradigms and techniques, is a more explicit and more sophisticated approach to the problem of what to control for when a conditional relationship has to be analysed. The main problem troubling both routine epidemiological research and the paradigms of elaboration and explanation in the social sciences, is the problem of selecting appropriate control variables for a given relationship. The number of possibilities is often astronomical and the final choice often appears in much practical work to be more or less arbitrary.

Graphical models suggest a solution to this problem that is at the same time both simple and complicated: *Control for all other variables at one and the same time excluding only consequent variables.* The argument against this proposal is that it will often be impractical to control for all possible variables at one and the same time. This, of course, is true in many cases, especially in high-dimensional cases with more than a handful of control variables, but graphical models have a solution to this problem as well: *A graph theoretical analysis of the independence graph may disclose so-called collapsibility properties of the statistical model informing us that the parameters of interest in many cases may be obtained by analysis of marginal tables from which some of the variables have been excluded.* This means that although we in principle want to control for everything at one and the same time, it is not always necessary to do so in practice. A quick look at the independence graph will in many cases tell us what may be disregarded, in connection with an analysis of a specific relationship between two variables. And if the graph is inaccessible, the network of interrelationships too complex, then graph theoretical algorithms are available which will procure the required information from the independence graph.

The usual way to introduce graphical models would be to focus on the statistical properties of the models and the special relationships between graphical models and other types of statistical models, such as log-linear models for multidimensional contingency tables (Bishop *et al.*, 1975) and covariance selection models for continuous data (Dempster, 1972). This, however, has already been done (Edwards & Kreiner, 1983; Whittaker, 1990, 1993; Wermuth, 1993) and will not be repeated here. The focus will instead be on some of the methodological relatives of graphical modelling in the social and epidemiological sciences. The definition and main results pertaining to graphical models will be presented, but the technical details of graphical modelling will be avoided here: They in any case follow well-trodden paths of model selection for log-linear models and variable selection for linear and logistic regression analyses.

Methodological prerequisites

Elaboration and explanation in the social sciences

When a researcher discovers a relationship between two variables, the first question implicitly or explicitly asked is whether this relationship is real or whether it is caused by some other variable(s). In other words, has the researcher observed a *spurious or indirect* relationship?

In order to answer this question it is necessary to introduce additional variables into the analysis. Typically one attempts to elaborate the crude relationship by stratification according to different levels of an 'explanatory' control variable. If the relationship disappears in all strata defined by the control variables, one concludes that the relationship is explained by the control variable. We refer to the original two-way table as the marginal table because it is found in the 'margins' of the multidimensional table including both control variables and the pair of variables of interest. The relationship observed in the marginal table is in the same way called a marginal relationship as opposed to the conditional relationships observed in different strata defined by control variables. The situation is illustrated in Table 10.1, which presents data from the Danish study of the social

Table 10.1. *Distribution of Dwelling and Work among 70-year-olds in 1967 and 1984*

Dwelling	Work (%)			
	Working	Retired	Never	Total
(a) *The marginal distribution*				
Good	14.8	69.4	15.8	1060
Bad	20.2	60.5	19.4	258
	$\chi^2 = 7.9$, d.f. $= 2$, $p = 0.02$			
(b) *1967*				
Good	24.3	54.3	21.4	383
Bad	23.9	54.2	21.9	201
	$\chi^2 = 0.0$, d.f. $= 2$, $p = 0.99$			
(c) *1984*				
Good	9.5	78.0	12.6	677
Bad	7.0	82.5	10.5	57
	$\chi^2 = 0.6$, d.f. $= 2$, $p = 0.72$			

situation of 70-year-olds. Table 10.1(a) shows the marginal relationship between working and quality of dwelling. There is a moderately significant association with the retired part of the population having somewhat better dwellings than those who are still working and those who have not been active on the labour market. Table 10.1(b) and (c) shows the same relationship stratified according to cohort year. It is immediately obvious that the association observed in the marginal table has disappeared completely. Test statistics are not even close to being significant. Cohort year has, in other words, explained the association apparent in Table 10.1(a). (The explanation should not come as a surprise: the general quality of life has, of course, improved from 1967 to 1984 both in terms of the quality of dwellings and in terms of the age at retirement.)

The special situation where elaboration with respect to a control variable uncovers the explanation of the relationship, is referred to by statisticians as a case of *conditional independence*.

Elaboration may also be useful in cases where the control variable does not completely explain the relationship between two variables. Table 10.2 elaborates the relationship between education and cohort year by stratifying with respect to gender.

Table 10.2. *Education among 70-year-olds in 1967 and 1984 by Gender*

Year	Education (%)			
	<9 years	9–12 years	13+ years	Total
(a) *The marginal distribution*				
1967	53.4	40.3	6.3	586
1984	43.6	43.7	12.7	730
	$\chi^2 = 21.1$, d.f. $= 2$, $p < 0.0005$			
(b) *Men*				
1967	35.5	55.1	9.4	287
1984	33.8	52.2	14.0	364
	$\chi^2 = 21.1$, d.f. $= 2$, $p = 0.13$			
(c) *Women*				
1967	70.6	26.1	3.3	299
1984	53.3	35.2	11.5	366
	$\chi^2 = 26.4$, d.f. $= 2$, $p < 0.0005$			

The marginal relationship between education and cohort year is shown in Table 10.2(a). It shows what one would expect: that the educational level of 70-year-olds has increased from 1967 to 1984. Elaboration with respect to gender tells us that it has only been the women (Table 10.2(c)) for whom the number of years in the educational system has increased. For the 70-year-old men (Table 10.2(b)) there is no apparent improvement. Gender is here playing the role of what is otherwise referred to as an *effect modificator* in epidemiological terms. In a statistical model this would be represented by interaction between the effects of cohort year and gender on the educational level, although this would be a rather imprecise expression that hides the fact that there is no association at all between cohort year and education for the male population of 70-year-olds. There is, in other words, only a local relationship between cohort year and education.

Elaboration is an intuitively appealing strategy with an obvious common sense face value. It does, however, have drawbacks. If several competing control factors are present there is an obvious problem of prioritising among these. Which control factor should be considered first? Should more than one control variable be introduced and how many and in which order? Should one stop once a 'good' explanation has been found or should other control factors be considered? And how should explanations be interpreted if more than one explanatory variable was found? Can we be sure that explanations given by different control variables are logically consistent and how do we guard against inconsistency?

The paradigm of elaboration and explanation has no general answers to these questions. Elaboration as described above remains – despite all its attractive features – an *ad hoc* trial-and-error procedure. It is for this reason that the popularity of the elaboration paradigm has declined since the advent of the log-linear models for contingency tables in the early 1970s (Hagenaars, 1990, pp. 23–4) even though the attractive straightforwardness of elaboration has been lost in the awkward bulk of hard-to-interpret log-linear parameters (Alba, 1988). The graphical models discussed in this chapter revitalise the notions of elaboration and explanation by placing them in a formal model-based context. In order to do this it is necessary to generalise the elaboration strategy, introducing both a simple and very broad notion association and a strategy of *complete elaboration* requiring that all other variables (excluding only consequent variables) are controlled for when a given relationship is examined. Two variables are *not associated* if they are conditionally independent given the rest of the variables (excluding only consequent variables according to a temporal and/or causal framework). Otherwise they are assumed to be associated.

Controlling for confounders and modificators in epidemiology

Even though the idiom of epidemiology differs somewhat from the social science language of elaboration and explanation it is obvious that epidemiological research has the same interest in conditional relationships as the paradigms of elaboration. Both are looking for the true relationships behind the effects of what epidemiology refers to as confounders and modificators. It is no particular surprise therefore, that the statistical techniques adhered to by the different disciplines are basically the same.

Epidemiology, however, puts a weaker emphasis on explanation (i.e. conditional independence) than does sociology. The primary aim of epidemiological methodology is to analyse and estimate exposure–outcome association, purged for confounding, that is for

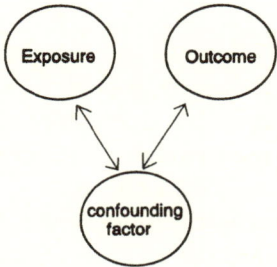

Fig. 10.2. An illustration of confounding.

the 'distortion . . . brought about by the association of another factor with both outcome and exposure' (Elwood, 1988, p. 85).

Fig. 10.2 shows a diagram adapted from Elwood (1988), illustrating the above definition of confounding. The diagram seems at first to be of the same type as the independence graph in Fig. 10.1. There are, however, important differences. One is that the double-headed arrows between the variables in Fig. 10.2 do not appear in Fig. 10.1, and cannot in fact appear in any independence graph. Another is that the missing connection between exposure and outcome in Fig. 10.2 does not mean that exposure and outcome are not assumed to be associated. Compared with an independence graph Fig. 10.2 is in fact a rather imprecise outline of a statistical model.

Notice also the reference to associations between the confounding factor and exposure and outcome mentioned above. To be of any use it should be clearly stated what is actually meant by association here. When one takes a closer look at the kind of distributions guiding the outcomes on the three variables one will find that it is not a question of marginal dependence. It is in fact possible to construct examples with three variables all of which are marginally independent but conditionally dependent.

For a definition like the one above to be useful, one must have a precise definition of what is meant by association and, given that, proceed to examine the possible effects of confounding.

Even though Fig. 10.1 and 10.2 are not the same kind of graphs it is clear that they have enough in common to consider the extent to which independence graphs and graphical models may be useful in epidemiology, and that the language of epidemiology may be useful in a discussion of the methodological foundation of graphical modelling.

Causal and recursive models

A block recursive model is a multivariate model in which the variables have been partitioned into an ordered sequence of subsets of variables according to some criteria usually related to either temporal or causal order in which causes occur before effects.

If each block contains only one variable the model is simply called a recursive model. The statistical model, the joint distribution of all variables, in this case reduces to a product of simple regression models, one for each conditional distribution of a variable given all its predecessors. This situation is shown in Fig. 10.3. Causal and recursive models have been given extensive treatment in the social sciences from Wright (1934) to Simon (1957) and Blalock (1964) and onwards.

Wright introduced so-called path diagrams for causal analysis of relations between normally distributed variables, where each conditional distribution was a standard linear regression model. A missing link in the path-diagram indicated that the corresponding regression parameter had to be equal to zero. The so-called Simon–Blalock technique for analysis of recursive models took exactly the same starting point, noting that missing edges in the path diagram implied vanishing partial correlation coefficients for those pairs of variables where a linkage had been omitted when the effects of all antecedent and intervening variables had been partialled out. The situation is illustrated in Fig. 10.4 by analysis of a path diagram for the recursive set-up shown in Fig. 10.3.

Graphical models

Definition

What, then, are graphical models? In what way are they related to the techniques and paradigms discussed in the preceding section? To what extent are they different, and what do they have to offer that is new?

The relationship between graphical models and the models behind the path analysis of Wright, Simon and Blalock is so close that one might prefer to talk about graphical modelling as generalised path analysis.

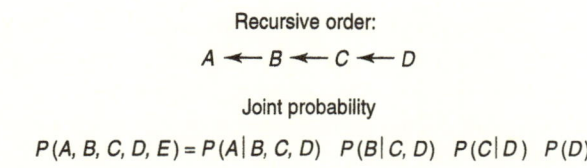

Recursive order:

$$A \leftarrow B \leftarrow C \leftarrow D$$

Joint probability

$$P(A, B, C, D, E) = P(A|B, C, D) \ P(B|C, D) \ P(C|D) \ P(D)$$

Fig. 10.3. Set-up of a recursive model for four variables.

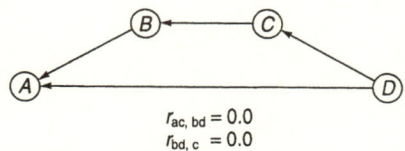

$$r_{ac, \, bd} = 0.0$$
$$r_{bd, \, c} = 0.0$$

Fig. 10.4. Simon–Blalock analysis of a path diagram for a recursive system with four variables.

The basic approach to path analysis is restricted in two ways. It is confined to recursive and not block recursive models, and it deals with multivariate normal distributions. Graphical models break both of these restrictions, preserving the possibilities inherent in path analysis.

The first restriction to be relaxed is the assumption of a completely recursive structure. Graphical models permit symmetrical relationships between variables in separate blocks, assuming only a recursive structure between blocks. The path analysis in this way generalises from a sequence of simple regression analyses to a complex of correlation analyses and regression analyses with multivariate dependent variables. The purely recursive structure of path analysis is still permitted within this framework of course, but it is treated as a very simple special case.

To relax the assumption on multivariate normal distributions we must replace the conditions on zero partial associations with the more general concept of conditional independence. The change may seem minor and is indeed inconsequential as long as one is dealing with normal distributions. In the general case – discrete variables and non-normally distributed continuous variables – conditional independence is the more general notion because conditional independence implies zero partial correlation, whereas partial correlations may vanish even though variables are conditionally dependent. The control variables of graphical models, the effect of which is partialled out by conditioning, are, however, exactly the same as in connection with the Simon–Blalock technique for path analysis: *Two variables must be conditionally independent given all prior and intervening variables if there is no linkage between them in the independence graph.*

A definition of graphical models, then, requires first a definition of conditional independence: Assume that A is a random variable. A and B are conditionally independent given C if and only if the conditional distribution of A given B and C does not depend on B. That is

$$P(A\,|\,B, C) = P(A\,|\,C) \tag{10.1}$$

for all values of A, B and C for which the conditional distributions are defined. P may be either probabilities, if A is a categorical variable, or a density function, if A is continuous.

We assume that B is a unidimensional variable, but apart from that make no special assumptions concerning the nature of B and C. They may be random variables or non-random explanatory variables with values that are fixed by the design of the study.

If B is a random variable the requirement for pairwise conditional independence may be rewritten in the following equivalent way:

$$P(A, B\,|\,C) = P(A\,|\,C)P(B\,|\,C) \tag{10.2}$$

for all possible values of A, B and C for which the conditional probabilities or densities are defined.

We will use the notation of Dawid (1979) to indicate conditional independence: $A \perp B\,|\,C$ where '$\perp$' is taken to mean 'independent' while '$|$' means 'conditionally given': A and B are conditionally independent given C.

The definition of conditional independence may without problems be extended to cover the situation where C is a multidimensional vector. Now, if C contains all the variables under consideration except A and B, we will for brevity write this as

$A \perp B\,|\,rest$

With this in place we may define graphical models. We will do this in three steps, looking first at the case with a multivariate set of random variables with no recursive structure, second at the situation where we have one set of random response variables and another set of explanatory variables, and third at the block recursive models.

The definition is simple: A graphical model of the joint distribution of a random set of variables is defined by a set of assumptions on pairwise conditional independence given *the rest*.

One assumes in other words that (10.1) and (10.2) hold for a limited number of *AB* pairs with *C* always alluding to the rest of the variables in the model.

If no assumption is made on recursive structure, the independence graph will be an undirected graph where variables are connected by edges. Arrows are for the recursive models to be defined below.

Consider next the situation where we have two sets of variables: a set of random response variables and a set of explanatory variables. The explanatory variables may be random or fixed by the design. It does not matter. The model we will consider is the model for the regression of the response variables on the explanatory variables.

A *regression* model is defined by the same type of assumptions as above with the additional constraint that at least one of the two variables *A* and *B* has to belong to the set of response variables. The conditioning set once again has to be the rest of the variables including all remaining response variables and all remaining explanatory variables.

The directed independence graphs of the recursive models defined hereafter serve two different purposes. The missing linkages between variables tell us which variables we take to be conditionally independent while the arrows tell us which variables we should include in the conditioning sets for specific pairs of conditional independent variables. As long as we are talking about graphical regression models, where it is assumed that we have no interest in the analysis of the associations among explanatory variables, we do not need the final piece of information because we already know that we are going to condition with respect to the complete set of variables. For this reason we do not have to include arrows in the independence graph of a regression model. We just have to make sure that all variables in the set of explanatory variables are connected to each other.

Block recursive models were defined above as a product of conditional distributions, one for each recursive block given the predecessors but not the descendants. Each of these conditional distributions, excluding only the ultimate set of explanatory variables, may be regarded as regression models, suggesting a very simple definition of so-called chain-graph models (Wermuth, 1993): A *chain-graph model* is a block recursive model where each component is a graphical regression model.

A chain-graph model is defined by assumptions on conditional independence of pairs of variables, but the conditioning set depends on the position of the variables in the recursive structure. For this reason we have to introduce arrows in the independence graphs.

This means that we have two types of graphs associated with chain-graph models. We have the directed independence graph showing the complete recursive structure, and we have the undirected graphs related to each of the separate graphical regression models.

The independence graph (Fig. 10.1) defines a chain-graph model for six variables partitioned into four blocks corresponding to three regression models and one non-random explanatory variable. The conditional distributions described by these models are:

1 The distribution of Dwelling (D) and Work (W) given Marriage (M), Education (E), Gender (G) and Cohort Year (Y)
2 The distribution of Marriage and Education given Gender and Cohort Year
3 The regression of Gender on Cohort Year

Fig. 10.1 implies four cases of conditional independence:

Dwelling $\perp$ Work | Marriage, Education, Gender and Year
Dwelling $\perp$ Gender | Work, Marriage, Education and Year
Work $\perp$ Marriage | Dwelling, Education, Gender and Year
Marriage $\perp$ Year | Education and Gender

and one case of marginal independence:

Gender $\perp$ Year

If the model includes continuous variables one will have to impose additional assumptions on the distribution of these variables to get to a workable model. When all variables are discrete, as in the above example, this will not be needed. We have enough information in the assumptions defining the graph to have a workable statistical model: A main result of graphical models connects graphical models to log-linear models. One has to look to the undirected graphs associated with the separate regression models. Darroch *et al.* (1980) show that these models may be represented as standard log-linear models with generators defined by the cliques – the maximally connected subsets of variables – of the graphs.

Fig. 10.1 in this way specifies three log-linear models that one may fit by most serious statistical packages:

Distribution	Log-linear model
$P(DW \mid MEGY)$	$DMEY, WEGY, MEGY$
$P(ME \mid GY)$	MEG, EGY
$P(G \mid Y)$	G, Y

Simon–Blalock techniques for graphical models: the separation theorem

The basic steps in the Simon–Blalock technique for causal modelling are first to construct a model and then generate to hypotheses that certain partial correlation coefficients are equal to zero.

Graphical modelling proceeds along the same lines. The path diagram of causal models and the zero partial correlation hypotheses are replaced by the independence graph and hypotheses on conditional independence, but apart from that there is no fundamental difference in the approach to the analysis of data and testing of models.

The graphical models, however, offer a wider range of conditional independence hypotheses than the Simon–Blalock approach for causal models, such as hypotheses generated by the so-called *separation theorem* (Whittaker, 1990, p. 67):

If *A*, *B* are two variables and *C* is a vector of variables disjoint from {*A*,*B*}, and if, in the undirected independence graph of the appropriate regression model, *A* is separated from *B* by the subset *C*, in the sense that any path from *A* to *B* has to go through at least one of the variables of *C*, then *A* and *B* are conditionally independent given *C*:

$$A \perp B \,|\, C$$

The separation theorem implies that Dwelling and Work are not only conditionally independent given the remaining four variables of Fig. 10.1, but that they are conditionally independent given Education, Gender and Cohort Year.

The separation theorem is a powerful tool for analysis of high-dimensional graphical models, reducing apparently inaccessible problems to a size which may be addressed by available standard programmes.

Complete elaboration and association in graphical models

The connection between graphical modelling and elaboration and explanation in the social sciences has been mentioned. The general principle forwarded by graphical models is one of complete elaboration. Graphical models assume that conditioning is always with respect to the rest of the variables. It is in this sense that the graphical model has explained the relationship between Work and Dwelling, and not by just controlling for the effect of Cohort Year as Table 10.1.

The principle of complete elaboration implies a very liberal view on what one should regard as association among variables. The association between Dwelling and Work has been broken down and analysed in 18 different groups according to Year, Gender, Marriage and Education. If strong evidence of association had been found in just one of the 18 groups one would have to conclude that some kind of association between the two variables is present. It follows that one must be prepared to expend considerable effort determining the characteristics of the association in question when a hypothesis of conditional independence has been rejected.

Although the graphical models cannot say much about a specific relationship, the independence graph may once again be of considerable help in connection with the analysis of the relationship. *Collapsibility* properties in the sense that parameters, estimates and test statistics can be recovered in marginal distributions of a subset of variables may be read directly off the graph. Analysis of the independence graph may therefore tell us first if there are some of the variables we do not have to control for when a given relationship is to be analysed, and second if higher-order interactions may exist between the variables in question and the variables we have not been able to exclude from the analysis. The reader is referred to Asmussen & Edwards (1983) and Agresti (1990) for further discussions of collapsibility.

In epidemiological terms it means that we are able to exclude variables both from the list of possible confounders and from the list of effect modificators by analysis of the independence graph, thereby reducing the amount of work otherwise spent on a more or less haphazard trial-and-error approach to the analysis of conditional relationships.

Computer programs for graphical modelling

Most major statistical packages, such as BMDP, SAS, SPSS, GENSTAT and GLIM, can be used for a statistical analysis by graphical models, but require that the user keeps track of the development of and analyses the independence graph him- or herself. To capitalise on the possibilities inherent in a proper integration of the graph theoretical analysis into the statistical analysis one has to use one of the programs developed for this purpose. There are now three programs available for such analysis: MIM by Edwards (1987),

DIGRAM (Kreiner,1989) and COCO by Badsberg (1991). The technical details of graphical modelling by DIGRAM are described at some length in Klein *et al.* (1995).

The case study

Summary

Fig. 10.1 shows the end result of the comparative analysis of the social situation for two different cohorts of 70-year-olds. The next subsection gives some details on the way the independence graph may be used in the final phase of the analysis aimed at a description of the conditional relationship between Cohort Year and Work.

The overall results on the differences between the two cohorts can be summarised as follows:

1 The educational level of the latter of the two cohorts is significantly higher than that of the earlier. Gender, however, plays the role of an effect modificator in the sense that this result only applies to women. For the 70-year-old men there is no significant evidence of a higher educational level in 1984 than in 1967.
2 Two trends are apparent with respect to work from 1967 to 1984: the generally earlier retirement from the workforce combined with a higher frequency of women who are or have been active on the labour market. Education and Gender are possible confounders and/or effect modificators. There is no apparent effect modification, however, and only slight confounding in the sense that the conditional relationship between Cohort Year and Work is a little stronger than the crude marginal relationship.
3 Dwellings are generally better in 1984 than in 1967. Marriage, Education and Gender are possible confounders/effect modificators but there is no evidence of either effect modification or confounding.

The Cohort Year–Work relationship

The above conclusions depend on an analysis of the collapsibility properties of the statistical model associated with the independence graph (Fig. 10.1).

To determine these properties for the relationship between Cohort

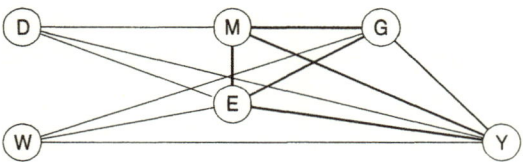

Fig. 10.5. The undirected independence graph associated with the conditional distribution P(DW|EMGY). D, dwelling; W, work; E, education; M, married; G, gender; Y, year. The mandatory edges between explanatory variables have been drawn as thick lines.

Year and Work, we must first look at the undirected graph associated with the conditional distribution of Dwelling and Work given the rest of the variables. This graph is shown in Fig. 10.5.

The separation theorem can hereafter be used to find the parametric collapsibility properties pertaining to the *WY*-relationship: Remove the *WY* edge from the graph and find the separators in the reduced graph. If one restates the conditions for parametric collapsibility (Agresti, 1990) in terms of the independence graph it follows that the table is parametrically collapsible onto the marginal table containing Work, Cohort Year, and the two separators, Education and Gender. The two other variables, Marriage and Dwelling, are linked to a completely connected subset of three variables: Education, Gender and Year. It follows from Asmussen & Edwards' (1983) condition for strong collapsibility, that estimates and test statistics calculated in the marginal table will be exactly the same as in the complete table. Marriage and Dwelling therefore cannot be confounders or effect modificators of the *WY*-relationship.

The collapsed model is saturated. The possibility that Gender and Education may be effect modificators and not only confounders therefore has to be taken into account. To exclude this possibility one would try to fit the log-linear model containing only a two-factor interaction between Work and Cohort Year (*WY, WEG, EGY*). The fit of this model is satisfactory ($X^2 = 8.77$, d.f. $= 9$, $p = 0.56$), suggesting that effect modification is absent. The final analysis of the confounding cause by Education and Gender has to be based on estimates of the *WY* interaction parameters in the (*WY, WEG, EGY*) model and the marginal table. As mentioned above there is some discrepancy present, suggesting that Education and Gender can not be completely acquitted.

Discussion

Graphical models do not represent a break with the past. It is in fact possible to argue that graphical models already existed as log-linear models for multidimensional contingency tables and covariance selection models for continuous data. What the graphical models represent is not so much a new type of statistical model as a different angle, a new perspective, on already established statistical methods for analysis of multivariate data. The graphical viewpoint has made it possible to integrate models for discrete and continuous data into one common framework, focusing on properties that these models share rather than the ways in which they differ.

Graphical models have been able to build on existing techniques and to a certain extent on existing software, that have been modified and adjusted in order to make use of the possibilities given by integration of network analysis of independence graphs with statistical analysis of data. For purely discrete or purely continuous data these methods can now be regarded as fully developed with very few loose ends to tie up. For mixed data with both discrete and continuous variables there are still a number of unsolved problems, but the MIM programme developed by Edwards (1987) has nevertheless turned these mathematically complicated models into a practical tool for data analysis. Future developments of graphical models will without doubt aim at solving the remaining problems for mixed data.

What, then, are the main advantages of graphical modelling compared with other standard techniques for multivariate data? First, by highlighting the collapsibility properties of log-linear models graphical models have permitted analysis of high-dimensional discrete data in a way that has not been conceivable before. Instead of selecting handfuls of variables for a large number of subanalyses, one may analyse a much larger number of variables in a way that is at one and the same time much less time-consuming and less prone to end up with inconsistent results.

The second advantage connects to the possibilities of analysing high-dimensional data. The graphical frame of inference permits construction of models more realistic than those based on standard methods. For discrete variables the standard solutions offered before the graphical models were either log-linear models with relatively few variables or logistic or logit regression models. Graphical models contain all of these possibilities to be used when appropriate, but have extended these boundaries.

For mental health service evaluation graphical models offer obvious possibilities. Data will be dominated by discrete variables, and contain several strongly correlated response variables the interrelationships between which can only be regarded as symmetrical, such that simple regression models are inappropriate.

References

Agresti, A. (1990). *Categorical Data Analysis*. New York: Wiley.

Alba, R.A. (1988). Interpreting the parameters of log-linear models. In *Common Problems/Proper Solutions: Avoiding Error in Quantitative Research*, ed. J.S. Long, pp. 258–67. Newbury Park: Sage Publications.

Asmussen, S. & Edwards, D. (1983). Collapsibility and response variables in contingency tables. *Biometrika*, **70**, 567–78.

Badsberg, J.H. (1991). *COCO: A Program for Analysis of Complete Contingency Tables*. Aalborg University, Denmark: Institute of Electronic Systems.

Bishop, Y.M., Fienberg, S. & Holland, P. (1975). *Discrete Multivariate Analysis*. Cambridge, Mass.: MIT Press.

Blalock, H.M. (1964). *Causal Inferences in Nonexperimental Research*. Chapel Hill: University of North Carolina Press.

Darroch, J.N., Lauritzen, S. & Speed, T. (1980). Markov fields and log linear interaction models for contingency tables. *Annals of Statistics*, **8**, 522–39.

Dawid, P. (1979). Conditional independence in statistical theory (with discussion). *Journal of the Royal Statistical Society*, B, **41**, 1–31.

Dempster, A.P. (1972). Covariance selection. *Biometrics*, **28**, 157–75.

Edwards, D. (1987). *A Guide to MIM*. Research report 87/1. University of Copenhagen, Denmark: Statistical Research Unit.

Edwards, D. & Kreiner, S. (1983). The analysis of contingency tables by graphical models. *Biometrika*, **70**, 553–65.

Elwood, J.M. (1988). *Causal Relationships in Medicine*. Oxford: Oxford University Press.

Hagenaas, J.A. (1990). *Categorical Longitudinal Data*. Newbury Park: Sage Publications.

Klein, J., Keiding, N. & Kreiner, S. (1995). Graphical models for panel studies, illustrated on data from the Framingham Heart Study. *Statistics in Medicine*, **14**, 1265–90.

Kreiner, S. (1989). *User Guide to DIGRAM: A Program for Discrete Graphical Modeling*. Research report 89/10. University of Copenhagen, Denmark: Statistical Research Unit.

Lazarsfeld, P.F. (1955). Interpretation of statistical relationships as a research operation. In *The Language of Social Research* ed. P.F. Lazarsfeld, A.K. Pasanella, & M. Rosenberg, pp. 115–25. New York: Free Press.

Lidegaard, Ø. (1993). Oral contraception and risk of cerebral thrombotic attack: results of a case–control study. *British Medical Journal*, **306**, 956–62.

Rosenberg, M. (1968). *The Logic of Survey Analysis*. New York: Basic Books.

Schultz-Larsen, K., Kreiner, S. & Avlund, K. (1993). Functional ability of community dwelling elderly: criterion-related validity of a new measure of functional ability. *Journal of Clinical Epidemiology*, **11**, 1315–26.

Simon, H. (1957). Spurious correlations: a causal interpretation. In *Models of Man*, pp. 37–49. New York: Wiley.

Suppes, P. (1984). *Probabilistic Metaphysics*. London: Basil Blackwell.

Wermuth, N. (1993). Association structures with few variables: characteristics and examples. In *Population Health Research*, ed. K. Dean, pp. 181–203. Newbury Park: Sage Publications.

Whittaker, J. (1990). *Graphical Models in Applied Multivariate Statistics*. New York: Wiley.

Whittaker, J. (1993). Graphical interaction models: a new approach for statistical modelling. In *Population Health Research*, ed. K. Dean, pp. 181–203. Newbury Park: Sage Publications.

Wright, S. (1934). The method of path coefficients. *Annals of Mathematical Statistics*, **5**, 161–215.

11

Meta-analysis

CLIVE ADAMS, NICK FREEMANTLE AND GLYN LEWIS

Introduction

Meta-analysis is the quantitative synthesis of the results of a systematic overview of previous studies. Systematic overviews are a method of collating and synthesising all the available evidence on a particular scientific question. For example, in making decisions about the most effective and efficient treatment for a condition, it is important to review *all* the previously generated evidence. On occasions it is appropriate to calculate some overall estimate of the effectiveness of the treatment. This can be done fairly simply by performing a stratified analysis of the available results, weighting the studies so that the larger, more statistically powerful studies are given more weight. However, the validity of such a quantitative approach will rest upon the method with which the studies have been selected and the completeness of the evidence collected in the systematic review.

It should be emphasised that the principles of the sytematic overview apply to many, perhaps all, areas of medical research. However, in the context of this book we shall concentrate almost exclusively on evaluations of the effectiveness of treatments, in particular using randomised controlled trials (RCTs). This is because the RCT is the most powerful research design available to assess the effects of health care, because of the random allocation of confounding variables between the groups to be compared (Altman, 1991).

Systematic reviews versus subjective reviews

The principle of systematic reviews is that the process of the review should be as scientific and systematic as the process of carrying out

176

Table 11.1. *Characteristics of Systematic Reviews*

Readers of review articles should ask:

1 Were the questions and methods clearly stated?
2 Were comprehensive search methods used to locate the relevant studies?
3 Were explicit methods used to determine which articles were included in the review?
4 Was the methodological quality of the primary studies assessed?
5 Were the selection and assessment of the primary studies reproducible and free from bias?
6 Were the differences in individual study results adequately explained?
7 Were the results of the primary studies combined appropriately?
8 Were the reviewers' conclusions supported by the data cited?

from Sackett *et al.* (1991).

new research studies. Systematic reviews and meta-analyses are a scientific endeavour, and to accomplish them properly requires considerable effort and attention to detail. One can reasonably enlarge this argument and claim that the design of new studies and the interpretation of results can only be done sensibly in the context of a comprehensive and systematic review of the literature. It seems that the medical profession has been rather late in accepting this principle and reviewing literature is often seen as a secondary process, in many ways qualitatively different from generating the research evidence itself. Systematic reviews have a key place in efforts to draw conclusions from research and thus influence clinical practice. As David Eddy described more than a decade ago:

> The profession has placed high value on developing the basic science of medicine; it has not emphasized the process by which the science is translated into practice ... When one considers the work involved in deciphering a complicated biochemical process, in designing a CT scanner, or in conducting a good clinical trial, it makes little sense to take such care in all the other steps that carry a medical procedure from idea to practice and not work as hard to analyze the last and most important step: determining how the procedure should be put to use.
>
> *(Eddy, 1982)*

In contrast with systematic reviews, subjective reviews (Mulrow 1987) rarely state a hypothesis, how relevant studies were identified, the reasons why studies were included or excluded, or how conclusions were reached (Table 11.1). Without standardising the criteria for inclusion it is easy for a biased sample of studies to be included in a review. Subjective reviews are neither objective nor reproducible and, even if they are conscientiously prepared, the results may lead to misleading recommendations for clinical practice (Antman et al., 1992). There is an urgent need to apply the process of systematic reviewing of RCTs in psychiatry. Currently, those responsible for providing care to people with mental health problems are, by and large, guided by reviews of treatments that are neither scientific nor objective. Where RCTs are comparable and of sufficient quality, formal meta-analyses may be undertaken, enabling a more accurate estimate on the treatment effect based upon weighted results from all suitable RCTs (Der Simonian & Laird, 1986; Peto, 1987; Thompson & Pocock, 1991).

Statistical power and the role of chance

One of the main problems in interpreting studies of treatment effectiveness is the random variation that occurs from studying small samples. There are still too many examples in the psychiatric literature of studies that report either 'positive' or 'negative' findings. The conventional 5% level of significance implies that 5% of all 'significant' findings are due merely to the random error introduced by sampling variation: type 1 errors (i.e. false positives). The interpretation of the primary result of a study is compounded by the tendency to 'trawl' or 'dredge' the data for significant findings. The possibility of type 2 errors, where a real difference between approaches is obscured by chance (i.e. false negatives), is less widely acknowledged and possibly a more common occurrence. These elementary statistical considerations alone introduce considerable problems in interpreting the findings of medical research, including RCTs. The greater numbers of subjects and events to be analysed in meta-analyses increases statistical power and reduces the chance of type 1 and type 2 errors. Meta-analysis narrows the confidence intervals, reflecting a more accurate estimate of the effect of treatment and allowing the possibility of testing more interesting hypotheses with the data. However, systematic biases such as reporting bias or publication bias may not neccessarily be avoided through meta-analysis.

Meta-analysis therefore ensures that the size of the treatment effect and the confidence intervals are given appropriate emphasis rather than considering results as positive or negative. Even those who are cautious about the statistical synthesis of results still point out that a table giving results with confidence intervals provides important information that helps to draw valid conclusions from the literature (Thompson & Pocock, 1991). For example, a study with a significant finding does not necessarily contradict one with a non-significant finding. The confidence intervals may overlap to such an extent that they are both consistent with the same study result.

Individual RCTs are therefore often too small to provide estimates of treatment differences of acceptable precision (DTB, 1992), and a single trial usually provides only limited guidance for clinical practice. There is now widespread recognition that the most reliable evidence is based on the results of systematic reviews of RCTs, rather than on the results of individual studies (Peto, 1987).

Citation and publication bias

A valid systematic review depends upon obtaining an unbiased estimate of the results of RCTs conducted in an area. This is a major problem as there is now considerable evidence of both citation and publication bias. 'Positive' results are more likely to be published and if published are more likely to appear in prestigious journals. 'Positive' results are more likely to appear in English-language journals and are more likely to be cited by other research workers (Easterbrook *et al.*, 1991). There are many circumstances when a new intervention is evaluated by a number of workers in small RCTs and those studies that reach publication are more likely to be those which report positive findings.

There are particular problems associated with interpreting the results of comparative phase III and IV clinical trials of new pharmaceuticals, typically compared with standard treatments and normally funded by the pharmaceutical industry. There are concerns that such funding leads to a bias in the design, publication and reporting of the results of such trials. Researchers who receive funding from the pharmaceutical industry may feel unwilling, or lack the motivation, to publish a negative finding for a new pharmaceutical agent. Peter Gøtzsche (1989) in an overview of 196 published RCTs comparing non-steroidal anti-inflammatory drugs, reported 22 factors which may increase the number and the proportion of significant results in favour of a new drug. He concluded:

> Doubtful or invalid statements were found in 76% of the conclusions or abstracts. Bias consistently favoured the new drug in 81 trials, and the control in only 1 trial.
>
> *(Gøtzsche, 1989)*

Similarly, in a further review of the outcome of manufacturer-supported RCTs Rochan *et al.* (1994) found that manufacturer-associated drugs were almost always reported as being equal or superior in efficacy and toxicity to the comparison drug. The authors conclude that: 'These claims of superiority, especially in regard to side effect profiles, are often not supported by trial data.' Similar problems could potentially arise when research is carried out under contract for government departments.

These phenomena would tend, on average, to overestimate the therapeutic efficacy of new interventions. To overcome this problem, a thorough and exhaustive ascertainment of relevant RCTs is necessary. This should ideally include unpublished material. In some areas researchers have started databases of RCTs in order to ensure that they are centrally notified, before they start, so that an unbiased sample of results is obtained for further analysis. If systematic reviews are to provide an unbiased estimate of treatment effectiveness, in addition to a more accurate estimate (Woolf *et al.*, 1990), then the available research evidence needs to be collated in an unbiased way. Rather than picking on a few RCTs which have the desired results, overviews enable a more balanced view of the literature to be formed.

Differences in the patients

The statistical issues discussed above are particularly important in considering efforts to study treatment effectiveness in sub-groups of patients. For example Paykel *et al*, (1988), in an effort to determine the group who responded best to tricyclic antidepressants, examined 18 different variables on five outcome variables. About 6% of the tests were significant and it is therefore difficult to decide which are type 1 errors. However, almost all the significant results were in the area of severity of illness and this suggests that severity may be an important determinant of treatment effectiveness with tricyclic antidepressants. Meta-analysis should, by increasing power, enable such hypotheses to be tested on existing data (e.g. Smith *et al.*, 1993), though access to the original data in addition to published results may also be necessary.

Analytical problems are introduced, though there are ways around them, if there are differences in the treatment effect between studies because of the different populations of patients that are studied. However, the increased statistical power provided by meta-analysis allows such hypotheses to be tested. One could also argue that by overviewing the results from a wide range of studies, on different groups and perhaps in different countries, much broader and more generalisable conclusions can be drawn.

Differences in the intervention

At first sight, it seems reasonable to assume that RCTs of pharmaceutical agents are using an identical intervention. However, different trials may be using different dosages or treatment regimens and sometimes a class of pharmaceutical agents is studied within a meta-analysis rather than a single compound. These interventions, though, seem less heterogeneous than a number of interventions of importance in psychiatry. Psychotherapy and case management are both areas where the interventions are difficult to specify and may depend upon idiosyncratic interpretation by local personnel. The influence of charismatic individuals may also obscure or overwhelm the overall effect of treatment. Some of the controversy surrounding the effectiveness of counselling in British general practice has been concerned with the poor specification of the nature of counselling (Corney, 1992). Systematic reviews of such interventions will therefore need to be clear about how the intervention is defined and what criteria will need to be used to determine inclusion in the study. Even if differences between interventions in different studies are suspected, these will usually alter the size of the effect rather than the direction of the effect. If this were true it should not dramatically affect the conclusions to be drawn from a meta-analysis. The increased power of meta-analysis should also allow hypotheses about the nature of the intervention or the characteristics of the group providing the treatment to be tested in a way which is impossible within individual randomised controlled trials.

An alternative approach could be adopted based upon the pragmatic argument that a systematic review of rather diverse interventions would still be of value as indicating the likely effectiveness of such an approach. For example, many British general practitioners (GPs) are providing 'counselling' for their patients, and a pragmatic review of the effectiveness of this intervention would still be of value in deciding upon the effectiveness of the policy of allowing GPs to provide such a service, even if one is not sure about what is going on in the counselling sessions themselves. Balestrieri *et al.* (1988) performed a meta-analysis on 11 studies which compared the effectiveness of mental health specialists based in general practice with the usual treatment given by the GP. This approach therefore examined the effectiveness of a wide variety of very different interventions, including counselling, behaviour therapy and general psychiatric management. The analysis compared these diverse interventions with 'usual GP treatment', which again is very varied. Though this approach can be criticised the study provided evidence to support the effectiveness of specialist mental health workers when attached to general practice – an important policy question.

As with all scientific endeavour the process of systematic reviewing requires a clear specification of the research questions and this will assist in determining the correct inclusion criteria for the study. Attention must also be paid to the quality of the studies to be included and criteria for inclusion on quality grounds must be specified beforehand.

Differences in the outcomes

In psychiatry there are often a large number of competing assessments for the clinical and social outcome of interventions. This poses potential problems in attempting to perform meta-analyses, but they can be overcome. For example in Effective Care in Pregnancy and Childbirth (Chalmers *et al.*, 1989) dichotomous outcomes are used throughout. This simplifies the analysis and allows diverse results to be combined. It also has the advantage that odds ratios can be used, which tend to be easier to interpret and have a more immediate presentational effect. This use of ratio measures of effect could be criticised, though, as absolute effects are usually more important in making decisions about treatments for individuals.

Meta-analyses of randomised controlled trials in mental health

The earliest meta-analyses of RCTs relevant to psychiatry were in the late 1970s (Smith & Glass, 1977; Smith *et al.*, 1980; Prioleau *et al.*, 1983), though the methodology of some of these early meta-analyses now looks inadequate. Until recently the technique has been applied more commonly to case–control studies than to RCTs. Meta-analyses relevant to mental health are, however, becoming increasingly frequent (Bond & Titus 1983; Buchan *et al.*, 1992; Byrne, 1989; Depression Guideline Panel, 1993; Dobson, 1989; Dush *et al.*, 1989; Eppley *et al.*, 1989; Janicack *et al.*, 1985; Jorm, 1986, 1989; Kavale & Mattson, 1983; Kim *et al.*, 1990; Mattick *et al.*, 1990; Moller & Huag, 1988; Parker *et al.*, 1992; Patten, 1990; Schneider *et al.*, 1990; Steinbrueck *et al.*, 1983; Balestrieri *et al.*, 1988).

In 1991 Wilkinson and colleagues evaluated the effects of antidepressants and benzodiazepines in patients with panic disorder (Wilkinson *et al.*, 1991). A meta-analysis comparing the effect of fluoxetine with tricyclic antidepressants on suicidality or death by suicide was also published in the same year (Beasley *et al.*, 1991). This meta-analysis, though influential, only included studies undertaken in North America, which reduced the statistical power of the study. Song *et al.* (1993; see below) examined the evidence for using selective serotonin reuptake inhibitors (SSRIs) instead of tricyclic antidepressants as the first line treatment of depression. A recent study examined the effectiveness of interventions designed to lower expressed emotion at preventing relapse of those with schizophrenia (Mari & Striener, 1994). As with RCTs in mental health, no definitive list of meta-analyses exists as yet, although the Cochrane Collaboration (see below) is working to remedy this.

The Cochrane Collaboration

Over a decade ago Archie Cochrane, a British epidemiologist, pointed out that 'it is surely a great criticism of our [medical] profession that we have not organised a critical summary, by specialty or subspecialty, updated periodically, of all relevant randomised controlled trials' (Cochrane, 1979). In the late 1970s, in the field of perinatal medicine, Chalmers and colleagues began to address this challenge. They searched 60 relevant journals and MEDLINE for all RCTs relevant to perinatology (Chalmers *et al.*, 1986). From this an electronic register was produced that contained over 6000 RCTs (Oxford Database of Perinatal Trials, 1992). This register continues to be updated from both journal and computer searches. A network of reviewers was established and trained. This network now produces over 500 systematic reviews on many aspects of perinatal care. These systematic reviews are incorporated in an inexpensive electronic publication that is updated and reissued every 6 months to reflect new evidence (Cochrane Pregnancy and Childbirth Database, 1995). The advantages of perinatal medicine's system for overviewing the effects of health care have recently been underlined:

> The work which [the perinatal register of RCTs and systematic reviews] has done in pointing the way towards evaluating the effects of different ways of organising maternity care cannot, we believe, be too highly praised. Their work has shown that many procedures and technologies have been introduced into intrapartum care over the last 30 years without adequate testing to ensure their efficacy and cost–benefit ratio.
>
> *(House of Commons Health Committee, 1992)*

In 1992 the first Cochrane Centre was established (Oxford, UK) as part of the Information Systems Strategy being developed to support the National Health Service Research & Development Programme. This initiative has now developed into the Cochrane Collaboration, an international network with centres in Australia, Canada, Denmark, Italy, the Netherlands, the United Kingdom and the United States. The Collaboration has the specific remit of facilitating systematic reviews of RCTs of all aspects of health care by helping specialists establish registers of RCTs, organising training for reviewers, and establishing systems by which the reviews will be easily updated and widely and inexpensively disseminated.

The need for systematic searching and widespread collaboration

The first phase of undertaking a meta-analysis is to identify all relevant RCTs in order to minimise the potential for the introduction of random error and selection bias into the review (Chalmers, 1992). MEDLINE is commonly used to search for trials by those undertaking meta-analyses (Depression Guideline Panel, 1993), but identifying RCTs in this database is not straightforward (Adams *et al.*, 1992). In specialties other than psychiatry, between 20% and 60% of RCTs are missed by skilled MEDLINE searches when compared with either hand-searching or searching a specialist RCT database (Dickersin *et al.*, 1994). Mental health RCTs are particularly difficult to identify. The most systematically constructed electronic search detects only 52% of reports (Adams *et al.*, 1994). Certainly those using electronic sources to identify data for a meta-analysis should not depend on one database alone. EMBASE has only a 37% overlap with MEDLINE and PsychLIT covers much psychological literature not indexed at all by the large medical databases. As with any scientific paper, a meta-analysis should state the exact methods by which data were identified so as to be both reproducible and as free from bias as possible.

The Cochrane Collaboration has persuaded the US National Library of Medicine to re-index MEDLINE entries as controlled trials when they have been identified as such by Cochrane collaborators. MEDLINE has offered to include RCTs identified in journals they do not currently index, so eventually MEDLINE should include a definitive list of RCTs.

The inadequacy of electronic searching would only be of importance if it identified RCTs that are systematically different in some way from those that are missed. As discussed above, this may well occur. There is therefore a clear need for full-text searching of journals. The first randomised trial was published over 40 years ago (Medical Research Council Streptomycin in Tuberculosis Trials Committee, 1948) so, in order to ensure an unbiased sample of RCTs, journals need to be hand-searched right back to 1948. Those wishing to help in this task have already hand-searched hundreds of journals, but much has yet to be done. Through the Cochrane Collaboration, researchers will be able to gain access to the results of the efforts of a world-wide network of hand-searchers in other specialties. Many of these RCTs are of direct relevance to those wishing to complete meta-analyses of mental health care (Silagy, 1993). The Herculean task of identifying all RCTs conducted in the past is of course a chore that once completed need never be undertaken again. Once this backlog has been cleared, the task of prospectively searching journals for new RCTs is relatively manageable.

The speed with which an acceptably high proportion of RCTs can be identified for any given meta-analysis will depend almost entirely on the resources and enthusiasm available. The Cochrane Collaboration can encourage enthusiasm, facilitate international links between like-minded individuals, and ensure there is no duplication of effort and that the task is done efficiently. Mental health specialists interested in investigating the efficiency and effectiveness of psychiatric care, however, must collaborate to find human and material resources necessary to establish registers of relevant RCTs (Adams & Gelder, 1994). From these systematically constructed registers high-quality reviews and meta-analyses will be possible. Reviewers will then have more confidence than is now possible that the potential for the introduction of bias into their results has been minimised.

An example: treatment of depression in primary care and selective serotonin reuptake inhibitors

The Universities of Leeds and York (UK) in conjunction with the Research Unit of the Royal College of Physicians, have been commissioned by the National Health Service (NHS) Management Executive to produce up-to-date reviews on the effectiveness and cost-effectiveness of key interventions in areas of controversy in which there is a high potential impact upon health status. The findings of these reviews are presented in the form of Effective Health Care bulletins, and widely distributed among decision-makers in the NHS.

The treatment of depression in primary care is an area of considerable importance, reflected by the recent publication of consensus guidelines on the recognition and treatment of depression by the Royal Colleges of Psychiatry and General Practice, under the banner of the Defeat Depression Campaign (Paykel & Priest, 1992). Most cases of depression are identified and treated in primary care by primary care physicians (Goldberg & Huxley, 1992). The importance of the topic, and in particular the absence of a formal systematic overview of the evidence of effectiveness of interventions, placed the treatment of depression in primary care high on the priority list for the Effective Health Care bulletins series. Examination of the data collected by the Prescriptions Pricing Authority indicated that the selective serotonin reuptake inhibitors (SSRIs) were being increasingly prescribed.

The SSRIs are a relatively new group of antidepressants which are almost 30 times more expensive than the equilavent dose of amitryptiline. Although there is controversy surrounding the place of the SSRIs in treatment (Edwards, 1992; British Association of Psychopharmacology, 1992), they are being heavily promoted as the routine first line treatment in depression. Fluoxetine, one of the SSRIs, is already the most commonly prescribed antidepressant in the United States (*Medical Letter*, 1992) and, since March 1992, SSRI prescribing increased in UK primary care from almost nothing to over 15% of the volume and 50% of the total cost of prescribing antidepressants in primary care in England (Effective Health Care, 1993).

Much of the evidence cited for the superior tolerance and thus effectiveness of these drugs comes from a limited number of RCTs and if correct would be an important and significant improvement in the treatment of a common and disabling disorder. For example, in one report paroxetine appeared to have around a 12% advantage as measured by drop-out from a RCT (Dunbar *et al.*, 1991). Although a switch to the use of SSRIs as routine first line treatment in depression may cost in excess of £100m in primary care prescribing in England (Effective Health Care, 1993) it has been argued that this additional spending may be cost-effective given the anticipated additional benefit to patients (Jonsson & Bebbington, 1993).

Reviewing the evidence

We undertook searches of the databases MEDLINE and Index Medicus, manually checked the reference lists of relevant publications and consulted with experts to identify published reports. Initial searches using Medical Subject Heading (MeSH) terms in MEDLINE proved disappointing, and many reports of RCTs were found through free-text searches using generic and proprietary drug names, followed by manual searching of the large number of abstracts to identify those which appeared to refer to RCTs. Two journals, *Acta Psychiatrica Scandinavica* and *International Clinical Psychopharmacology*, contained several reports and appeared to be poorly coded, so were hand-searched through recent years to aid detection of RCTs. Many of the reports appeared in relatively obscure journals which were hard to access. Several reports appeared to duplicate results of RCTs which were published elsewhere, and great care was taken not to include duplicate publications in the overview (Leizorovicz *et al.* 1992).

In all, 64 RCTs were located by this pragmatic search strategy (Song *et al.*, 1993). Results from these RCTs were examined in order to attempt to answer two key questions: the comparative efficacy of the SSRIs and other commonly prescribed antidepressants; the comparative tolerability of the SSRIs.

The only efficacy outcome measure commonly reported in the RCTs was the Hamilton Depression Rating Scale (HAMD), which was reported in 61 of the RCTs (though slightly different versions were used in some studies). The HAMD is a commonly used assessment and provides adequate estimates of efficacy, although it is particularly weighted towards and sensitive to change in somatic symptoms rather than psychological and cognitive factors (Mann & Murray, 1987). The mean difference in Hamilton scores between the patients treated with SSRIs and those treated with tricyclic or related antidepressants was calculated for each trial. A pooled estimate of the treatment difference was calculated by averaging all the treatment differences, and weighting each by the inverse of the individual squared standard errors (Der Simonian & Laird, 1986). This gave larger studies with tighter confidence intervals more influence in the pooled estimate of difference in efficacy than the smaller ones (Peto, 1987).

Only 20 RCTs presented the standard deviation of HAMD scores needed to calculate the weights. A test for heterogeneity (non-random differences) of standardised treatment difference between the studies showed no significant heterogeneity, so a fixed effects method was used to estimate the pooled difference in efficacy. To avoid the potential bias from using only 20 studies, a standard deviation was ascribed for the remaining trials which used the 17 and 21 item versions of the scale. For each scale a weighted average of these standard deviations was used to calculate a standard error for each of the studies. The analysis of 20 trials which presented the standard deviation, together with the larger comparison including those trials to which a standard deviation was ascribed, indicated that there was no significant difference in the efficacy of the SSRIs when compared with the other available and commonly used antidepressant agents (Song *et al.*, 1993).

Acceptability was measured using the proxy of drop-out from RCTs. This measure goes some way to avoiding potential reporting bias, and could be calculated from the data presented in the published studies. Given the strong likelihood of publication bias (Easterbrook *et al.*, 1991), especially in reporting side-effects in RCTs of this kind (Gøtzsche, 1989; Rochan *et al.*, 1994), it might be expected that some differences in measures of tolerability would have been found in the trials. However, no clinically or statistically significant differences in drop-out between the SSRIs and the comparison drugs was found. Three further RCTs identified later made no important difference to the results presented in the initial analysis.

There were a number of limitations to the conclusions that were possible from this systematic review and meta-analysis. The examination of efficacy was limited by the use of different versions of the HAMD, and the standard deviation was often not reported. Generally the follow-up time was short (median 6 weeks) in relation to the commonly accepted treatment period in this population. Perhaps any influence of drop-outs would not be apparent in the artificial circumstances of a randomised clinical trial with follow-up over a relatively short period? In addition the population in the RCTs was heterogeneous, containing some patients who had experienced only short-lived mood disorder and so were more likely to recover spontaneously, along with others who had a more persistent disorder. Spontaneous resolution is likely to reduce the ability of any trial to show differences in the effect of treatment and it is possible that sub-groups of patients may benefit from this class of compounds. On the other hand, the fact that some patients had already failed to respond to tricyclics before entering the trial might have introduced a bias against this class of drug and effects on drop-outs may be more apparent early on in treatment than later. The increased power of the meta-analysis would have been expected to pick up clinically significant effects if they had been present. Better-designed studies with more complete reporting of data should enable more reliable estimates of efficacy of treatment. This is essential for the translation of research findings into clinical practice, and should be mandatory in reports in clinical journals.

Implementing the results from the systematic overview of randomised controlled trials

Perhaps predictably the publication of the meta-analysis led to a wave of criticism from enthusiasts for the SSRIs and from elements of the pharmaceutical industry. The debate was played out in the correspondence pages of the *British Medical Journal* (BMJ, 1993) and the *Drug and Therapeutics Bulletin* (DTB, 1993). The meta-analysis published in the *British Medical Journal* was abstracted in the US ACP Journal Club, and led eventually to the publication of an alternative meta-analysis (Montgomery *et al.*, 1994).

The SSRIs initially appeared to be a promising new intervention in an area where drop-out from treatment is known to be a real problem. Unfortunately the results of the meta-analysis suggest that this initial enthusiasm may have been misplaced and current evidence does not support the use of SSRIs as the routine first line treatment of major depression. Further questions on the likely impact of prescribing SSRIs to reduce suicide from antidepressant overdose have been raised since the publication of the original meta-analysis. Because suicide is a rare event it may not easily be examined in RCTs, or in overviews of those trials. However, the meta-analysis has raised further important issues for evaluation in this important area.

Conclusions

Meta-analyses of randomised controlled trials are, like any research activity, difficult to undertake and will often arouse controversy and criticism. There is a constant need for continual review and updating if they are to remain relevant. With the advent of electronic publication and the systems established within the Cochrane Collaboration the process of reviewing and updating is becoming easier. Even with its limitations this technique of evaluation is very widely applicable to investigate the effectiveness of interventions in mental health, an area where small randomised controlled trials with low statistical power are commonplace. Well-conducted, regularly maintained systematic reviews are a powerful guide for clinicians, researchers, managers, funding bodies and users who are interested in the best available evidence for the effectiveness and efficiency of care.

References

Adams, C.E. & Gelder, M.G. (1994). The case for establishing a register of randomized controlled trials of mental health care. *British Journal of*

Psychiatry, **164**, 433–6.

Adams, C.E., Lefebvre, C. & Chalmers, I. (1992). Difficulty with MEDLINE searches for randomised controlled trials. *Lancet*, **340**, 915–6.

Adams, C.E., Power, A., Frederick, K. & Lefebvre, C. (1994). An investigation of the adequacy of MEDLINE searches for trials of the effects of mental health care. *Psychological Medicine*, **24**, 741–8.

Altman, D.G. (1991). *Practical Statistics for Medical Research*. London: Chapman & Hall.

Altman, D.G. (1994). The scandal of poor medical research. *British Medical Journal*, **308**, 283–4.

Antman, E.M., Lau, J., Kupelnick, B., Mosteller, F. & Chalmers, T.C. (1992). A comparison of results of meta-analyses of randomized control trials and recommendations of clinical experts. *JAMA*, **268**, 240–8.

Balestrieri, M., Williams, P. & Wilkinson, G. (1988). Specialist mental health treatment in general practice: a meta-analysis. *Psychological Medicine*, **18**, 711–17.

Beasley, C.J., Dornself, B., Bosomworth, J., Sayler, M., Rümpey, A.J., Heiligenstein, J., *et al.* (1991). Fluoxetine and suicide: a meta-analysis of controlled trials for depression. *British Medical Journal*, **303**, 685–92.

BMJ (1993). Correspondence. *British Medical Journal* **306**, 1124–6.

Bond, C.J. & Titus, L. (1983). Social facilitation: a meta-analysis of 241 studies. *Psychological Bulletin*, **94**, 265–92.

British Association for Psychopharmacology (1992). *Guidelines for Treating Depressive Illness with Antidepressants*. London: British Association for Psychopharmacology.

Buchan, H., Johnstone, E., McPherson, K., Palmer, R.L., Crow, T.J. & Brandon, S. (1992). Who benefits from electro-convulsive therapy? *British Journal of Psychiatry*, **160**, 355–9.

Byrne, M.M. (1989). Meta-analysis of early phase II studies with paroxetine in hospitalised depressed patients. *Acta Psychiatrica Scandinavica*, **350**, 138–9.

Chalmers, I., Hetherington, J., Newdick, M., Mutch, L., Grant, A., Enkin, M., Enkin, E. & Dickersin, K. (1986). The Oxford Register of Perinatal Trials: developing a register of published reports of controlled trials. *Controlled Clinical Trials*, **7**, 306–24.

Chalmers, I., Dickersin, K. & Chalmers, T.C. (1992). Getting to grips with Archie Cochrane's agenda. *British Medical Journal*, **305**, 786–8.

Cochrane, A.L. (1979). 1931–1971: a critical review, with particular reference to the medical profession. In *Medicines for the Year 2000*, pp. 1–11. London: Office of Health Economics.

Cochrane Pregnancy and Childbirth Database (1995). [Derived from The Cochrane Database of Systematic Reviews.] Disk Issue 1. London: BMJ Publications.

Corney, R. (1992). The effectiveness of counselling in general practice. *International Review Journal of Psychiatry*, **4**, 331–8.

Depression Guideline Panel (1993). *Depression in Primary Care*, vol. 2, *Treatment of Major Depression*. Clinical Practice Guideline 5. Rockville, MD: US Department of Health and Human Services. Public Health

Service. Agency for Health Care Policy and Research. AHCPR Publication no. 93-0551.

Der Simonian, R. & Laird, N. (1986). Meta-analysis in clinical trials. *Controlled Clinical Trials*, **7**, 177–88.

Dickersin, K., Scherer, R. & Lefebvre, C. (1994). Identification of relevant studies for systematic reviews. *British Medical Journal*, **309**, 1286–91.

Dobson, K.S. (1989). A meta-analysis of the efficacy of cognitive therapy for depression. *Journal of Consulting and Clinical Psychology*, **57**, 414–19.

DTB (1992). Systematic overviews of controlled trials help clarify treatment effects. *Drug and Therapeutics Bulletin*, **30**, 25–7.

DTB (1993). Selective serotonin reuptake inhibitors for depression? *Drug and Therapeutics Bulletin*, **31**, 57–8.

Dunbar, G.C., Cohn, J.B., Fabre, L.F., Feighner, J.P., Fieve, R.R., Mendels, J. & Shrivastava, R.K. (1991). A comparison of paroxetine, imipramine and placebo in depressed out-patients. *British Journal of Psychiatry*, **159**, 394–8.

Dush, D., Hirt, M. & Schroeder, M. (1989). Self-statement modification in the treatment of child behaviour disorders: a meta-analysis. *Psychological Bulletin*, **106**, 97–106.

Easterbrook, P.J., Berlin, J.A., Gopalan, R. & Matthews, D.W. (1991). Publication bias in clinical research. *Lancet*, **337**, 867–72.

Edwards, J.G. (1992). Selective serotonin reuptake inhibitors. *British Medical Journal*, **304**, 1644–6.

Eddy, D.M. (1982). Clinical policies and the quality of clinical practice. *New England Journal of Medicine*, **307**, 343–7.

Effective Health Care (1993). *The Treatment of Depression in Primary Care*. Bulletin no. 5. Leeds: University of Leeds.

Eppley, K.R., Abrams, A.T. & Shear, J. (1989). Differential effects of relaxation effects on trait anxiety: a meta-analysis. *Journal of Clinical Psychology*, **45**, 957–74.

Goldberg, D.P. & Huxley, P. (1992). *Common Mental Disorders*. London: Routledge.

Gøtzsche, P.C. (1989). Methodology and overt and hidden bias in reports of 196 double-blind trials of nonsteroidal antiinflammatory drugs in rheumatoid arthritis. *Controlled Clinical Trials*, **10**, 31–56.

House of Commons Health Committee (1992). *Maternity Services (2nd report)*, vol. 1. London: HMSO.

Janicack, P., Davis, J., Gibbons, R., Ericksen, S., Chang, S. & Gallagher, P. (1985). The efficacy of ECT: a meta-analysis. *American Journal of Psychiatry*, **142**, 297–302.

Jonsson, B. & Bebbington, P. (1993). Economic studies of the treatment of depressive illness. In *Health Economics of Depression: Perspectives in Psychiatry*, vol. 4. ed. B. Jonsson & J. Rosenbaum, pp. 35–48. Chichester: Wiley.

Jorm, A. (1986). Effects of cholinergic enhancement therapies on memory function in Alzheimer's disease: a meta-analysis of the literature. *Australian and New Zealand Journal of Psychiatry*, **20**, 237–40.

Jorm, A. (1989). Modifiability of trait anxiety and neuroticism: a meta-analysis of the literature. *Australian and New Zealand Journal of Psychiatry*, **23**, 21–9.

Kavale, K. & Mattson, P. (1983). 'One jumped off the balanced beam': meta-analysis of perceptual motor training, *Journal of Learning Disability*, **16**, 165–73.

Kim, H., Delva, N. & Lawson, J. (1990). Prophylactic medication for unipolar depressive illness: the place of lithium carbonate in combination with antidepressant medication. *Canadian Journal of Psychiatry*, **35**, 107–14.

Leizorovicz, A., Haugh, M.C. & Boissel, J.P. (1992). Meta-analysis and multiple publication of clinical reports. *Lancet*, **340**, 1102–3.

Mann, A. & Murray, R. (1987). Measurement in psychiatry. In *Essentials in Postgraduate Medicine*, 2nd edn, ed. P. Hill, R. Murray & A. Thorley, pp. 55–80. London: Academic Press.

Mari, J. & Striener, D.L. (1994). An overview of family interventions and relapse on schizophrenia: meta-analysis of research findings. *Psychological Medicine*, **23**, 565–78.

Mattick, R., Andrews, G., Hadzi, P.D. & Christensen, H. (1990). Treatment of panic and agoraphobia: an integrative review. *Journal of Nervous and Mental Disorder*, **178**, 567–76.

Medical Letter on Drugs and Therapeutics (1992). Sertraline for treatment of depression. *Medical Letter on Drug and Therapeutics*, **34**, 47–8.

Medical Research Council Streptomycin in Tuberculosis Trials Committee (1948). Streptomycin treatment for pulmonary tuberculosis. *British Medical Journal*, **II**, 769.

Moller, H.J. & Huag, G. (1988). Secondary and meta-analysis of the efficacy of non-tricyclic antidepressants. *Pharmacopsychiatry*, **21**, 363–4.

Montgomery, S.A., Henry, J., McDonald, G., Dinan, T., Lader, M., Hindmarch, I., Clare. A. & Nutt, D. (1994). Selective serotonin reuptake inhibitors: meta-analysis of discontinuation rates. *International Clinical Psychopharmacology*, **9**, 47–53.

Mulrow, C.D. (1987). The medical review article: state of the science. *Annals of International Medicine*, **106**, 485–8.

Oxford Database of Perinatal Trials (1992). Oxford Electronic Publishing. OUP: Oxford.

Parker, G., Roy, K., Hadzi-Pavlovic, D. & Pedic, F. (1992). Psychotic depression: a meta-analysis of physical treatments. *Journal of Affective Disorders*, **24**, 17–24.

Patten, S. (1990). Propranolol and depression: evidence from the antihypertensive trials. *Canadian Journal of Psychiatry*, **35**, 257–9.

Paykel, E.S. & Priest, R.G. (1992). Recognition and management of depression in general practice: consensus statement. *British Medical Journal*, **305**, 1198–202.

Paykel, E.S., Hollyman, J.A., Freeling, P. & Sedgwick, P. (1988). Predictors of therapeutic benefit from amitryptiline in mild depression: a general practice placebo-controlled trial. *Journal of Affective Disorders*, **14**, 83–95.

Peto, R. (1987). Why do we need systematic overviews of randomized trials? *Statistical Medicine*, **6**, 233–40.

Pocock, S.J. (1983). *Clinical Trials: A Practical Approach*. Chichester: Wiley.

Prioleau, L., Murdock, M. & Brody, N. (1983). An analysis of psychotherapy versus placebo studies. *Behavioral and Brain Sciences*, **6**, 275–310.

Rochan, P.A., Gurwitz, J.H., Simms, R.W., Fortin, P.R., Felson, D.T., Minaker, K.L. & Chalmers, T.C. (1994). A study of manufacturer-supported trials of nonsteroidal anti-inflammatory drugs in the treatment of arthritis. *Archives of Internal Medicine*, **154**, 157–63.

Sackett, D.L., Haynes, R.B., Guyatt, G.H. & Tugwell, P. (1991). *Clinical Epidemiology: A Basic Science for Clinical Medicine*. Toronto: Little, Brown.

Schneider, L., Pollock, V. & Lyness, S. (1990). A meta-analysis of controlled trials of neuroleptic treatment in dementia. *Journal of the American Geriatric Society*, **38**, 553–63.

Shapiro, D.A. & Shapiro, D. (1982a). Meta-analysis of comparative therapy outcome studies: a replication and refinement. *Psychological Bulletin*, **92**, 581–604.

Shapiro, D.A. & Shapiro, D. (1982b). Meta-analysis of comparative outcome therapy research: a critical appraisal. *Behavioural Psychotherapy*, **10**, 4–25.

Silagy, C. (1993). Developing a register of randomized controlled trials in primary care. *British Medical Journal*, **306**, 897–900.

Smith, G.D., Song, F. & Sheldon, T.A. (1993). Cholesterol lowering of mortality: the importance of considering the initial level of risk. *British Medical Journal*, **306**, 1367–73.

Smith, M.L. & Glass, G.V. (1977). Meta-analysis of psychotherapy outcome studies. *American Psychologist*, **32**, 752–60.

Smith, M.L., Glass, G.V. & Miller, T.I. (1980). *The Benefits of Psychotherapy*. Baltimore, MD: Johns Hopkins University Press.

Song, F., Freemantle, N., Sheldon, T., House, A., Watson, P., Long, A. & Mason, J. (1993). Selective serotonin reuptake inhibitors: meta-analysis of efficacy and acceptability. *British Medical Journal*, **306**, 683–7.

Steinbrueck, S., Maxwell, S. & Howard, G. (1983). A meta-analysis of psychotherapy and drug therapy in the treatment of unipolar depression with adults. *Journal of Consulting and Clinical Psychology*, **51**, 856–63.

Thompson, S.G. & Pocock, S.J. (1991). Can meta analysis be trusted? *Lancet*, **338**, 1127–30.

Wilkinson, G., Balestrieri, M., Ruggeri, M. & Bellantuono, C. (1991). Meta-analysis of double-blind placebo-controlled trials of antidepressants and benzodiazepines for patients with panic disorders. *Psychological Medicine*, **21**, 991–8.

Woolf, S.H., Battista, R.N., Anderson, G.M., Logan, A.G., Wang, E. and the Canadian Task Force on the Periodic Health Examination (1990). Assessing the clinical effectiveness of preventive manoeuvres: analytic principles and systematic methods in reviewing evidence and developing clinical practice recommendations. *Journal of Clinical Epidemiology*, **43**, 891–905.

World Health Organization Scientific Group on Treatment of Psychiatric Disorders (1991). *Evaluation of Methods for the Treatment of Mental Disorders*. Geneva: WHO.

PART IV

SYSTEM-LEVEL RESEARCH

12

Sectorised services outcome research

Lars Hansson

Sectorised services

The main trend in the development of mental health care systems has, during the last decades, been the replacement of care in psychiatric hospitals with care in community-based settings. This deinstitutionalisation movement has been defined as (1) the prevention of inappropriate mental hospital admission through the provision of community alternatives for treatment, (2) the release to the community of all institutionalised patients who have been given adequate preparation for such a change, (3) the establishment and maintenance of community support systems for non-institutionalised people receiving mental health services in the community (Bachrach, 1977). There has been a continuing debate concerning the success of this transformation of the care system, and a number of research reports concerning the failure of coordination between the depopulation of hospitals and the building up of adequate community-based services. The result has been increasing burdens on, in particular, long-term patients and their relatives (Braun *et al.*, 1981; Lehman *et al.*, 1982).

A number of principles have evolved, guiding the building up of care systems directed towards care in the community. Some of these principles have been related to the organisation of care, while others have expressed public policy, care ideology or a philosophy of care, relying on social values which have been seen as consistent with, or as a base for, the development of these new services. Important goals and principles identified in this change process have been that psychiatric services should be comprehensive, coordinated, accessible, acceptable, accountable, efficient and effective (Huxley, 1990). These principles refer to both structure and content of services, and have also been seen as a means to increase effectiveness.

The concept of sectorisation or a sectorised service has been used as a description of an organisational framework which would facilitate the establishment of a community-based service system according to the above principles. However, the concept has become ambiguous since it has also been associated with many of the principles directing the content of community-based services. To avoid confusion, especially when we are discussing the evaluation of sectorised services, the term 'sectorisation' should be limited to the depiction of a way of formally organising a local service system which has a proposed potential for supporting the development of community-based care models. A sectorised service is recognised by the following characteristics:

1 The psychiatric care organisation is related to a specific geographic area: *the catchment area principle*.
2 The psychiatric care organisation is responsible for care of the total population within the catchment area: *the population responsibility principle*.
3 The psychiatric care organisation is specified in a range of differentiated services covering all levels of mental health services for the population under its responsibility: *the comprehensiveness principle*.

According to this a sectorised psychiatric service might be seen as an important but not sufficient prerequisite for the implementation of a community-based service system, and should not be confused with locally and culturally differing principles and objectives which have been seen as important in the deinstitutionalisation process and the development of effective community care models.

The advantages of sectorisation both from the point of view of the clinical development of a community care model, and from a systems research viewpoint, are that it is a population-based system with a defined responsibility as a comprehensive care organisation. This may have a relevance for the effectiveness of care in that it may increase accessibility, availability and cooperation with other agents within the local community. A sectorised service system may also counteract the demonstrated risk of fragmentation of community-based services. From a research point of view a sectorised service enables population-based studies of the service system, that is the evaluation and monitoring of the mental health of a defined population which is encountering a defined psychiatric service system, thereby also increasing the possibility of drawing inferences on an epidemiological and system level from studies of outcome, performance and use of services. Some disadvantages of services organised according to the above principles have also been put forward (Lindholm, 1983; Johnson & Thornicroft, 1993). A sectorised service limits the patient's choice of services and caregiver, and it may also promote generalist rather than specialist services.

Objectives of sectorised services

In view of the fact that sectorisation of psychiatric services has been linked with the objective of putting the emphasis on care in the community, the objectives of the sectorised services have been intertwined with objectives of the deinstitutionalisation process. The general objective of a sectorised service, as for any other model of organisation of a psychiatric service, is to improve the mental health in the population, focusing on prevention and the reduction of prevalence and incidence of mental illness. Objectives related to this are the reduction of needs for care in the population and that care should be delivered in a cost-effective way.

However, these health-related objectives are seldom stated clearly or operationalised by the services in a way that makes an evaluation of outcome of services possible in this respect (Falloon, 1987). In changing to a sectorised service system there has been a reliance on operational and intermediate objectives which at best have a potential relationship with the mental health in the population. Common objectives used have been to reduce inpatient treatment, stated as number of admissions, length of stay, and number of readmissions. A linked objective has been to keep the patient in the community and to avoid inpatient treatment for patients staying in the community (Häfner & an der Heiden, 1991). Another set of outcome objectives has related more to the qualitative aspects of performance and the care process, where objectives such as promotion of the continuity of care, coordination of care and integration of the patient in the community have been put forward. It is therefore, with regard to the evaluation of sectorised services, a high priority that clinically developed and locally based sets of operationalised objectives relating to the mental health of the population being served are developed.

Evaluating the outcome of sectorised services

A sectorised service has a general objective of delivering comprehensive services, either through its own care activities or through cooperation with other community services such as primary care services, social services, and voluntary and relatives organisations. An evaluation of such a service should therefore be comprehensive in at least two ways. As an evaluation at a local system level it should include all levels of intervention managed by the specialist psychiatric services. It should also be comprehensive with reference to the population it is serving, and include the whole network of services outside the specialist psychiatric services dealing with mental health care or support in the target population. This may be seen as one of the major differences compared with programme evaluations (Bachrach, 1982), which deal with specific components of the system without an explicit reference to, or consideration of, the interaction of components of the service system, or the total impact on the population being served.

Outcome research of sectorised services on a system level is concerned with the efficacy and effectiveness of the local service system as a whole. It is concerned with outcome regarding both the patient population and the total population being served. It should ideally be performed against stated objectives of specific services. However, since objectives of services are often vaguely stated and poorly operationalised (Bachrach, 1982) it is important as a first step in the evaluation process to clarify and operationalise implicit and unstated objectives which may be considered crucial in an outcome evaluation. It is also important to distinguish between objectives relating to the transition process or change in organisation of services towards a sectorised model, and outcome objectives of a sectorised service in operation.

The general objective of improving mental health in the population may as a first step be operationalised as a reduction of the incidence and prevalence of mental illness. It is of course important to be conscious of the difference between measuring treated incidence and prevalence and true incidence and prevalence in the population. The interventions corresponding to these objectives may be defined as primary and secondary prevention efforts, treatment and rehabilitation interventions, and all activities securing continuity, coordination and integration of interventions, e.g. cooperative activities, supervision and assessment procedures.

Outcome measures

Outcome of the services in operation is reflected in the mental health situation in the population, or in indicators of mental health. Health outcome in relation to mental illness is multidimensional and contains aspects of symptoms, distress, ability for self-care, and social and occupational skills. Health outcome measures must reflect this and may be divided into measures of symptoms, social functioning and quality of life. On a population level epidemiological measures such as mortality rates and suicide rates may be used in addition to incidence and prevalence rates. Consumer ratings of the quality of services, used as a measure of outcome, have also become of increasing importance. Measurements of outcome must also incorporate different perspectives on outcome. The views of patients, relatives, staff, independent observers, the surrounding network of services, and the local community should be included.

It is not within the scope of this chapter to evaluate the great number of scales measuring aspects of mental illness such as symptoms, discomfort or psychosocial stress. The development of psychiatric treatment and programme evaluation research has led to the development of a variety of internationally published scales with an acceptable reliability and validity, and a tested sensitivity and specificity. A differentiation between objective measures performed by professionals or independent raters and self-rating scales may be done. The use of subjective measures is stressed since the subjective experience of illness has been shown to be more related to actual use of health resources than are objective measures (Hunt, 1988; Borgquist *et al.*, 1993). For reviews of psychiatric rating scales measuring mental illness see Thompson (1989), Wetzler (1989) and Malt *et al.* (1990).

Concerning measures of social functioning or social adjustment an overview is found in Weissman *et al.* (1981). Quality of life measures have received increasing interest, although this field is younger and still struggling to a greater extent with both validity and reliability issues. Quality of life measures are discussed further elsewhere in this volume by Peter Huxley. One of the advantages of using measures of social adjustment or quality of life in this context may be that they have a better correspondence with goals, intentions and strategies of interventions in a sectorised service system as opposed to mere symptom or illness ratings.

A second approach to measuring indicators of health in the

population is the needs assessment approach (Brewin, 1987; Wing, 1990; Thornicroft *et al.*, this volume). Although the content and understanding of the concept of need has been under debate (McLachlan, 1974), the most appropriate view in this context is that a need for care or support is existent when a disability exists in terms of lowered physical, psychological or social funtioning and there exist accepted methods of care or support which might reduce or eliminate this disability. In accordance with this, need is not a measure of health or illness but is seen as valuable in terms of outcome research since it enables measures of unmet needs as well. A combination of measures of met and unmet needs might be used as measures of the capacity of the services to care for mental illness in the population, and as a link between problem, demand for care, utilisation, evaluation and outcome.

Outcome measures of a third category are the satisfaction of users, relatives and professionals with the services delivered. The best developed part of this field is user satisfaction measures, although a number of methodological and empirical problems have been raised (Lebow, 1982; Kalman; 1983, Berger 1983; Hansson, 1989a, b). Of special concern have been issues concerning validity and reliability, which have seldom been tested in a thorough way, and problems concerning sampling and attrition. A few recent publications dealing with these matters have, though, shown satisfactory results (OTA, 1988; Thornicroft *et al.*, 1993; Ruggeri & Dall'agnola, 1993). There have also been diverging opinions on which aspects of the services delivered users may evaluate (OTA, 1988).

Outcome research so far

In an review article Bachrach (1982) stated six major methodological problems concerning studies of community support programmes:

1 The goals of the community support programmes were not clearly stated.
2 The major outcome measure used was recividism.
3 If other outcome measures were used they were largely unstandardised and of questionable adequacy (which could be seen in connection with the goal problem).
4 Interactive and combined effects of multiple interventions were not studied, which excludes conclusions concerning the impact of interventions at a system level.

5 Study groups were inadequately standardised with regard to diagnosis, psychopathology, symptomatology, institutional history and other patient characteristics.
6 The time frame of the studies was not adequate.

This critique still holds for much of the research on a programme level and is also valid for research done at the system level. Outcome research of sectorised services may be divided into two kinds of studies: those which are concerned with outcome in relation to changes of the service system into a sectorised service, and those which evaluate the outcome of a service in operation. In studies related to the changes into a sectorised service it is also of great importance to differentiate methodologically between research on effects of the organisational change as such, and research on outcome of delivered care and support.

Strict outcome research in term of studies investigating health-related outcome is lacking, both concerning studies of organisational change and regarding studies of sectorised services in operation. This implies that after several decades of this continuing transitional process we still lack basic scientific evidence of the efficacy and effectiveness of sectorised services in terms of impact on the mental health status of the target population (Johnson & Thornicroft, 1993), and in terms of other health-related outcome measures and quality of care.

Studies concerning the implementation of a sectorised service have to a large extent been occupied with intermediate operational objectives of reducing inpatient care in favour of the use of alternative services, and have consequently been discussing 'outcome' in terms of changes in utilisation rates at different care levels. These studies have used utilisation rates, which strictly speaking are measures of performance and care processes, as proxies for outcome, and have reported changes in bed-days used, rates of admission, length of inpatient treatment, readmission rates, survival measures such as time in the community, and changes in day- and outpatient contact patterns. There has been a clear tendency to view these measures as outcome measures, sometimes clearly stated, and sometimes implicitly. However, there is some rationale for using these kinds of measures in monitoring the system change if the change in service model is associated with objectives concerning changes in the distribution of care between care levels and in patterns of care. But utilisation is not cure or necessarily related to need, and the above measures have been strongly criticised as measures of outcome with a relationship to changes in psychopathology or mental health status (Rosenblatt & Mayer, 1974; Turner, 1979; Bachrach, 1982; Falloon, 1984). As far as the inpatient treatment indices are concerned, the best predictor of being admitted to hospital has been shown to be a record of earlier admissions rather than level of symptoms or psychopathology. These measures are also strongly influenced by a number of other variables such as bed capacity, availability of alternative services, social characteristics of the patients, level of tolerance in the community, administrative and discharge policies (Brandon, 1975; Zohar *et al.*, 1987; Häfner & an der Heiden, 1991). Furthermore, since bed usage is so highly correlated with beds available it is quite astonishing that so much interest and effort has been put into demonstrating that a decrease in the number of beds leads to a diminished use of beds.

A number of studies reporting on the transition into a sectorised service have shown changes in utilisation rates. Results have been diverging but generalisable results have been that total rate of utilisation as well as rates of outpatient utilisation have increased (Tischler *et al.*, 1972; NIMH, 1977; Babigian, 1977; Häfner & Klug, 1982; British Psychiatric Register Group, 1984). Concerning bed use there have generally been reports of a decrease in admissions (Babigian, 1977; Stefansson, 1985; Tyrer *et al.*, 1989; Hansson, 1989c) although an increase has also been reported (Holsten & d'Elia, 1984). An initial increase in admissions has been demonstrated (Babigian 1977; Hansson 1989c). In these instances it was shown to be related to an increased geographical accessibility of outpatient services, and discussed in terms of earlier unmet or cumulated needs for care. Readmissions have been shown both to increase and to decrease. Concerning changes in patterns of clinical characteristics of admitted patients the findings are also diverging. In some instances there has been an increase for patients with non-psychotic disorders and in others an increase for patients with psychotic disorders. The point of departure in changing the service system and the specific accessibility and availability of care facilities in the new services seems crucial for the results in this respect.

Outcome studies of sectorised services in operation are also noticeably lacking. The studies performed in this area have, rather, been process studies analysing care utilisation data. The increased treated prevalence or incidence in sectorised services has raised the question of utilisation of resources when the patient has entered the service system. This has to be studied in individual patient-linked studies of utilisation of care or of individual patterns of care. Patterns of care reflect the interaction of features of the psychiatric care organisation and the help-seeking behaviour of the patient. The concept of pattern of care is central to the analysis of resource utilisation and is composed of several dimensions such as type of care, setting, intensity and duration of care (Sytema *et al.*, 1989). The utilisation of care may then be weighted, classified and/or categorised, resulting in individual patterns of care or consumption scores. A review of eight system-level studies of psychiatric services revealed that these utilisation studies in no instance included outcome measures pertaining to mental health (Hansson & Sandlund, 1992). The results from these studies show that a small proportion of patients use a large proportion of resources. Social characteristics, such as living alone or having no occupation, in some of the studies predicted a higher utilisation. Only one study reported sex differences, male patients being more common among heavy users. In most of the studies a diagnosis of psychosis predicted a higher utilisation. It is notable that the only multicentre study performed, the WHO multicentre study of mental health in a pilot study area (Giel *et al.*, 1987), which could have been a useful framework for the evaluation of outcome, did not derive generally interpretable and meaningful analyses of the utilisation data gathered. Its merits lie rather in the important effort regarding methodological development of information systems, care episode/patterns of care classification models, and the empirical description of incidence cohorts and their utilisation of care in settings of different kinds.

An analysis of the effectiveness of utilisation and of specific patterns of care requires measurement of the benefits or outcome of care. A strict analysis of the optimality of resource allocation/utilisation requires an analysis of the relationship of costs to the effectiveness and benefits of care. Since no comprehensive studies of utilisation have related individual care patterns to costs or outcome/benefits of care, conclusions cannot at present be drawn concerning efficiency or effectiveness of specific patterns of care for specific groups of patients. However, in studies defining a group of high users there seems to be an implicit notion of the ineffectiveness or 'burden' of these high users to organisation and staff, which is not appropriate, since no measures of health-related outcome have been used.

Cost and cost-effectiveness studies

Ultimately all utilisation of the resources of the psychiatric services should be evaluated with respect to the health effects, without which the optimality or effectiveness of resource utilisation cannot be evaluated. Investigations of utilisation of care have a major merit in the description and analysis of quantitative aspects of care processes. They have a secondary merit in that utilisation data are indispensable in investigations of efficiency of sectorised services. Comprehensive data concering utilisation and health-related outcome of interventions together constitute the basis for cost-effectiveness analysis. Cost-effectiveness studies are scarce within psychiatry, and lacking at a system level. So far there have mainly been attempts to evaluate cost-effectiveness of specific programmes for targeted groups of patients within sectorised or community-based service systems. Cost analyses are also highly relevant, cost being seen as a common unit in summarising, describing and comparing resource allocation between settings and systems. However, cost measurement without outcome measurement and outcome measurement without cost measurement is, in a way, the blind leading the blind. In order to accomplish an effective allocation of resources, outcome of service use must in the end be evaluated against its costs.

Further research

Methodological matters of measurement and design strategies in this field of research are dealt with elsewhere in this volume. I will therefore sum up with some comments and proposals concerning priorities for further system-level research:

1. Outcome studies at the system level of sectorised services, using health-related measures of outcome, are noticeably lacking, and therefore have a high priority. This lack of studies is in great contrast to the longlasting and continuing trend towards the clinical development and implementation of sectorised services. The scientific evidence regarding the effectiveness and efficiency of these services must become a guide for further development of such services.

2. A full-scale outcome evaluation of a sectorised service in many ways requires a very great and cumbersome effort, which probably

can be performed only in a few instances. To increase the feasibility of system-level research, defined homogeneous cohorts of patients could be used. These cohorts could be made homogeneous with respect to illness or need of care, and chosen to reflect important objectives regarding patient groups prioritised by the sectorised service in question. These cohorts could be viewed as tracer groups of the effectiveness of the services. This approach is to be separated from studies at the programme level, where specific components of the services are under study; the approach suggested follows patients through all interventions during a defined period. A second useful approach would consist of a dismantling procedure, where certain parts of the sectorised service are withheld for some defined groups of patients, and differences in outcome are evaluated. This would be a preferable approach when the effectiveness of specific parts of the sectorised services are also under study, and there are research questions dealing with 'what works for whom in which setting?' In a further development of sectorised services it is not enough to get an overall picture of effectiveness. Issues of effectiveness of specific components of the services and, above all, the interaction of components of the services are of great interest.

3. System-level outcome studies should make efforts to include and link utilisation data to health outcome data. There are too few studies which have attempted this at a system level. As shown, utilisation data have been used as proxies for outcome, which is not appropriate. Studies should use both kinds of data in order to evaluate the effectiveness of use of services. This would greatly enrich the scientific and clinical value of studies in the area. A further reason for including both kinds of data in studies is that this is the only way to enable evaluations of cost-effectiveness, which might be viewed as the ultimate evaluation of the outcome of services.

4. Concerning outcome measures, they should reflect several dimensions and perspectives of outcome. Central dimensions are changes in symptomatology, social functioning, quality of life and level of social disablement, to what extent needs of care are met, and the satisfaction of users, relatives and professionals with services. In some of these dimensions there is a long tradition of instrument development, while others have a rather short history. In the future, the use of needs assessment approaches and user satisfaction approaches should be stressed for several reasons. The most obvious of these are that both have the benefit of being links between problem, action and

outcome, and both have an apparent connection to the general objectives of community-based care within sectorised services. The perspectives of outcome measurement should also be several. The perspective of the patient, the relatives, the profession, the surrounding network of services and the local community should be included in outcome measurement. In research so far, the perspectives of the care organisation and the profession have been predominant. Corresponding to the transition from provider-led servicers to needs-led services, we may state a transition to user-led services. Accordingly future studies should make greater efforts to include the user or patient perspective, in both the measurement of health and quality of care.

5. There has been improvement in the standardisation of outcome measures. However, this is not the case concerning descriptive measures of services and care organisations. Since the structure and content of sectorised service systems may differ greatly, these should be described in detail in connection with system-level outcome research. Without comparable and standardised descriptions of the structure and content of the different components of the services it is hard to make analyses and comparisons of the role of organisational characteristics and components of the system in evaluations of outcome. This is a neglected field, although there is some developmental work being performed, such as the WHO study on classification of mental health care (ICMHC), which aims at producing a model for the classification of structure and content of mental health care services.

6. System-level outcome research of sectorised services should be comprehensive. It should take into consideration all levels of interventions of the sectorised services, and also all interventions from outside the sectorised psychiatric services directed towards the target population. Concerning outcome research on the system level of sectorised services there are two major research questions. The first deals with the outcome of a change into a sectorised service, and the second with the evaluation of outcome of an operational service. A discussion of the research questions at hand inevitably involves the question of research design and the problem of control. The experimental design is most often put forward as the ideal solution to the design question in evaluating outcome of health care. If this is not feasible a quasi-experimental or a naturalistic descriptive design might be used.

Concerning changes into a sectorised service, the research design alternatives are to use a control or comparison catchment area, or to use a pre–post design. The use of a comparison catchment area puts great responsibility on the researcher to choose this catchment area in a way that makes comparisons with the service under study meaningful, insofar as the influence of population differences and other extraneous and intervening variables could make differences with respect to outcome hard to interpret. However, the use of multivariate statistical techniques, such as covariance analysis, could make up for some of these difficulties. A pre–post design is not afflicted with these kinds of control problems. The usefulness of this design could also be strengthened by using a time series design, with an appropriate time frame of outcome measurement. In many cases the problems of control are easier to handle with this kind of design, and it is also in most cases a more feasible design, which is of great importance in a research field where studies are so scarce.

Considering studies of services in operation, the research problem is somewhat different. A comparison catchment area design could be used, but there are other options available. Two such options are, firstly, to evaluate outcome against preset standards of care and health targets concerning the target population and catchment area population. Secondly a dismantling design can be used in which the interventions of the sectorised service are offered in controlled components to parts of the target population.

References

Babigian, H. M. (1977). The impact of community mental health centers on the utilisation of services. *Archives of General Psychiatry*, **34**, 385–94.

Bachrach, L. (1977). *Deinstitutionalization: An Analytical Review and Sociological Perspective* Rockville, MD: National Institute of Mental Health, Division of Biometry and Epidemiology.

Bachrach, L. (1982). Assessment of outcomes in community support programs: results, problems and limitations. *Schizophrenia Bulletin*, **8**, 39–60.

Berger, M. (1983). Toward maximising the utility of consumer satisfaction as an outcome. In *The Assessment of Psychotherapy Outcome*, ed. M. J. Lambert, E.R. Christensen & S.S. DeJulio. New York: Wiley.

Borgquist, L., Hansson, L., Nettelbladt, P., Nordström G. & Lindelöw G. (1993). Perceived health and high consumers of care: a study of mental health problems in a Swedish primary health care district. *Psychological Medicine*, **23**, 763–70.

Brandon, R.N. (1975). Differential use of mental health services: social pathology or class victimization? In *Handbook of Evaluation Research*, ed. M. Guttentag & E.L. Struening. Beverly Hills, CA: Sage Publications.

Braun, P., Kochansky, G. & Shapiro, R. (1981). Overview: deinstitutionalization of psychiatric patients, a critical review of outcome studies. *American Journal of Psychiatry*, **138**, 736–49.

Brewin, C. (1987). Principles and practice of measuring needs in the long-term mentally ill: the MRC needs for care assessment. *Psychological Medicine*, **17**, 971–81.

British Psychiatric Register Group (1984). *Psychiatric Care in Eight Register Areas: Statistics from Eight Psychiatric Case Registers in Great Britain, 1976–1981*. Southampton: British Psychiatric Register Group, Knowle Hospital.

Falloon, I. (1984). Relapse: a reappraisal of assessment of outcome in schizophrenia. *Schizophrenia Bulletin*, **10**, 293–9.

Falloon, I. (1987). Evaluation in psychiatry: planning, developing and evaluating community based services for adults. In *Evaluating Mental Health Practice: Methods and Applications*, ed. J. Milne, pp. 196–238. Beckenham: Croom Helm.

Giel, R., Hannibal, J.U., Henderson, H.H. & ten Horn, G.H.M.M. (eds.) (1987). *Mental Health Services in Pilot Study Areas*. Copenhagen: WHO.

Häfner, H. & Klug, J. (1982). First evaluation of the Mannheim community mental health service. In *Epidemiological Research as Basis for the Organization of Extramural Care*, ed. E. Strömgren, A. Dupont & A. Nielsen, pp. 67–78. *Acta Psychiatrica Scandinavica Supplementum*, 285.

Häfner, H. & an der Heiden, W. (1991). Methodology of evaluative studies in the mental health field. In *Evaluation of Comprehensive Care of the Mentally Ill*, ed. H. Freeman & J. Henderson, pp. 1–23. London: Gaskell.

Hansson, L. (1989a). Patient satisfaction with in-hospital psychiatric care: a study of a 1-year population of patients hospitalized in a sectorized care organization. *European Archives of Psychiatry and Neurological Sciences*, **239**, 93–100.

Hansson, L. (1989b). The quality of outpatient psychiatric care: a survey of patient satisfaction in a sectorised care organisation. *Scandinavian Journal of the Caring Sciences*, **3**, 71–81.

Hansson, L. (1989c). Utilization of psychiatric inpatient care: a study of changes related to the introduction of a sectorized care organization. *Acta Psychiatrica Scandinavica*, **79**, 571–8.

Hansson, L. & Sandlund, M. (1992). Utilization and patterns of care in comprehensive psychiatric care organizations: a review of studies and some methodological considerations. *Acta Psychiatrica Scandinavica*, **86**, 255–61.

Holsten, F. & d'Elia, G. (1984). Sectorized psychiatry: some characteristics of patient population after reorganization. *Nordic Journal of Psychiatry*, **38**, 603–11.

Hunt, S.M. (1988). Subjective health indicators and health promotion. *Health Promotion*, **3**, 23–4.

Huxley, P. (1990). *Effective Community Mental Health Services*. Aldershot:

Avebury/Gower.

Johnson, S. & Thornicroft, G. (1993). The sectorisation of psychiatric services in England and Wales. *Social Psychiatry and Psychiatric Epidemiology*, **28**, 45–7.

Kalman, T.P. (1983). An overview of patient satisfaction with psychiatric treatment. *Hospital and Community Psychiatry*, **34**, 48–54.

Lebow, J. (1982). Consumer satisfaction with mental health treatment. *Psychological Bulletin*, **91**, 244–59.

Lehman, A.F., Ward, N.C. & Linn, L.S. (1982). Chronic mental patients: the quality of life issue. *American Journal of Psychiatry*, **139**, 1271–6.

Lindholm, H. (1983). Sectorized psychiatry: a methodological study of the effects of reorganization on patients treated at a mental hospital. *Acta Psychiatrica Scandinavica Supplementum*, 304.

Malt, U.F., Bech, P., Dencker, S.J., *et al.* (1990). Skalaer for diagnostikk og sykdomsgradering ved psykiatriska tillstander. II. Udvalg av skalaer. *Nordic Journal of Psychiatry*, **44**(2), 103–238.

McLachlan, G. (1974). The pursuit of research objectives. In *Positions, Movements and Directions in Health Services Research*, ed. G. McLachlan, pp. 148–58. London: Oxford University Press.

National Institute of Mental Health (NIMH) (1977). *Psychiatric Services and the Changing Institutional Scene*, 1950–1975. DHEW Publication no. 77–433. Washington, DC: US Government Printing Office.

Office of Technology Assessment (OTA) (1988). *The Quality of Medical Care: Information for Consumers*. Washington, DC: Congress of the United States.

Rosenblatt, A. & Mayer, J.E. (1974). The recividism of mental patients: a review of past studies. *American Journal of Orthopsychiatry*, **44**, 697–706.

Ruggeri, M. & Dall'agnola, R. (1993). The development and use of the Verona expectations for care scale (VECS) and the Verona service satisfaction scale (VSSS) for measuring expectations and satisfaction with community based psychiatric services in patients, relatives and professionals. *Psychological Medicine*, **23**, 511–23.

Stefansson, C.G. (1985). *A Case Register as a Tool for Studies in Sectorised Psychiatry*. Doctoral thesis, Karolinska Institute, Department of Social Medicine, Stockholm.

Sytema, S., Giel, R. & ten Horn, G.H.M.M. (1989). Patterns of care in the field of mental health: conceptual definitions and research methods. *Acta Psychiatrica Scandinavica*, **79**, 1–10.

Thompson, C. (ed.) (1989). *The Instruments of Psychiatric Research*. New York: Wiley.

Thornicroft, G., Gooch, C., O'Driscoll, C. & Reda, S. (1993). The TAPS project. IX. The reliability of the patient questionnaire. *British Journal of Psychiatry*, **162** (Supplement 19), 25–9.

Tischler, G.L., Henisz, J., Myers, J.K., *et al.* (1972). Catchmenting and the use of mental health services. *Archives of General Psychiatry*, **27**, 389–92.

Turner, A.J. (1979). Readmisson rates to community mental health centers as a measure of programme effectiveness. *Evaluation and the Health Professions*, **1**(5), 20–31.

Tyrer, P., Turner, R. & Johnsson, A. (1989). Integrated hospital and community psychiatric services and use of inpatient beds. *British Medical Journal*, **299**, 298–300.

Weissman, M.M., Sholomskas, D. & John, K. (1981). The assessment of social adjustment: an update. *Archives of General Psychiatry*, **38**, 1250–8.

Wetzler, S. (ed.) (1989). *Measuring Mental Illness: Psychometric Assessment For Clinicians*. Washington, DC: American Psychiatric Press.

Wing, J.K. (1990). Meeting the needs of people with psychiatric disorders. *Social Psychiatry and Psychiatric Epidemiology*, **25**, 2–8.

Zohar, M., Hadaz, Z. & Modan, B. (1987). Factors affecting the decision to admit mental patients in a community hospital. *Journal of Nervous and Mental Disease*, **175**, 301–5.

13

Dynamic analysis of patterns of care

SJOERD SYTEMA AND TINEKE OLDEHINKEL

Introduction

For a few decades now, the development in mental health care has been guided by two main principles, which are based on humanitarian as well as financial factors. The first principle is that patients should be kept and treated in the community as much as possible. The second is that 'continuity of care' should be provided as a flexible response to variations in need of care in a patient career. The realisation of these goals necessitates restructuring of mental health care, in which three processes can be distinguished: *deinstitutionalisation* (decreasing the number of beds in mental hospitals, increasing day- and outpatient care); *sectorisation* (the establishment of mental health regions) and *integration* of in-, day- and outpatient services.

To evaluate these processes properly we should take into account that:

1 the whole system of mental health care should be studied and not just specific programmes or new facilities, because changes in one part of the system will often affect others;
2 to evaluate the development of the mental health care system long-term longitudinal studies are needed, because these processes evolve very slowly; and
3 the functioning of mental health care is reflected in patterns of service utilisation. This is the care that has come to function within a given period of time.

Ultimately, planning is directed towards altering these patterns. Therefore, we can evaluate restructuring processes aimed at reaching certain goals by studying patterns of service utilisation. In order to obtain unbiased data about service utilisation the use of a psychiatric case register is indispensable. Until now, each patient's career in care tends to be described in register studies in terms of one summary statistic (Sytema *et al.*, 1989). Yet, a patient's career in modern mental health care is a dynamic process in which several 'transitions' to and from various types of care may occur. Moreover, new statistical techniques, known as hazard models, have become available allowing the study of 'change' in patients' careers. In this chapter we will outline a simple approach to a dynamic analysis of patterns of care. First the basic concepts will be described, then the Cox's proportional hazards model will be introduced, and finally an example, using the data of a cohort of schizophrenic patients, will be given. In the Appendix the reader will find an example of how to organise the data.

Patterns of care: from classification to dynamic model

Basically, a pattern of care is a record of consecutive contacts with mental health facilities during a fixed follow-up period. But in order to obtain relevant information, variables have to be constructed based on these data. Usually, a distinction is made between three *types of contact*: outpatient; day-care or partial day-care; and admission to an inpatient facility. It is very important to be clear about which contacts are included in each type. For example, sheltered housing may be assigned to semimural or day-care, but also to inpatient care.

A second important concept is the *episode*. This can be defined as a continuous series of contacts. Some researchers restrict the definition to a continuous series of the same type of contacts (Tricot, 1986). The length of an episode is determined by the point at which there is a break in continuity. The existence of a break can be designated by the formal termination of a series of treatments or by establishing a criterion for the maximum number of days intervening between two contacts. If this criterion is exceeded, then the episode is considered to have come to an end. The latter criterion might be different for different types of care (for example: 90 days for outpatient care; 8 days for day-patient care).

One way to put order in all individual patterns of care is to classify them into a limited number of categories. This is not an easy task, because a number of dimensions are involved.

Patterns can be grouped according to:

1 the setting of the treatment (in-, day- or outpatient);
2 the intensity of the treatment (i.e. the number of contacts or inpatient days);
3 the duration of the treatment.

It very much depends on the concepts of interest or the aim of the study which dimensions should be included in the classification and which classes should be distinguished. Various methods have been applied, which have been critically reviewed elsewhere (Sytema *et al.*, 1989).

Although classifications are intuitively appealing and useful for many purposes, they can be denoted 'static' because processes of change within patient careers remain unstudied. To take into account these change processes, one has to apply 'dynamic' models, which will be described in the following sections.

Key concepts in dynamic models

Dynamic models require information about the *timing* of events. An *event* is a transition from one state to another. A *state* in our case is the type of care a patient is consuming at some point in time. The *state-space* is the classification of states distinguished: for example, the in-, day- and outpatient state. An episode is the duration of a state. A risk set is the number of patients at risk of event occurrence at each point in time.

Tuma & Hannan (1984) distinguish between four observation plans providing information about the timing of events. With increasing precision, this information is available in:

• panel data: the state of a patient at a number of timepoints.
• event count data: the number of events during an observation period.
• event sequence data: the sequence of different types of events during an observation period.
• event history data: the sequence of different types of events as well as their exact timing during an observation period.

Only in event history data is the exact timing of events known, allowing the use of survival analysis. For this reason survival methods are often denoted as event history analysis. Case-register data allow the construction of event histories.

An important concept traditional methods are not able to deal with is *censoring*. This means that we witness the starting event but fail to witness the terminating event. One main reason for this is that the observation period ends while the patient is still occupying a state. For example, the patient may still be in hospital when the observation period ends. Therefore the duration of a censored episode is unknown. As a consequence, it is impossible to calculate the mean duration of episodes when there are censored observations and therefore traditional methods (linear regression, ANOVA, etc.), based on the mean of a dependent variable, can not be used unless the censored observations are removed.

Now let us consider the basic statistical concepts of event history analysis. For simplicity's sake, the one-episode situation (with given initial and final state) without covariates is regarded here. Broadly speaking, models including covariates, repeated episodes and/or competing risks are merely extensions of this simple model; many of the principles developed for the one-episode case may be applied to more complex situations as well.

The duration of the episode is represented by the random variable T, which can be any number equal to or greater than zero. Any specific value for the variable T is denoted by t. The probability that an individual remains in the state (survives) until time t is expressed by the *survival function*, $S(t)$. In mathematical notation:

$$S(t) = P(T \geqslant t)$$

Another important concept in event history analysis is the *hazard rate* or hazard function, $\lambda(t)$, defined as:

$$\lambda(t) = \lim_{\Delta t \to 0} \frac{P(t \leqslant T < t + \Delta t / T \geqslant t)}{\Delta t}$$

Hazard rates, also called transition or mortality rates, are difficult to explain in practical terms. It is important to realise that they are not probabilities: although hazard rates are always non-negative, they can take values greater than 1. For small Δt, $\lambda(t) \times \Delta t$ can be interpreted as an approximation of the conditional probability $P(t \leqslant T < t + \Delta t \,|\, T \geqslant t)$, which is the probability that the event (i.e. the transition to the destination state) takes place in the time interval

$[t, t + \Delta t]$, given that the individual 'survived' until time t. The survival and hazard function can be derived from each other.

Goals of the analyses usually are to estimate, interpret and compare survival and/or hazard functions (distributional approach), and to assess the relationship of explanatory variables (covariates) to the duration of the episode (regression approach). At present, most attention is focused on regression models in which the occurrence of an event depends on a linear function of explanatory variables.

Cox's proportional hazards regression model

Until now, we have discussed 'some' hazard rate, $\lambda(t)$, and 'some' survival function, $S(t)$. Usually, some kind of mathematical modelling of these functions is required or desirable. To specify the actual functions, one can choose from a variety of models, each with its own characteristics, advantages and drawbacks. One of the most famous parametric specifications is the exponential model, which defines the hazard rate to be constant over time. A more complex parametric model is the Weibull model, which is quite flexible and adaptable to a variety of situations. In this chapter, however, we will discuss a so-called semi-parametric approach: Cox's proportional hazards regression model. This model is called semi-parametric because the actual form of the hazard function (and thus the actual form of the survival function) remains unspecified. In other words, the effect of covariates can be established without knowing the formula of the 'baseline' hazard function $\lambda_0(t)$. The Cox regression model is very popular. One of the reasons for this is that, even though the baseline hazard is not specified, fairly good estimates of regression coefficients can be obtained for a variety of data. Hence, when one is in doubt about the goodness of fit of a parametric model, the Cox model is a 'safe' alternative which in a majority of cases will give sufficiently reliable results.

The Cox proportional hazards model is usually written in terms of the formula:

$$\lambda(t \mid X) = \lambda_0(t) e^{\sum_{i=1}^{b} \beta_i X_i}$$

In this formula, X denotes a collection of covariates ($X = X_1, X_2, \ldots, X_p$), and the β_i values are the corresponding regression coefficients.

$\lambda_0(t)$ is the arbitrary, unspecified baseline hazard rate, which depends on time but not on the covariates. On the other hand, the exponential expression e to the sum of $\beta_i X_i$ involves the covariates but not the time t. Considering the quotient (*hazard ratio*) of two individuals with the respective covariates X_1 and X_2, i.e.

$$\frac{\lambda(t\,|\,X_1)}{\lambda(t\,|\,X_2)}$$

we can see that it is not dependent on time. Because of this characteristic the model is called proportional. Dividing a regression coefficient by its standard error gives the Wald test statistic, the square of which can be compared with a chi-square distribution with one degree of freedom to obtain a p value.

Cox regression: example

Above we described the single-state single-episode case. However, a pattern of care is a multi-state multi-episode data record. It is multi-state because we distinguish between (at least) three states (in-, day- and outpatient) and it is multi-episode because each of these states is repeatable in a patient career. The following procedure may be adopted to prepare the data for the multi-state multi-episode analyses (see Allison 1984, p. 59):

1. break down each individual's event history into a set of intervals (episodes) between events;
2. group episodes with equal origin state and destination state;
3. estimate models for each type of episode.

In the Appendix, an example is given of an event history data set organised in this way.

For this example, patterns of care have been analysed of a cohort of 52 schizophrenic patients, who were first registered in the case register with an admission in 1987. The follow-up period was 2 years starting with the date of the first admission. In total, the patients of the cohort were admitted 82 times during the 2-year observation period and there were 50 outpatient episodes. Inpatient episodes included admissions to mental hospitals as well as to psychiatric units in general hopsitals. Outpatient episodes included contacts with polyclinics and with the Regional Institute for Outpatient Care (denoted as

Table 13.1. *Calculation of survival and hazard function of the first admission of 52 schizophrenic patients at fixed intervals of 14 days. The terminating event is discharge (= 'failure' in survival terms)*

Time interval (days after first contact)	At risk	Failure	Survival function	Hazard
14	52	10	0.808	0.192
28	42	4	0.731	0.095
42	38	3	0.673	0.079
56	35	5	0.577	0.143
70	30	3	0.519	0.100
84	27	5	0.423	0.185

RIAGG). Day-patient episodes were neglected, because there were only a few.

The analyses were performed using the computer program EGRET, a package for epidemiological computing, which is particularly suitable for several kinds of event history analyses.

A more practical insight into the concepts at risk, survival and hazard function may be obtained from Table 13.1, which shows the process of discharge ('failure' in survival terms) of the first admission at six time intervals. The survival function is calculated by dividing the number still in hospital at the end of each interval by those at risk at the beginning of the process (all 52 patients). In the first interval 10 patients 'failed' (because of a discharge from hospital), giving a survival function of 42/52 = 0.808. During the second interval 4 more patients 'failed', so the survival function at the end of this interval was 38/52 = 0.731. Hence, the survival function is simply the proportion of patients still in hospital at each point in time. The hazard function is calculated by dividing those who 'failed' during an interval by those at risk at the beginning of that interval. Thus, the hazard function at the end of the first interval is 10/52 = 0.192 and after the second interval is 4/42 = 0.095. Hence, the hazard function is an expression of the speed of discharge in time.

To obtain a first insight into the data, the Kaplan–Meier (K–M) model may be applied. This model estimates the survival function, allowing the use of one or more stratification variables. In Figs. 13.1 and 13.2, the K–M estimates are displayed for the 82 inpatient episodes.

Fig. 13.1 shows the survival curves for four strata: first admission to a mental hospital (MH), first admission to a psychiatric ward (PW) of

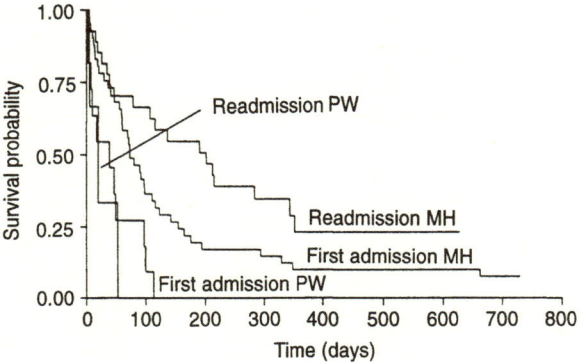

Fig. 13.1. Survival curves stratified on type of admission (inpatient episodes, n = 82). PW, psychiatric ward of a general hospital; MH, mental hospital.

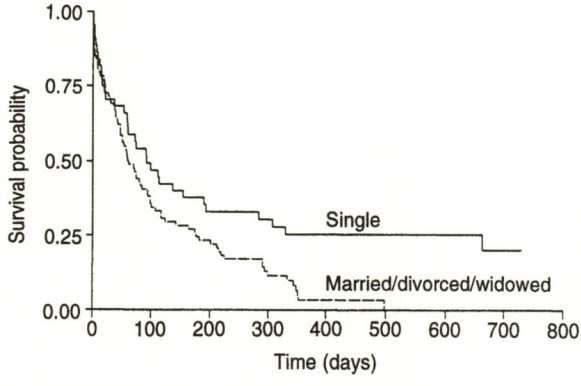

Fig. 13.2. Survival curves stratified on marital status (all episodes, n = 132).

a general hospital, readmission in a MH, and readmission in a PW. The survival functions simply represent the proportion of patients still admitted at a certain point in time, starting with the day of admission. The figure shows that all patients admitted in psychiatric wards of general hospitals (PW) were discharged within 120 days of admission. Inpatient episodes in mental hospitals (MH) tended to last much longer. This is not surprising, because psychiatric wards in general hospitals only provide short-term admissions. Furthermore, the graph seems to indicate that readmission episodes generally last longer than first admission episodes. Fig. 13.2 shows the survival curves for the unmarried and for the married, divorced or widowed patients. Patients belonging to the latter category tended to have shorter episodes of inpatient care.

Stratification has a number of drawbacks. First, in order to have a reasonable number of observations in each stratum, only a limited number of strata can be used simultaneously. Moreover, only categorical variables can be used as stratification variables. Therefore, when more sophisticated analyses are required, it is often expedient to apply regression models.

In our example, we used Cox's proportional hazards model to examine whether the hazard rates (and accordingly the survival curves) differed significantly between certain groups of patients, as defined by a number of explanatory variables.

The results of the analyses are presented in Tables 13.2 and 13.3. One of the outcomes of Cox's regression is the *hazard ratio*. The hazard ratio of a certain category should be interpreted as the hazard rate of that category divided by the hazard rate of the so-called baseline category, which in EGRET is the first category of a variable. A hazard ratio of 1 means that the hazard rates of both categories are equal. Table 13.2 reveals that the hazard ratio of readmissions related to first admissions (the baseline category) in mental hospital episodes is 0.44. The hazard function may here be described as the speed of discharge in time. Hence, the speed of discharge of readmissions is lower and therefore the duration of readmissions tends to be longer than the duration of first admissions. In psychiatric wards the reverse seems to be true, although the effect is not statistically significant. We have seen this already in the survival functions plotted in Fig. 13.1. The duration of outpatient episodes after readmissions and after first admissions are almost equal (hazard ratio 1.06). An outpatient episode before a mental hospital admission seems to reduce the length of stay (hazard ratio 1.27), but the difference is not statistically significant. Mental hospital episodes and outpatient episodes tend to be longer for females because the hazard ratio is less than 1, but again the difference was not significant. The hazard ratio of the married/ divorced/widowed compared with the single patients (the baseline category) in mental hospital episodes exceeded 3 (significant). Hence for the latter category the duration of these episodes tends to be longer. From this it may be concluded that those who are or have been married have a better prognosis. Marriage might be an indicator of social functioning (the ability to attract and bind a partner). Then a higher level of social functioning would explain the

Table 13.2. *Estimated hazard ratios according to Cox's regression for three types of episodes consumed by a cohort of 52 schizophrenic patients during a 2-year observation period*

| | | Type of episode (hazard ratio) | | |
| | | Mental Hospital ($n = 68$) | Psychiatric ward ($n = 14$) | Outpatient episode ($n = 50$) |
Variable	Value			
Admission	'Readmission'	0.44*	1.33	1.06[a]
Previous outpatient episode	'Yes'	1.27	—	1.04
Gender	'Female'	0.69	1.54	0.60
Age		0.98*	1.03	0.99
Marital status	'Mar–div–wid'[b]	3.10*	—	2.02

[a]This is the hazard ratio of outpatient episodes after a readmission versus after a first admission
[b]'Mar–div–wid', married–divorced–widowed.
*$p < 0.05$

difference. The final variable in the model – age – is a continuous variable. It may seem strange that the hazard ratio is so close to 1 but still significant in mental hospital episodes. However, hazard ratios of continuous variables have to be interpreted differently from those of categorical variables. The hazard ratio of 0.98 means that the chance of discharge for those at risk in a certain time interval is 0.98 times the chance of someone who is only 1 year younger. In other words, the duration of episodes in mental hospital increases with age.

Another outcome of Cox's regression is the *likelihood ratio statistic*. The likelihood ratio statistic is the difference between the likelihood (or deviance) of two nested models with the number of parameters which are included in one but not in the other model as the degrees of freedom. This statistic has approximately a chi-square distribution. Its use will be illustrated below in testing the proportionality assumption of parameters in a Cox model.

Recall that the hazard ratio expresses the difference between the hazard functions of two categories of a variable, one of which is the baseline category. The Cox model assumes that this ratio is constant in time (the proportionality assumption). In other words, this assumption implies that the hazard ratio is independent of time. Model 1 in Table 13.3 includes the variables which are significantly

Table 13.3. *Testing the proportionality assumption of the variable 'admission' in a Cox model of mental hospital episodes (n = 68) consumed by a cohort of 52 schizophrenic patients during a 2-year observation period*

| Variable | Value | Hazard ratio | |
		Model 1	Model 2
Type of admission	'Readmission'	0.49*	0.47*
Age		0.98*	0.98*
Marital status	'Mar–div–wid'	2.43*	2.47*
Readmission	*Log(time)		0.88

*$p < 0.05$.
Likelihood ratio (model 2/model 1) on 1 degree of freedom: 0.331, $p = 0.565$.

related to the duration of mental hospital episodes. In model 2 we test whether the hazard ratio of 'type of admission' (readmission versus first admission) is proportional by including the interaction term of the latter variable with a function of time (here the logarithmic transformation of time) in the model. If the inclusion of this interaction term significantly improves the model, we have to conclude that the hazard ratio is not independent of time. The likelihood ratio of models 1 and 2 is 0.331 with 1 degree of freedom, giving a p- value of 0.565 (this can be found in a chi-square table). As this is far from significant, it can be concluded that the proportionality assumption of 'type of admission' is not violated. Moreover, the hazard ratio of the interaction term is not significant, which leads to the same conclusion. The same procedure may be applied to test this assumption for the other variables in the model. In case the assumption does not hold, the interaction term needs to be included in the model.

Conclusion

In the evaluation of the functioning of the mental health care system, the study of patient careers is of utmost importance. Objectives in the planning process of the mental health system are directed towards changing patterns of service utilisation. Therefore, these patterns have to be studied in such a way that the effectiveness of the planning goals can be evaluated properly. Elsewhere in this volume Eaton stresses the importance of the concept *continuity of care* as an outcome measure in health system research. If we define this concept as 'the delivery of the type of care according to the need of care of patients continuously in time', what pattern of care would we expect to see? Assuming that the need of care of most patients will vary in time between inpatient, day- and outpatient care and no care, we expect to see a dynamic pattern of episodes of care, in which most, if not all, types of care are included in the sequence of episodes. In this sense *flexibility of care*, expressed in the number of transitions between types of care, would be an indicator of continuity of care. Hence, dynamic methods seem to be particularly useful in mental health system research related to this concept.

Until now the research into patterns of care has been dominated by descriptive and 'static' methods. Most studies used an *a priori* classification of patterns of care. The consequence of this technique is that the available information on a patient is reduced to one score (for example, high user). However, in reality a pattern of care is a dynamic process in which transitions between various states may take place. In order to make full use of the quality of the data, dynamic models have to be applied. Nevertheless, until now this approach has seldom been found in this research area. One of the reasons might be that many researchers do not know how to use methods of dynamic analysis. The structure of the data is certainly rather complex, and statistical programs that can handle censored data are not yet universally well known.

In this chapter, we briefly discussed some strategies to deal with event history data. From a broad range of continuous-time event history analysis techniques, we chose Cox's proportional hazards model to be treated in more detail, because of its popularity and relative simplicity. We by no means claim to have been exhaustive; this chapter is meant merely to serve as an introduction and illustration of these techniques. The interested reader is referred to statistical textbooks for further details (e.g. Tuma & Hannan, 1984; Allison, 1984; Blossfeld *et al.*, 1989; Yamaguchi, 1991).

Appendix. An example of a pattern of care

In Fig. 13.3 an example is given of an event history which has been broken down into episodes. Note that the definition of Tricot (1986)

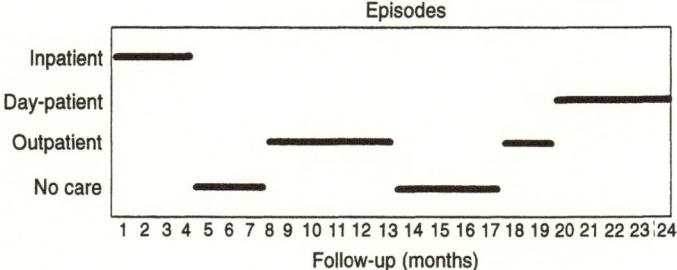

Fig. 13.3. *An event history of episodes of care during 24 months of follow-up.*

was used to define the episodes. The pattern starts with an admission. This episode ends with a discharge, which is the beginning of the second episode ending with an outpatient contact. Recall that an outpatient episode ends when the interval to the next contact exceeds 90 days. Therefore the outpatient contacts after the eighteenth month are not included in this episode. The last episode is censored, because the patient was still in day-care at the end of the follow-up period of 24 months.

The data set prepared to analyse patterns of care with Cox's regression may be organised as in Table 13.4 (see Blossfeld *et al.*, 1989, p. 111).

Each episode is fully characterised by the state at the beginning of the episode and the state at the end of the episode. Duration is the dependent variable in event history analysis. The censoring variable indicates either that the episode was terminated because of a transition to a new state (censoring = 1) or that the observation period ended before the endpoint of the episode (censoring = 0).

A number of things might complicate the procedure described above. For example, a patient might be in day- and outpatient care at the same time. One solution would be to assume a hierarchy in which inpatient care is at the highest level and outpatient care at the lowest. When a patient is in two states at the same time, the higher level counts. Or in other words, as long as a patient is in a state, states ranked lower in the hierarchy are neglected. Another solution would be to allow for overlapping states. In the example given above, this patient would have two episodes, a day- and an outpatient episode, consumed (partly) in the same time-frame. Finally, one might create a new state: day-patient care including outpatient contacts.

Table 13.4. *An event history data set of episodes of care*

Case no.	Episode	Start time (days)	End time (days)	Duration (days)	State at start	State at end	Censoring[a]	Explanatory variables Gender	Age
1	1	0	138	138	3	0	1	1	28
1	2	138	230	92	0	1	1	1	28
1	3	230	411	181	1	0	1	1	28
1	4	411	564	153	0	1	1	1	28
1	5	564	610	46	1	2	1	1	28
1	6	610	730	120	2	2	0	1	28

[a] 1, no; 0, yes.

References

Allison, P.D. (1984). *Event History Analysis: Regression for Longitudinal Event Data*. London: Sage Publications.

Blossfeld, H.P., Hamerle, A. & Mayer, K.U. (1989). *Event History Analysis: Statistical Theory and Application in the Social Sciences*. New Jersey: Lawrence Erlbaum Associates.

Sytema, S., Giel, R. & ten Horn, G.H.M.M. (1989). Patterns of care in the field of mental health. *Acta Psychiatrica Scandinavica*, **79**, 1–10.

Tricot, L. (1986). An example of the standardization of terminology: defining episodes of care. In: *Psychiatric Case Registers in Public Health*, ed. G.H.M.M. ten Horn, R. Giel, W.H. Gulbinat & J.H. Henderson. Amsterdam: Elsevier.

Tuma, N.B. & Hannan, M.T. (1984). *Social Dynamics: Models and Methods*. New York: Academic Press.

Yamaguchi, K. (1991). *Event History Analysis*. Newbury Park, CA: Sage Publications.

14

Social indicators of outcome at the system level

PETER HUXLEY

Introduction

This chapter considers the evaluation of service systems, with particular reference to non-health outcomes. The nature of the mental health service system is considered and system-level analysis is subdivided into idiographic, normative and legislative types. Examples of measures developed for this kind of evaluation are given. The mental health service system interacts with many other social systems, and illustrations are given from the interfaces with work, criminal justice, housing and health care systems, together with some suggested measures.

The evaluation of system-level outcomes involves the assessment of what Rossi & Freeman (1993) call 'fully saturated' services which are intended to provide for the whole population. In this situation there are limited opportunities to undertake evaluative comparisons, because there is no other provider with which to compare results. We shall return to the question of what constitutes a mental health service system below, but if we assume for a moment that the system provides services to the whole population but in a predetermined geographical location, then we do have the possibility of comparing different service systems. The geographical location, or unit of analysis, can be a sector within a district (Thornicroft, Knudsen, this volume), whole districts (Huxley, 1993), or even whole countries. Cultural issues arise in connection with the last form of analysis, but recent developments in standardised assessments have made meaningful interstate and international comparisons possible (see for example Warner & Huxley, 1993). Finally, and this will also be discussed in more detail later, it is possible to examine changes within the same service system over time; this is known as the reflexive control technique, and requires regular repeated measures over a long time period in order to produce credible results (Rossi & Freeman, 1993). The major comparative study of service systems in the United States, the Robert Wood Johnson initiative, has recently begun to produce findings based upon results from the major study sites, and the comparison service in Colorado Springs (H. Goldman, personal communication). An adapted version of the key informant approach to the evaluation of service systems has been used in North Wales, permitting an attempt at cross-cultural comparisons using similar methodologies (W. Barr, personal communication).

What is the mental health service system?

What do we mean by a mental health service system? I think that we need to distinguish between the total mental health system, which includes every form of statutory service, independent sector service and informal care, and the mental health service system, which is the mandated part. For the purpose of the present chapter we wish to confine examples to the formal services provided for psychiatric patients and funded especially for them. In this sense we neglect all other 'mental health' provision, whether this be informal care or care provided by non-mental health agencies such as voluntary organisations for non-psychiatric patients. This may seem arbitrary or unnecessary, but the quality of the information available to describe non-statutory services and audit their contribution is sadly lacking. The absence of systematic information is indeed unfortunate when one considers the research which shows that the burden of care falling on families and communities is substantial. Moreover, changes in the formal mental health services can have a major impact, for better or worse, upon this burden.

Examples of system-level analysis within the system or between mental health systems

Idiographic analysis

The idiographic approach involves comparison of the mental health service system with itself at different points in time, or with another mental health service system. Within-systems evaluations use outcome or output measures such as: patient flows; service locations; interventions offered; information provided; costs incurred; and staffing patterns. Patterns and flows (or pathways) refer to the number of patients coming into the system, the number leaving and the pattern of care over time of those who are treated. For instance, one can look at numbers assessed compared with numbers treated, and numbers who have to be reassessed within a particular period of time.

It is also possible to examine aspects of the efficiency of a service in terms of technical efficiency, and target efficiency. How do the cost–benefit or cost-effectiveness aspects of the service change over time, and to what extent does the service reach all those people in the community who are in most need? Gater and his colleagues (1993) were able to show that a community-based team consisting of a psychiatrist, social worker, community nurse and occupational therapist improved the efficiency of psychiatric care. The team operated in one of two comparable districts in South Manchester (UK). They continued to use hospital beds when required. The results of the comparison of the standard service and the service provided by the community team showed that there was a close association between the assessed needs of the patients and the amount of care expended on them in the index service. In the control service, based largely on a traditional District General Hospital service, there was no such association between assessed need and expended resources. There is increasing interest in the development of instruments to assess need, and there are now a number of such questionnaires in operation in service evaluations; the Camberwell Assessment of Need (CAN) is being extensively used.

A similar question would be: To what extent are patients users of multiple services and to what extent is multiple service use reduced by different types of engagement with the mental health service system? In a small study conducted in children's services in Boulder, Colorado (Huxley & Warner, 1993), a comparison group of untreated cases at high risk for child abuse were found to use more services than the index group which received the innovative specialist early intervention service. Both groups were using a similar range and frequency of services at inception. The two groups differed significantly in the use they made of emergency room services in the study period ($p < 0.01$), and the comparison group presented the only cases of traumatic injury ($p = 0.07$), as well as more cases of vomiting, dehydration and diarrhoea ($p < 0.01$).

Within-system offsets refers to the impact on another part of the mental health service system when one of the existing components is altered, removed or added. The opening of a new community mental health facility or service will inevitably have an impact on other parts of the service. In the United Kingdom, assessment and care planning (the care programme approach: CPA) has been introduced for all patients of the psychiatric services. Pierides and his colleagues (1993) have been able to assess aspects of the introduction of the CPA in terms of its effects on service provision. The preliminary findings suggest that longer initial in-hospital assessment may be related to shorter stay subsequently. An index group of admitted patients who were subject to the CPA remained in hospital longer for their initial assessment (56% stayed longer than 28 days) compared with controls (46% stayed longer than 28 days). However, the length of stay on subsequent admissions was reduced in the index group but increased or remained the same in the controls.

At the system level continuity of care as an outcome variable is an important consideration. Eaton (1993) has argued that this is the most important strategic measure of outcome because volume of service is too crude, hospitalisation only appropriate for those likely to be hospitalised, and satisfaction inappropriate for involuntary patients. He argues strongly that in order to judge the continuity of care in the mental health service system it is critical to have record linkage which covers a large geographical area, extends for several years, and covers at least 70% of the population and service events. He advocates the use of graphical presentations of treatment history. Records of this sort could facilitate our understanding of system features such as the frequency of reassessments. The impact of organisational changes and changes in staffing levels and patterns would be more easily evaluated if this type of continuity information were available on all patients in the system.

Normative analysis

In the National Health Service (NHS) in the United Kingdom in the early 1990s there was an increase in the requirements for health services to provide information about their performance and a number of these requirements were formally incorporated into standards. The service might establish standards for itself to achieve, and these might be used as assessments of the performance of the service system. For example, Tameside and Glossop Health Authority's

(1993) care programme approach documentation includes criteria for the review of performance in care planning (p. 96). All professionals involved in the client's care are to be sent a copy of the care plan, and the plan is to be reviewed at least annually. These requirements can be translated into service standards by recording the percentage of completed care plans and reviews which are sent out to the relevant professionals, and the percentage of reviews completed within the specified time periods. The service managers might alter the requirements, or specify that higher levels of achievement are to be attained.

However, as well as making judgements about somewhat arbitrarily defined standards, it is sometimes useful to compare the extent of activity in the mental health system with characteristics of the population in which that service operates. For instance, figures show that the proportion of assessments for action under the Mental Health Act 1983 differs by local authority in the United Kingdom. For some services the proportion of people from ethnic minority groups, and the proportion who are elderly, are identical in the population and the service assessments. In others there is a distinct tendency for a greater proportion to be assessed than the proportion in the population. Difficulties with this type of analysis are: what the larger proportion means and at what magnitude the difference assumes importance; and whether the proportion in the assessments reflects the proportion in the population anyway – we know that there is an increase in certain forms of illness in old age, and an associated increase in the amount and cost of health care delivered, for instance. However, one then has to explain why some services assess a smaller proportion of elderly people than exists in the population. It is probable that socio-demographic and socio-economic differences explain some of these findings, since, as we have reported elsewhere (Huxley & Kerfoot, 1993), requests for mental health assessments vary according to the Jarman index of social deprivation. Districts with more social deprivation produced a greater number of requests for assessment that those with less social deprivation. Jarman *et al.* (1992) have advocated the use of the index as a straightforward predictor of the level of admissions in different districts.

Legislative analysis

One could argue that governmental guidelines on service standards should be included under normative analysis. However, they are included here because they are normative standards in formal governmental guidance and so are perhaps more like legislative requirements. As time goes on these requirements may become more and more specific, and may ultimately be the subject of legislation. At the moment, there are ten rights under the Patient's Charter (including access to records, clear explanation of treatment, and not waiting for admission for more than 2 years), nine national standards (including maximum waiting times in outpatient clinics, and named nurses for each patient), and five prescribed local standards (including waiting times for first appointments, and waiting time for NHS transport after treatment) (Ham & Haywood, 1993). One imagines that it will not be long before league tables are prepared showing the performance of different service systems. The problem with this type of service performance measure is that, taken in isolation, they tell us nothing about the outcome for the service users. In some cases a longer waiting time might facilitate the resolution of a problem by the user's own resources, or those of his or her social network, and this outcome might be preferable to the user and the service. Without considerable investment in understanding the relationship between these service indicators and actual outcomes, it would be unwise to assume that all is well when particular targets are achieved.

It is possible to compare different service systems in respect of their use of sections of the mental health legislation. If, for the moment, one assumes that it is preferable to conduct a mental health assessment without resort to an emergency admission, and, at the same time one recognises that there will always be a small number of very urgent admissions, one indicator of the outcome of the service is the proportion of emergency to other forms of admission undertaken. In the United Kingdom Section 4 of the Mental Health Act 1983, is used in an emergency and requires the signature of only one medical practitioner. Section 2 requires two practitioners and is therefore usually regarded as preferable. The proportion of Section 4 admissions fell between 1990 and 1991 and the reduction was sustained into 1992. An interesting feature of this figure is that it is the Section 3 admissions (for treatment rather than observation) which have increased. Several explanations can be proffered, including a general increase among professional staff of the tendency to recognise the right to treatment when it is needed. There is also the tendency for more patients to be readmitted, and therefore more are already known to the services; it is possible that it is easier for staff to arrive at a firm decision about the need for treatment rather than for

observation when they have come to know the patient well. A simple
analysis of the figures will tell us whether the increase in the use of
Section 3 in 1992 occurs in respect of known patients. In order to
undertake this kind of analysis one needs a routinely applied measure
of activity under the mental health legislation. There is no national
requirement for these data to be collected in this way in the United
Kingdom.

Finally, when supervised discharge into the community is enacted
in legislation, then services can be compared in terms of their use of
these powers, the balance of use of community and hospital powers,
how this changes over time, and the relative success of the use of the
powers in different settings.

System-level analysis between mental health and other social systems

We can now turn our attention to the interface between the mental
health services system and other social systems. Society consists of a
number of interacting and interrelated social systems. The mental
health service system is one such system, and it interacts with a
number of other systems. One way of describing and then discussing
the interface between social systems is to use the life domains widely
used in quality of life profiles. This gives a reasonable coverage of
important systems and permits us to limit the discussion to those most
central to the lives of seriously mentally ill people.

The mental health service system is often involved with the other
social systems as people make transitions into or out of them. The
matrix in Table 14.1 illustrates some of the points of contact where
transitions (or life-events) occur, and where there may already be a
formal association between the mental health service system and the
other social systems.

The social systems in Table 14.1 can be divided into two groups.
The first five (health, work/education, criminal justice, income
maintenance and housing/social care) are those which have specific
service systems provided by the state, and where, broadly speaking,
participation in the system is not really voluntary. The final four do
not involve the state in making service provision to the same extent
and involve a greater degree of choice and freedom to participate.
Mechanisms for participation in the latter group are, on the whole,

Table 14.1. *Transition points between social systems*

Social system	Entrances	Exits
Health	Consultation for illness	Discharge from care
Work and education	Beginning school, work or higher education	Redundancy; leaving school
Criminal justice	Criminal proceedings	Leaving prison
Income maintenance	Bankruptcy; poverty	Poverty trap
Social care and housing	Residential homes; community care	Leaving residential care
	Moving house	Homelessness
Religion	Baptism or equivalent	Leaving church
Leisure	Joining association	Withdrawal
Marital/family relations	Marriage	Divorce
Friendships/social relations	Developing networks	Breaking partnerships

informal rather than formal, although some involve formal and legal contracts of various sorts (e.g. marriage). It is possible to produce local or national norms in respect of the participative systems, but it is more difficult to use these in normative comparisons with patient samples. The reason is that although normative levels can be determined in the population it is not necessarily good for the individual's mental health to approximate normative behaviours. Social interaction is one example, and participation in religion is another. For some patients more social interaction with the wrong people can be damaging to their mental health, and in some extreme cases an individual's participation in a fundamentalist or extremist religious organisation might feed and be fed by their psychotic experiences. Extreme forms of social isolation are generally bad for one's mental health but for some psychotic patients, and some others with serious and long-lasting problems, the opportunity to choose to withdraw from social contacts may be an important aide to the maintenance of their mental health.

Examples of social systems outcomes and measures

All the information in the following examples comes from application of the Lancashire Quality of Life Profile (Oliver, 1991). The Profile

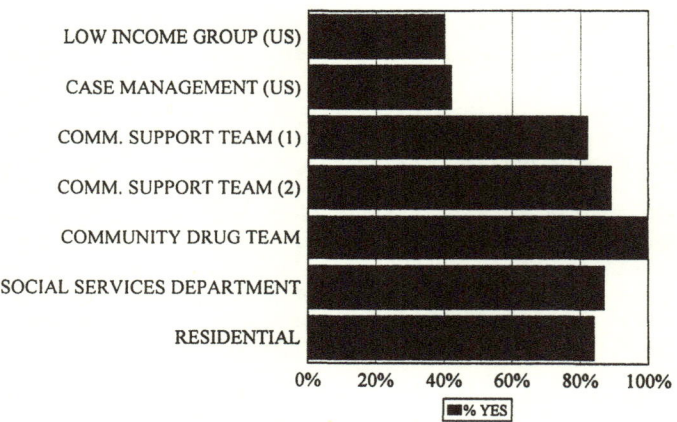

Fig. 14.1. Unemployment rates in different patient samples.

covers all of these major life domains, and is one of several instruments which are designed to assess quality of life (QOL). There is some debate about the content of QOL scales, with some people arguing that the concept is entirely subjective (Orley, 1994), while others argue that it includes personal characteristics and material circumstances (Oliver *et al.*, 1995). This debate is beyond the scope of the present chapter, but it is important to observe that if we had only subjective well-being data, few if any of the outcome assessments presented below would have been available to us.

Social systems outcomes

Work

Fig. 14.1 shows a comparison of the proportion of patients who are unemployed in different patient samples and a low income group from a study in the United States (Huxley & Warner, 1992). The low income group and case management group have similar levels of unemployment because the case management service utilised the sheltered workshops and clubhouse. In this sense the mental health system outcome approximated that of the low income group in that society. The community support teams, the social services group and the residential group are all provided by social care agencies rather than the mental health services. The community drug team is part of

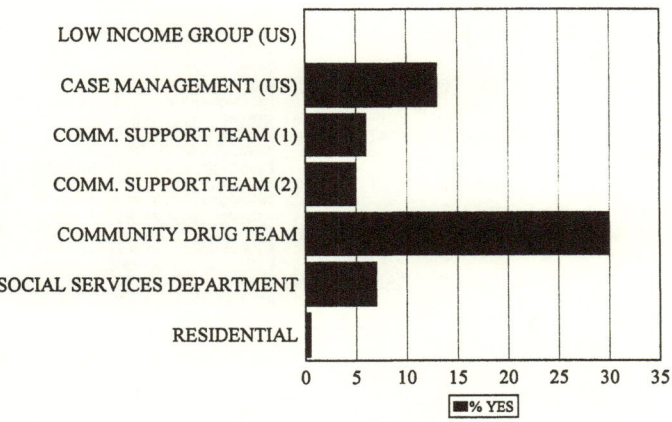

Fig. 14.2. Accusations of crime in different patient samples.

a mental health service provision. All their clients are unemployed, and 80% of the social care agency clients are too. In this respect the US case management service, working with similar if not more difficult clients, has a better outcome.

Criminal justice

Using the same samples as in the previous example we can see (Fig. 14.2) that the US low income group has no problems with the law, and that the community drug team have the most. Mentally ill people in residential care also have limited problems, while the three local authority samples approximate the rate in the community. So far as being a victim of crime is concerned (Fig. 14.3), the residential group are protected to a considerable extent, and the drug addicts have the most problems. The community support teams and the social services sample are again closer to UK national norms.

Social security

The service might aim to ensure that the patients receive their entitlements from the social security system. In Fig. 14.4 the findings are consistent in that the drug addicts have access to most resources, and the three local authority samples are receiving the same level of state benefit. In the two US samples the low income group are only marginally better off than the case management clients.

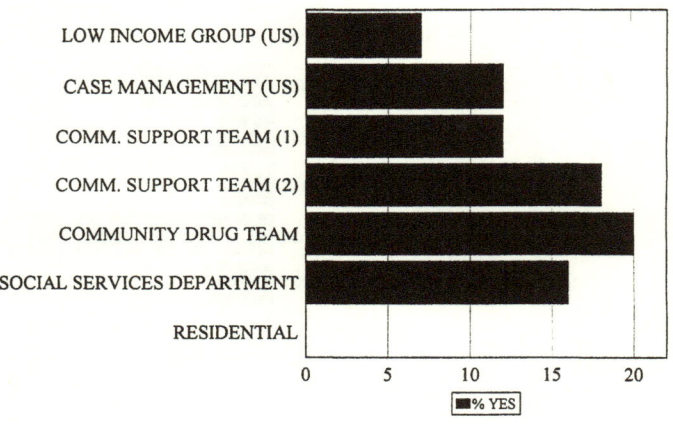

Fig. 14.3. Victims of crime in different patient samples.

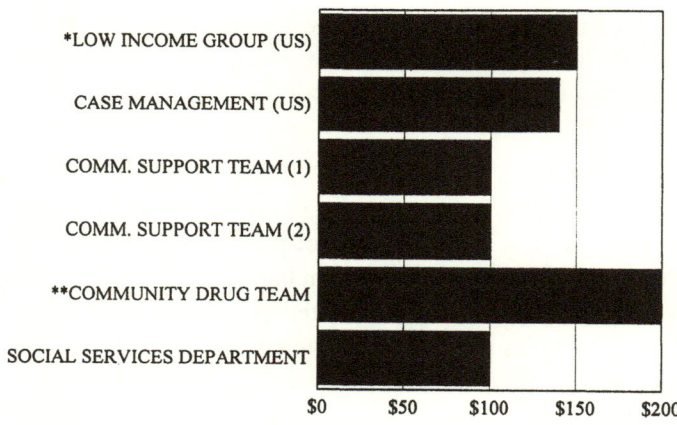

* LOW INCOME GROUP WITH OUTLIER = $175   ** OVER $330 PER WEEK

Fig. 14.4. Weekly income in different patient samples.

Living situation

A mental health service system might use as an outcome measure the extent to which clients who are homeless when they come to the service are successfully housed when they are discharged.

Fig. 14.5 shows samples of chronic patients living in the community in Yorkshire, Wales and Lancashire (UK). The Yorkshire sample

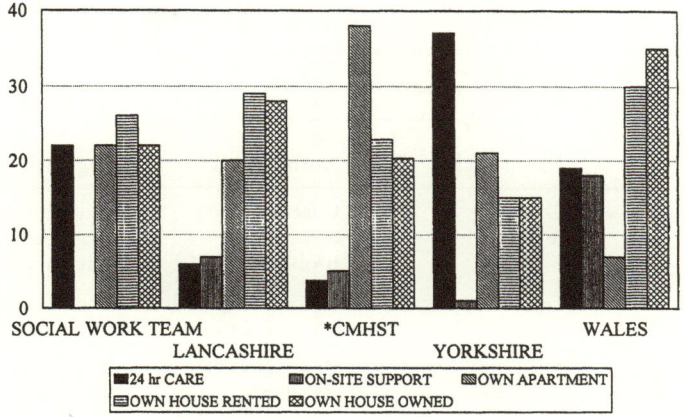

*Fig. 14.5. Living situations in different patient samples. *Community mental health support team.*

lives in accommodation with 24-hour care in almost 40% of cases, compared with less than 5% in the community support team sample. Many of the community support team clients live in their own apartments, suggesting either that they have adequate support to provide care out of hours, or that they are not such a disabled group as those being cared for by the social work teams. Over 60% of the Welsh sample live in their own house, which is partly a reflection of the local housing stock. The question of what constitutes appropriate living arrangements depends, of course upon the nature of the patient population and their individual needs. Services clearly need a range of types of accommodation, and patients may progress from needing more supervision to less, over time. A high frequency of unplanned changes of accommodation is not, generally, an indication of a good outcome. In a study of people with learning disability (MHSWRU, 1993) residents who were moved from home to home showed greater levels of anxiety and depression than those who were not moved. On the whole the moves were made for administrative reasons and not because of the clinical condition of the resident.

Health

Although this chapter is concerned with non-health outcomes it is worth reminding ourselves that the mental health service system interacts with the general health system. Some of the outcomes from the mental health system have cost implications for general health

Table 14.2. *Community services evaluation matrix*

Level of analysis	Type of evaluation/analysis		
	Idiographic	Normative	Legislative
Individual level	Compare interventions	Cases with comparable problems	Detention type; formal review; statutory aftercare
	Examples of outcome units for the individual level: clinical; social; QOL; satisfaction; due process		
Programme	Compare programmes for comparable groups	Programme standards	Proportion detained; proportion with plans and reviews
	Examples of outcome units for the programme level: aggregated individual (clinical, etc.); unit costs; vertical target efficiency; mandatory services provided		
System level	Compare service systems; within-system 'offsets'	Population norms; service standards	Mandatory requirements; mandatory standards
	Examples of outcome units for the system level: costs; volumes; throughput; patterns of utilisation; horizontal target efficiency; social indicators; unmet need; legal changes		

services. The failure to recognise mental health components when physical illnesses are presented can certainly affect outcomes, and prolong treatment unnecessarily (Goldberg & Huxley, 1992). There are many evaluation instruments available to assess physical and psychological aspects of health and these are presented elsewhere in this volume.

A framework for evaluation

This chapter has examined the use of outcome measures in mental health service evaluation. The matrix in Table 14.2 is presented in order to assist in understanding the nature and range of evaluation in this field. For comparative purposes the matrix includes the two other levels of analysis used in the remainder of the book; however, for the purpose of this chapter the system level is the focus. The matrix is presented by level and by type of evaluation analysis. There may be other (and perhaps more obvious) examples than the ones given, but these have been omitted in the interests of brevity and clarity.

Idiographic analysis involves comparing two separate mental health systems with one another, at national or more probably local levels, or comparing the same mental health service system at two or more points in time. 'Within-system offsets' refer to the evaluation of the same service system at more than one point in time (and so is a reflexive control technique) and the identification of the impact of changes within the system upon other parts of the system. The most obvious example is the effect on other parts of the service of a reduction in the number of psychiatric inpatient beds. The units of analysis tend to arise out of the concerns of service users and professionals providing the service; these are often couched in terms of ideas about what constitutes 'good practice'.

Normative analysis involves setting the service against some agreed normative standards, produced by professional bodies or district, regional or national bodies (but not governments). The units of analysis arise from population or census data, or from standards produced by the professional bodies or service organisations themselves.

Legislative analysis involves setting the service system against standards or requirements laid down by the legislation of the state or nation. The units of analysis arise from the legislation itself or the official publications such as circular or Codes of Practice (such as the Patient's Charter in the United Kingdom).

Conclusion

A framework has been offered for considering system-level outcome measurement in mental health service systems. This framework includes three levels (individual, programme and system levels) and three types of evaluation/analysis (idiographic, normative and legislative). Examples have been given in each area, and these do not necessarily represent a comprehensive range of possibilities, nor necessarily the most economic or efficient examples. There is growing interest, particularly in the United Kingdom, in establishing service standards, but the same caveat applies to these efforts; we are still not sure that the items selected are the best ones for mental health services, and may simply be focusing on the measurable rather than on the most important patient outcomes.

The mental health service system is one of a number of social systems which interact with one another. These social systems cover the main life domains used in the Lancashire Quality of Life Profile. Five of them – health, work/education, housing/social care, criminal justice and income maintenance – are also major areas of statutory service provision. On the whole, normative experiences for mentally ill people in these domains can be regarded as good system-level outcome indicators. It is possible to examine outcomes from the mental health service system which affect these other systems, and several examples have been given. The other four social systems – religion, family, social relations and leisure – while having formal aspects are more participative in nature. It is harder to assess the impact of the mental health service system in these areas because of their reciprocal relationship with mental health. Greater participation and less participation can both have positive and negative impacts on an individual's mental health. It is more difficult to identify normative behaviours in these areas which one can equivocally regard as good system-level outcome indicators.

Before closing, a word of caution. It is my view that system-level outcome indicators are just that: indicators. An evaluation of a service should use outcome measurements from individual and programme levels and not rely exclusively on system-level indicators. The main purpose of the mental health service system is to improve the lot of the person with mental illness, and that of his or her carer, not to demonstrate the superiority of one system of care over another in terms of variables which have no meaning or impact at the individual level.

Finally, in order to make a meaningful contribution future research in this area has to address a number of issues. The first of these is that system evaluation relies heavily upon the adequacy of routine data collected by the service systems. These data need to be improved in terms of their comprehensive coverage, their accuracy and reliability. It is vitally important for service research and evaluation that basic demographic and clinical data are available in sufficient detail to be sure that like is being compared with like. This is a great challenge but is one which must be successfully addressed. The second, and related challenge, is to develop operational assessment and outcome measures of non-health items which can be used to assess service impact. There are a number of valid and reliable measures available, but nowhere near enough which have been adequately tested in the field. One of the sets of measures of significance will be that which attempts to capture continuity of care, since this is of central importance in personal and policy terms. Another will be the assessment of user satisfaction with services, using that term to include other agencies and service systems, as well as individual patients and their families. There is somewhat greater progress in respect of the latter.

All these attempts to understand the nature of service provision and outcome will have to include an understanding of service costs, and of the costs which fall outside the mental health service system. Systems which can understand the relationship between costs and outcomes will be those which survive and develop.

References

Eaton, W. (1993). *Strategies of Measurement.* NATO Advanced Research Workshop on Research Evaluation of Community Psychiatric Services, 3–7 September, Il Ciocco, Italy.

Gater, R. (1993). *The South Manchester Pathway Project.* Paper presented to Mid-Glamorgan Health and Social Services day conference, 2 March 1993.

Goldberg, D.P. & Huxley, P.J. (1992). *Common Mental Disorder: A Bio-social Model.* London: Routledge.

Ham, C. & Haywood, S. (1993). *The NHS: A Guide for Members and Directors of Health Authorities and Trusts.* Health Services Management Centre, University of Birmingham, UK: National Association of Health Authorities and Trusts.

Huxley, P. (1993). Improving health and social care in mental illness services: a survey of health service managers in one region of the UK. *Journal of Management in Medicine,* **7**(3), 5–11.

Huxley, P.J. & Kerfoot, M. (1993). Variation in requests to social services departments for assessment for compulsory psychiatric admission. *Social Psychiatry and Psychiatric Epidemiology,* **28**, 71–6.

Huxley, P.J. & Warner, R. (1992). Case management for long term psychiatric patients: a study of quality of life. *Hospital and Community Psychiatry,* **43**, 799–802.

Huxley, P.J. & Warner, R. (1993). Primary prevention of parenting dysfunction in high risk cases. *American Journal of Orthopsychiatry,* **63**, 582–8.

Jarman, B., Hirsch, S., White, P. & Driscoll, R. (1992). Predicting psychiatric admission rates. *British Medical Journal,* **304**, 1146–51.

Oliver, J.P.J. (1991). The social care directive: development of a quality of life profile for use in community services for the mentally ill. *Social Work Social Sciences Review*, **3**, 5–45.

Oliver, J.P.J., Huxley, P.J., Bridges, K. & Mohamad, H. (1995). *Quality of Life and Mental Health Services*. London: Routledge.

Orley, J. (1994). The WHOQOL project. Paper presented at the Quality of Life Conference of European Psychiatrists, 6–9 April, Vienna, Austria.

Pierides, M., Craig, T. & Roy, D. (1993). An evaluation of the care programme approach: preliminary results. Paper presented at the First Prism Conference, Institute of Psychiatry, London, 16 November 1993.

Rossi, P.H. & Freeman, H.E. (1993). *Evaluation: A Systematic Approach*, 5th ed. London, Sage Publications.

Tameside and Glossop Mental Health Service (1993). *The Care Programme Approach*. Tameside General Hospital, Tameside, Greater Manchester, UK.

Warner, R. & Huxley, P. (1993). Psychopathology and quality of life among mentally ill patients in the community: British and US samples compared. *British Journal of Psychiatry*, **163**, 505–9.

15

Psychiatric admission rates: the relationship with health and social factors and the effects of confounding variables

BRIAN JARMAN

Background

As long ago as 1939 Faris and Dunham drew attention to the higher rate of psychiatric admissions of people living in inner city areas. Hare in 1956 confirmed the high admission rate from schizophrenia in electoral wards with a high proportion of people living alone. There are higher proportions of people living alone in inner city areas but these studies do not prove that the stress of inner city life or the problems of social isolation are the cause of the associated higher psychiatric admission rates. Since these early studies other social factors, such as higher proportions of ethnic minority groups, and of working class, poor and unemployed people have similarly been shown to correlate with higher usage of psychiatric inpatient services (Thornicroft, 1991). It is possible to suggest a number of hypotheses: that social isolation, poverty and social disruption cause the psychiatric illnesses, or that the greater availability of services is associated with their higher usage, or that people with these social problems tend to drift into inner city areas, and so on. The aim of this chapter is to examine the relationship between psychiatric admission rates on the one hand and health, social and demographic factors on the other and to attempt to disentangle the possible influence of confounding variables.

Confounding

As an example of the influence of a confounding variable, suppose that the incidence of a disease is elevated in a population living near a factory which employs a high proportion of working class people and a research study is being designed to investigate whether proximity to the factory is associated with the increased incidence of the disease near the factory (Jolley *et al.*, 1993). The population living around the factory are not a random sample of the general population but are more likely than average to be of working class status. Members of the working classes are known to have a higher than average incidence of many diseases (Department of Health and Social Security, 1980). Social class factors are therefore likely to confound the relationship between disease incidence in the population and proximity to the factory. In the case cited an increased incidence of carcinoma of the lung, for example, could be due entirely to socio-economic factors, which in themselves may be related predominantly to smoking rates. If, in this instance, the incidence of the disease were considered as the outcome measure and proximity as a predictor variable, then social class might be considered as a confounding variable which could affect the outcome, and which should therefore be taken into account in the research design. An analysis of the potential effects of confounding can be particularly relevant in mental health services research where, for example, it may be of interest to study the relationship between the provision of psychiatric services in the community and the hospital admission rate from mental illnesses: the provision of services may vary with, for instance, the predominant social class or ethnic group of the area, which themselves may independently be related to mental illness admission rates.

For individuals a number of social factors have been shown in numerous studies, particularly in Britain, the United States, Scandinavia, France, Germany and Australia, to be associated significantly with morbidity and mortality (Department of Health and Social Security, 1980; Fox & Goldblatt, 1982; Wilkinson, 1986; Bunker *et al.*, 1989), the commonest factors being occupation, employment status (unemployment), social class and income. For households, similar results have been found for density of accommodation (persons per room), housing tenure (council/local authority housing), lack of basic amenities, lack of a car, and family income. For neighbourhoods, population density has been used.

The underprivileged area score and other deprivation indices

In the United Kingdom, a score, known as the underprivileged area or UPA score, has been developed which has been used to form a composite index of factors which general practitioners nationally consider are likely to increase their workload or pressure on their services (Jarman, 1983, 1984, 1990). The UPA score is based on a combination of eight social variables derived from the decennial census. The 1981 census was the first to be used. The score is most often applied at the electoral ward level – a geographical area containing approximately 5000 people on average. The variables used to form the score are those which a survey of 1 in 10 national sample of general practitioners in the United Kingdom considered to be associated with increased workload or pressure on their services. In recognition of the increased workload associated with the care of socially and materially disadvantaged patients, the Department of Health pays a deprivation allowance to general practitioners for those on their list of patients who live in electoral wards identified as deprived by having high values of the UPA score (the cut-off between deprived and non-deprived being decided by the Department of Health).

To calculate the score, the eight social variables used (all from the census) are first transformed with an angular transformation to give them a more normal, symmetrical distribution. The standardised values are then calculated for these transformed values of the eight variables, using the means and standard deviations of the transformed values of the approximately 10 000 electoral wards of England and Wales. The standardised transformed values are then weighted by the average weighting given to each variable in the survey of 1 in 10 general practitioners in the United Kingdom. The sum of the weighted, standardised transformed values gives the UPA score.

The eight variables, and their weightings, are the proportions of the ward population who are:

	Weighting
Elderly living alone	6.62
In one-parent families	4.62
Children under 5 years old	3.01
Social class V (unskilled workers)	3.74

Unemployed (as a % of the economically active population)	3.34
In overcrowded households	2.88
Have changed house within the last year	2.68
In ethnic groups (born in New Commonwealth or Pakistan)	2.50

In many countries in which good social statistics are recorded it would be possible to calculate UPA scores using the above variables. It would not be essential for the definition of each variable to be exactly the same as that used in the United Kingdom because the variables are standardised in order that the relative values of the UPA score between areas may be compared. Exact definitions would, however, be needed in order to make comparisons between countries. In this instance it would also be necessary to use the same means and standard deviations of the variables (e.g. for the electoral wards of England and Wales for 1981 or 1991) for the comparison.

A number of similar composite indices have been developed in the United Kingdom. Two of them, the Townsend (Townsend *et al.*, 1986) and Carstairs (Carstairs & Russell, 1989) indices, use variables which are particularly associated with material deprivation (unemployment, social class, overcrowding of households, housing tenure, lacking a car), whereas the other, the Department of the Environment index (Department of the Environment, 1983), resembles the UPA score in that it also includes factors related to family composition (single-parent households, elderly living alone, ethnic group) in addition to the material deprivation variables.

Several studies have linked these composite social indices of deprivation with measures of mortality, morbidity, and other factors such as general practitioner workload (Carstairs & Russell, 1989; Jarman, 1990).

Adjusting for the effects of confounding

Various methods can be used to adjust for confounding variables. A regression analysis can be used to introduce the variable as a covariate for each unit of analysis (e.g. a small geographical area) in order that trends can be examined by examination of the residuals after adjustment for selected variables. Another possibility is to extend the normal method of indirect standardisation for age to include the confounding variable, such as social class (Jolley *et al.*, 1993). Using the indirect standardisation method to control for age and another variable, say social class, involves knowing the overall population variation of the outcome variable with age and social class together with the age and social class structure of the population in each area used as the unit of analysis. Normally 5-year or 10-year age group stratifications and five or six social class groups would be used in this example. Similar variations within bands of the social deprivation indices or other variables can also be used.

Psychiatric hospital admission rates

Psychiatric admission rates have been shown to be strongly correlated with several demographic and social variables (Thornicroft, 1991; Jarman *et al.*, 1992). An example of the application of the methodology described above for taking account of confounding variables in an analysis of the relationship between psychiatric admission rates and the provision of psychiatric services was a study which we carried out to examine the variation of psychiatric admission rates to hospital for the approximately 190 district health authorities in England (Jarman *et al.*, 1992).

Data were collected from the Mental Health Enquiry (MHE) records of all psychiatric admissions for 1986, by district of residence of the patients admitted. Of all psychiatric admissions recorded by the MHE, those for mental handicap (18%) and psychogeriatrics (11%) were excluded from further study as were any other admissions with a diagnosis of senile dementia (ICD code 290) – leaving a total of 168 652 admissions in England in 1986 (Department of Health and Social Security, 1986).

A wide range of data is available from other sources regarding the demographic, social and health status of the residents of these districts and the extent and availability of services from hospitals, general practitioners and community psychiatric and non-psychiatric services and nursing homes (a total of about 160 factors for each district).

An initial analysis was carried out of the variation of crude admission rates (psychiatric admissions per 10 000 resident population) with the other district variables by calculating the Pearson correlation coefficients between the crude admission rates and the other factors

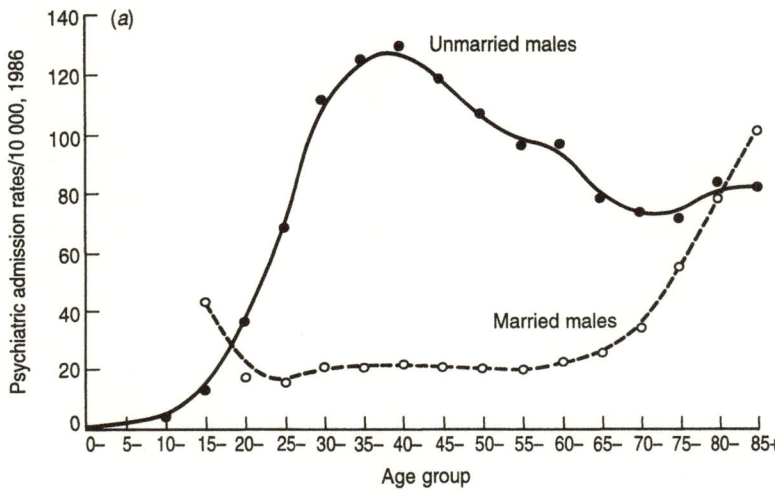

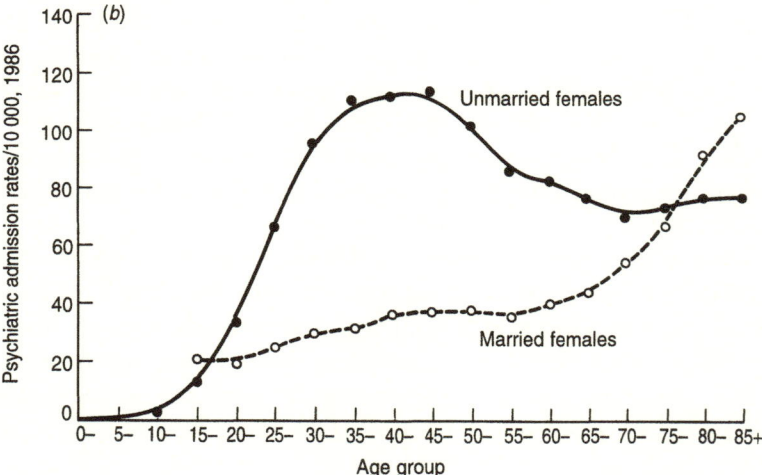

Fig. 15.1. Psychiatric admission rates by age and marital status for (a) males and (b) females. (Source: Mental Health Enquiry, 1986.)

for the 190 districts. Strong correlation coefficients were found between crude psychiatric admission rates and marital status and several social factors (Jarman *et al.*, 1992).

Individual, anonymised data were available for each hospital admission which included the age, sex and marital status of each patient. This enabled us to control for these three confounding variables by indirect standardisation. We calculated, for the whole population of England, the variation of psychiatric admission rates with age, sex and marital status (Fig. 15.1). These national admission rates by age, sex and marital status were multiplied by the numbers of residents in each age, sex and marital status group of each district to calculate the numbers of admissions in each district which would have been expected if the national rates had applied in that district. The actual number of admissions for the residents of each district divided by the expected number of admissions based on national rates and district age, sex and marital status structures, calculated in this manner, gave the indirectly standardised psychiatric admission ratio based on age, sex and marital status.

Correlations with psychiatric admission rates

The strongest correlations between the age, sex and marital status standardised admission ratios for 1986 were with: the standardised mortality ratio (SMR) to age 65 years (SMR65) for each district for 1986, various measures of material deprivation (both composite indices and individual variables such as unemployment), illegitimacy levels, and the levels of notified drug misusers. The deprivation variables, which inter-correlate strongly with the SMRs, were not significant when included with the SMRs.

In order to examine the relationship between the psychiatric admission rates, as the outcome variable, and the provision of psychiatric services (hospital, general practice and other community services, doctors and nurses: see Appendix), taken as the predictor variables, it was important to adjust for the influence of other confounding variables in addition to age, sex and marital status (which had been controlled for by the indirect standardisation). It was not possible to use the method of indirect standardisation for SMRs, levels of illegitimacy and drug addiction because the national variation of admission rates with these variables, as well as age, sex and marital status, was not known, and so stepwise regression analyses were carried out to control for the effects of these important confounding variables, after indirectly standardising the admission rates for age, sex and marital status as described above.

The only psychiatric service provision variables which were found to explain variations in district admission rates significantly, after

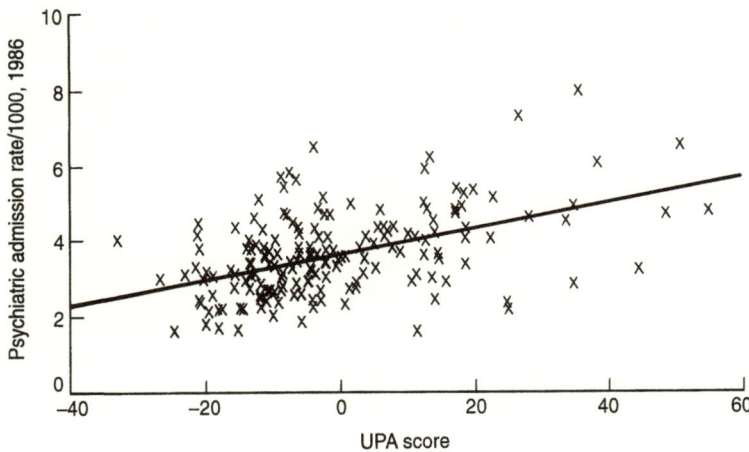

Fig. 15.2. Psychiatric admission rate versus UPA score for the district health authorities of England.

adjusting for the confounding variables, were the proportions of community psychiatric nurses in a district working in the community (a higher proportion was significantly associated with lower admission rates) and the proportion of psychiatric nurses in training (higher values associated with higher admission rates). Their explanatory powers were considerably lower than those of the confounding variables.

In order to arrive at an approximate analysis which could be applied at the district or electoral ward level, regression analyses were also carried out using the crude psychiatric admission rates per 10 000 resident population for each district health authority or electoral ward as the dependent variable and the UPA score as the independent variable, without the indirect standardisation for demographic factors. Fig. 15.2 shows the relationship between these two variables for the district health authorities of England. The correlation coefficient between the number of admissions predicted by this method and the actual number per district is 0.84. The district UPA score explains 23% of the variation of district crude psychiatric admission rates. A similar result was found using the crude psychiatric admission rates for the electoral wards in one regional health authority with a population of about 3.5 million.

This type of analysis provides a tool for identifying resource needs. However, when interpreting the results of regression analyses of the relationship between psychiatric admission rates and social factors the problems of multi-colinearity and linearity of the model must be borne in mind. Furthermore, studies based on the relationship between variables which are the averages for populations in geographical areas (as opposed to those based on individuals) suffer from the possibility that the relationships found between the area-based averages may not exist to the same degree between individuals within the populations in the areas on which the averages are based (the ecological fallacy) (Royal College of Psychiatrists, 1988; Jarman *et al.*, 1992; Jarman & Hirsch, 1992).

Conclusions

These findings suggest that, after taking into account the important confounding variables (age, sex and marital status by means of indirect standardisation, and SMRs, illegitimacy and drug addiction by means of regression analysis) the provision of psychiatric services appears to have only small influences on psychiatric admission rates in the 190 district health authorities in England in 1986. The results of the analysis indicate that, after adjusting for confounding variables, admission rates are slightly higher in districts which have higher proportions of psychiatric nurses in training and lower in districts which have higher proportions of community psychiatric nurses. Even though the predictor variables used in this study (factors related to the provision of psychiatric services) appear to have less influence on the outcome variable (psychiatric hospital admission rates) than the confounding variables, it may still be worth following up this finding with field studies.

The model, based on demographic and social factors – age, sex, marital status (which may be acting as a proxy for social isolation), levels of overall mortality (as measured by SMRs), drug addiction and illegitimacy (which correlates strongly with ethnicity) – may be used to predict the psychiatric admission rates in each district health authority area. If, however, the model is used at smaller area levels, such as electoral wards, it is not possible to use the indirect standardisation method to adjust for the effects of confounding variables because the population breakdown for each electoral ward by age, sex and marital status is not known for inter-census years.

Summary

It is difficult to measure the prevalence of mental illnesses. This makes it difficult to plan and evaluate services or to measure outcomes on much more than an individual basis. The model described could be useful for predicting the likely admission rates to hospital for psychiatric illness in small areas.

This chapter has attempted to illustrate the importance of adjusting for the influence of various demographic and social confounding variables in a study of the relationship between psychiatric admission rates and the provision of psychiatric services.

Appendix. Supply variables

Hospital services: non-psychiatry

Bed availability index
Hospital doctors: ratio of juniors to consultants
Consultants per bed
Consultants per 100 000 population
Consultants + juniors per bed
Consultants + juniors per 100 000 population
Average waiting list in weeks, total and by age group
Thames region district
Outer London district
Inner London district
Teaching district

Hospital services: psychiatry 1985/6

% Psychiatry admissions with no fixed abode (homeless + temporary resident)
% Psychiatry admissions with temporary address
% Psychiatry admissions who are homeless
Psychiatry beds available per 1000 population
Senior doctors in mental illness per 100 000 population
Consultants in mental illness per 100 000 population
% Mental illness nurses in hospitals
% Mental illness nurses in day hospitals
% Mental illness nurses in the community
% Mental illness nurses in training
% Mental illness nurses who are learners
% Mental illness nurses who are auxiliaries

Mental illness nurses per occupied bed
Mental illness nurses per available bed
Community psychiatric nurses and day hospital mental illness nurses per resident population

General practice

% GPs single-handed
% GPs aged 65 or more
Average GP list size
District resident population per GP

Community health services

Community health service expenditure 1984/5 per 1000 population

Nursing homes

Private beds as % non-psychiatric NHS beds 1984
Nursing home beds per 100 000 population 1984
Nursing home elderly beds per 10 000 elderly population 1984

References

Bunker, J.P., Gomby, D.S. & Kehrer, B.H. (1989). *Pathways to Health*. Menlo Park, CA: The Henry J. Keiser Family Foundation.

Carstairs, V. & Russell, M. (1989). Deprivation: explaining differences in mortality between Scotland and England. *British Medical Journal*, **299**, 886–9.

Department of the Environment (1983) Urban Deprivation. Information Note no. 2. London: Inner Cities Directorate.

Department of Health and Social Security (1980). *Inequalities in Health: Report of a Research Working Group* (the Black Report). London: Department of Health and Social Security.

Department of Health and Social Security (1986). *In-patient Statistics from the Mental Health Enquiry for England*. London: HMSO.

Faris, R. & Dunham, H. (1939). *Mental Disorders in Urban Areas*. Chicago: University of Chicago Press.

Fox, A.J. & Goldblatt, P.O. (1982). *Longitudinal Study: Socio-demographic Mortality Differentials, 1971–1975*. Series LS No. 1. London: HMSO.

Hare, E. (1956). Mental illness and social conditions in Bristol. *Journal of Mental Science*, **102**, 349–57.

Jarman, B. (1983). Identification of underprivileged areas. *British Medical Journal*, **286**, 1705–9.

Jarman, B. (1984). Underprivileged areas: validation and distribution of scores. *British Medical Journal*, **289**, 1587–92.

Jarman, B. (1990). *Social Deprivation and Health Service Funding*. Papers in Science, Technology and Medicine no. 22. London: Imperial College.

Jarman, B. & Hirsch, S. (1992). Statistical models to predict district psychiatric morbidity. In *Measuring Mental Health Needs*, ed. G. Thornicroft, C.R. Brewin & J. Wing. London: Gaskell.

Jarman, B., Hirsch, S., White, P. & Driscoll, R. (1992). Predicting psychiatric admission rates. *British Medical Journal*, **304**, 1146–51.

Jolley, D., Jarman, B. & Elliott, P. (1993). Socio-economic confounding. In *Geographical and Environmental Epidemiology: Methods for Small Area Studies*, ed. P. Elliott, J. Cuzick, D. English & R. Stern. Oxford: Oxford University Press.

Royal College of Psychiatrists (1988). *Psychiatric Beds and Resources; Factors Influencing Bed Use and Service Planning*. Report of a Working Party of the Section for Social and Community Psychiatry. London: Gaskell.

Thornicroft, G. (1991). Social deprivation and rates of treated mental disorder. *British Journal of Psychiatry*, **158**, 475–84.

Townsend, P., Phillimore, P. & Beattie, A. (1986). *Inequalities in Health in the Northern Region*. Northern Regional Health Authority and the University of Bristol.

Wilkinson, R.G. (ed.) (1986). *Class and Health*. London: Tavistock Publications.

PART V

PROGRAMME-LEVEL RESEARCH

16

Randomised controlled trials of programmes

Herman Kluiter and Durk Wiersma

Introduction

The objective of this chapter is to provide a functional frame of reference to those who want to familiarise themselves with the basic ideas behind randomised controlled trials (RCT), and with the practical problems and technicalities involved. Emphasis is on RCT of treatment programmes in a clinical context (RCT-P: P for such programmes) rather than on single interventions in the laboratory or laboratory-like situations. The chapter should be of help to those who want to evaluate published randomised clinical trials and research proposals, and to those intending to conduct such a trial.

Underutilisation of non-medication RCT in psychiatry will be discussed. Basic terms are introduced and defined. The aims pursued by the randomisation procedure are described. Several technical issues are addressed: the number of patients required as implied by power analysis, allocation of equal or unequal numbers of patients to the control and experimental condition, schemes of randomisation, and blinding. The differences between so-called management trials (RCT-P are such trials by nature) and explanatory trials are explicated. Specific problems of analysis in RCT-P as reflected by the concepts of 'intention-to-treat analysis' and 'as treated analysis' are referred to. Attention is drawn to two criteria by which each RCT should be judged: internal validity and generalisability. The chapter ends with a general appreciation of the position of RCT-P in psychiatry.

Underutilisation of randomised controlled trials in psychiatry

RCT are the scientific standard to settle claims concerning the superiority of one intervention over another (e.g. Pocock, 1987). There is a growing consensus in medicine that new major therapies should be tested rigorously, preferable by RCT. Their application in psychiatry is, however, extremely limited, excepting the evaluation of psychotropic medication. The number of trials in which, for example, inpatient psychiatric care for the acutely mentally ill has been soundly tested against alternative interventions is surprisingly small. Up till now no more than eight randomised trials have been conducted in which inpatient care for the acutely mentally ill stood the test against day treatment. Between the first and last trial in this series nearly 30 years elapsed. The total number of patients involved in the trials is about 1000; the generalisability of most studied samples was very limited (Kluiter *et al.*, 1992). The day treatment RCT were restricted to only three countries: the United States, Great Britain and the Netherlands. Corresponding figures concerning trials on home treatment versus inpatient treatment for the acutely mentally ill are even lower. Psychiatry is still in urgent need of properly controlled tests of much of its intervention repertoire.

Several reasons might account for this state of affairs. Much has for a long time been taken for granted in many areas of psychiatry. Unproven 'theories' and beliefs dominated the field and barriers were created against potential empirical falsifiers. Neither the orthodox psychoanalytic-oriented workers nor those representing anti-psychiatry, anti-institutionalism or institutionalism were interested in studies that could undermine fostered beliefs or 'theories'. When much of the deinstitutionalisation in the United States, which profoundly affected the lives of thousands of patients and their relatives, had already taken place Braun *et al.* (1981) had to conclude that the reformers had only two randomised studies of sufficient quality to go by. The Italian reform has yet to produce experimental proof of the efficacy of the treatment methods applied.

Apart from an essentially anti-scientific attitude or a lack of understanding of what science is meant to be there are more down-to-earth reasons for not applying RCT. 'The idea that patients should be randomly assigned to one or other form of treatment is not intuitively appealing to the medical profession or the layman. Superficially, randomized comparison of treatments appears contrary to the need to give every patient the best possible care' (Pocock, 1987, p. 50). McKhann (1989), evaluating his research experiences in neurology, found the organisation and execution of randomised trials outside the laboratory extremely complicated and time-consuming. McKhann's conclusions are certainly also valid for RCT-P in psychiatry. In particular, the recruitment of a sufficient number of patients for trials may take an inordinately long time. (It took us, for example, 17 months to assemble 160 patients from a catchment area of 100 000 inhabitants for a day treatment trial; hardly any selection criteria were applied (Wiersma *et al.*, 1991; cf. Kluiter *et al.*, 1992).) Short follow up-periods are usual trivial in psychiatry. Experts on schizophrenia recommend a follow-up period of at least 1 year and preferably much longer for intervention studies concerning that illness. Given the long time before results are publishable and the prevailing culture of 'publish or perish', one could speculate that RCT are not popular with many researchers (Fletcher & Fletcher, 1979).

Terminology

In medicine the terms 'randomised controlled trials', 'randomised controlled clinical trials' and 'randomised clinical trials' may be used interchangeably. We follow the definitions of Pocock (1987): the term clinical trial 'may be applied to any form of planned experiment which involves patients and is designed to elucidate the most appropriate treatment of future patients with a given medical condition' (p. 1). 'Controlled clinical trials ... are comparative. That is, one needs to compare the experience of a group of patients on the new treatment with a control group of similar patients receiving a standard treatment. If there is no standard treatment of any real value, then it is often appropriate to have a control group of untreated patients. Also, in order to obtain an unbiased evaluation of the new treatment's value one usually needs to assign each patient randomly to either new or standard treatment ... Hence it is now generally accepted that the randomised controlled trial is the most reliable method of conducting clinical research' (pp. 4–5).

In RTC-P in psychiatry assignment is mostly to one control

condition and one experimental condition. 'Condition' stands for treatment, programme or treatment programme. More complicated designs with, for example, more than one experimental condition are of course possible though often not practicable or feasible. The control condition is in most cases a standard treatment programme; the experimental condition is usually a newly developed alternative to this standard. The patients assigned to the experimental condition are the experimental patients (or experimentals); together they form the experimental group. Corresponding terms are applicable for the patients assigned to the control condition; the control group is sometimes also called the comparison group. We do not follow the rather confusing proposal by some authors to call a group a control group if there is no treatment or a placebo treatment, and to call a group a comparison group if there is a standard treatment.

In psychiatry, outside the field of specific medication studies, control groups on placebo or a control group denied all treatment are nearly always out of the question. The mental state of psychiatric patients, especially those in the acute phase of one of the major mental disorders, urges generally for one intervention or another.

RTC-P in psychiatry are rarely about mono-therapy. In psychiatry, treatment programmes, experimental or not, usually consist of several ingredients, such as crisis intervention followed by medication therapy, individual therapy, group therapy and occupational therapy.

Outcome variables (also known as end points or effect variables) are measured in order to assess which programme has more favourable effects. In a properly designed RTC-P these variables, such as psychopathology, social functioning and burden on the family, should be measured before the patients are enrolled into the programme or very shortly after the programme has commenced (pretest). That measurement should be repeated at least once after a fixed and sufficiently long period following enrolment or at the time the programme is completed (posttest). A design with these qualities is called a 'pretest–posttest follow-up design' (Campbell & Stanley, 1966; Cook & Campbell, 1979). Combined with random assignment to a control and experimental condition it is about the strongest design possible.

The target population is the population one wants to generalise to, e.g. all patients presenting for admission in a country. All patients who are within reach for the study constitute the study population, e.g. the patients presenting for admission at the hospital where a trial

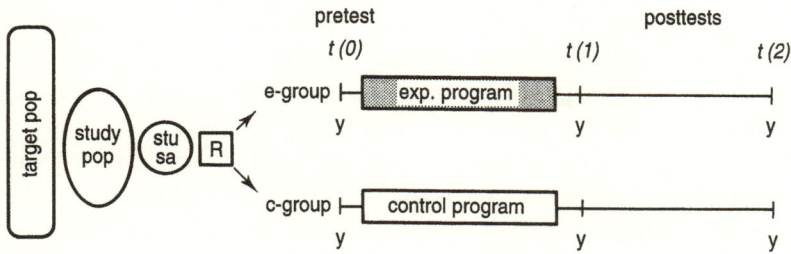

Fig. 16.1. Diagram of a randomised controlled trial with a pretest-posttest follow-up design; two conditions. pop, population; stu sa, study sample; R, random assignment; e, experimental; c, control; t(0), outcome measures in null situation (pretest); t(1), outcome measures directly after intervention (first posttest); t(2), outcome measures at end of follow-up (second posttest); y, outcome variables (e.g. psychopathology, social functioning).

is to be conducted. The members of the study population actually recruited for the trial form the study sample.

For reasons of simplicity we assume throughout the rest of this chapter that only one control and one experimental programme are compared. This does not imply loss of generality.

Fig. 16.1 illustrates the pretest–posttest follow-up design with random assignment.

Why randomise?

Randomisation serves two essential functions. The first function is the creation of control and experimental groups that only by chance differ in entry characteristics, i.e. are prognostically balanced. The line of thought is simple: initial differences between the groups to be compared ought to be ruled out as an explanation for the outcomes of the trial. Ruling out such differences is one of the meanings of the rather imprecise term 'control(led)' in RCT. Randomisation is a lottery procedure that prevents human interference which could easily lead to assigning patients to the condition thought (by their doctors, relatives, themselves, sometimes even researchers) to be most suitable for them, thus introducing bias which in its turn might lead to a confounding of the effects resulting from the contrasting programmes and the differential characteristics of the assigned groups. This function of randomisation is meant to promote the internal validity of the trial. The latter concept indicates the degree of validity of cause–consequence conclusions that can be derived from the observed effects within an experiment. Causes other than the differences between experimental and control intervention, i.e. confounding variables, ought to be excluded as much as possible.

The danger of non-randomised studies, such as those based on matching or quasi-experiments, is that in the end one has to conclude that observed effects are only a consequence of pre-existing differences between the study samples. Of course, there are techniques such as analysis of covariance to correct for such initial differences. From a mathematical-statistical and practical point of view the results stemming from such techniques are not unchallenged (Neter *et al.*, 1985). Moreover variables in psychiatric research more often than not are in conflict with the statistical conditions required for this technique.

The second function of randomisation is to secure the applicability of statistical techniques of comparison that in principle are based on chance fluctuations (Hays, 1977; Pocock, 1987; McKhann, 1989). For those techniques to be applicable it is a necessary condition that all patients recruited for the trial have the same chance of being placed in either the control or one or more experimental groups. This condition is violated if those chances fluctuate during the recruitment of the patients. This, for instance, might be the case if management wants to avoid underutilisation of hospital wards that are involved in the research project or wants to avoid waiting lists. Such violation may yield incorrect estimates of the probabilities of observed differences and thus may lead to unwarranted conclusions.

The number of patients required

Numerous trials have been conducted that should not have been. Cohen had to draw this conclusion in 1969 and was compelled to repeat it in 1992 by looking simply at the sample sizes. He found that in many trials sample sizes were so low that only huge effects were likely to be detected, i.e. could reach statistical significance. Huge effects are not common in psychiatry or in medicine in general. At the heart of the argument is the concept of statistical power. Power is the probability that an effect will be detected if there is one. If there is a real effect and the applied statistical test generates the result 'not significant', i.e. the null hypothesis of no relation cannot be rejected, a wrong conclusion is drawn. To give a real effect a fair chance, i.e. an acceptable amount of power, to show up statistically implies determining the number of subjects required to create such a chance by means of power analysis.

It is not possible to go into the technicalities of power analysis here. However, a short outline might be useful. To determine the minimum number of subjects required the following components are needed:

1 An outcome variable.
2 Relevant statistical properties (distribution, average, standard deviation) of the outcome variable as assessed in or estimated from previous research. The properties entered into the power equation depend on the index at stake; e.g. for differences between averages an estimate of the standard deviation is imperative.
3 The statistical technique appropriate to test (in)equality between the experimental and control group on this outcome variable in terms of averages, proportions, etc.
4 The level of significance (usually 5% or 1%), i.e. the risk one wants to take that an observed inequality is not a false inequality caused by influences having nothing to do with the differences in the experimental and control condition.
5 The direction of the test of significance: one- or two-tailed.
6 The minimum effect thought to be a realistic success (effect size).
7 The desirable power, i.e. the probability one wants to have that this minimum effect also shows up statistically, in other words leads to rejection of the null hypothesis of no relation.

The following relations exist:

- the lower the level of significance, the more patients are needed;
- the smaller the effect size, the more patients are needed;
- the higher the power, the more patients are needed.

Cohen (1988) provides clear explanations of the principles involved in power analysis and many tables for deriving the number of required patients under given circumstances. There are now also computer programs available to conduct power analyses.

An example

An experimental treatment programme aims at reducing the readmission rate within 1 year to 20% compared with 29% in a standard programme. The level of significance is 5%, one-tailed. To have a fair chance of 4:1 (i.e. power = 80%) that an observed difference of 29% − 20% = 9% actually exceeds this level of significance, 392 patients are needed in each condition. If a reduction of 29% to 10% were aimed at, the same power would be reached with only 63 patients in each condition. With 63 patients in each condition an actual 'real' reduction of 29% to 20% readmissions hardly stands a chance of reaching significance as power would be a mere 30%, i.e. 3:7.

In psychiatric RCT-P two complicating factors not often mentioned in statistical texts should be accounted for: loss to follow-up and the fact that usually many outcome variables are of interest and included in the design. In trials, especially with the severely mentally ill, considerable numbers of patients may be lost to follow-up. For the purposes of power analysis a non-conservative estimate of this loss should be made for obvious reasons. Different outcome variables require different sample sizes, depending on the statistical properties of the variable and the statistical index (proportion, mean, etc.) one wants to calculate. An efficient procedure might be to identify the outcome variable most critical to the trial and then determine the sample size needed given the desired specifications outlined above. After this the procedure is turned around by answering the question: Is this sample size sufficient to generate an acceptable level of power for the next most critical outcome variable, and if not, how many more patients are needed? When all important outcome variables have passed the review in this way, a sample size should be chosen. In this choice the associated durations of the recruitment phase and the differential costs involved are of course weighted heavily.

In medicine in general, and in psychiatry in particular, special attention should be given to trials that aim at establishing the value of therapies less intrusive than standard therapies or treatment modalities less restrictive than is common practice. The (statistical) equivalence of some less restrictive alternative to, say, inpatient treatment is readily shown if the sample size is small enough to prevent virtually any difference from reaching significance level, even if the observed differences are large and in favour of inpatient treatment. Such practice is unacceptable from a scientific and an ethical point of view. What we would like to stress by this argument is that if one wants to demonstrate that two therapies are equivalent in outcome, but different in intrusion or implied restriction, the sample size should be large enough to let any difference shine if it is there.

Should equal or unequal proportions of patients be allocated to the conditions?

It is a common misunderstanding that randomisation requires the allocation of equal proportions of patients (0.50/0.50; 0.33/0.33/0.33; etc.) to the two or more research conditions (Peto *et al.*, 1976; Pocock, 1979). Especially in psychiatry it may be of advantage to allocate more patients to the experimental condition(s) than to the control condition. In RCT-P in psychiatry it is not uncommon that patients are not suited for the treatment programme they are allocated to according to the randomisation scheme. Patients allocated to a day treatment programme may, for example, not be fit to follow such a programme because their condition requires a level of protection that can only be given in inpatient treatment which was the control condition. In such a situation a higher number of patients in the experimental condition(s) contributes to, among other things, a better estimation of the proportion of patients who can be treated with the experimental programme. In methodological literature one important advantage is not mentioned. Patients actually receiving the experimental treatment tend to differ in their response to this treatment. Within the classical framework of experimentation and analysis of variance such differences are seen as errors, as they are in agricultural research from which analysis of variance originates. In human research such 'errors' may contain useful information as they will, at least in part, reflect true differences between the subjects. It would be a waste not to analyse which qualities of the patients or subgroups correlate with differences in outcome. Such analysis may lead to important clues concerning subgroups of patients for whom the programme is especially effective or particularly ineffective. The adequacy of response prediction depends on the number of subjects available: the more the better.

A disadvantage of unequal randomisation is the loss of statistical power compared with a design with equal randomisation. This disadvantage does not, however, need to take dramatic forms. Pocock (1979, p. 191) compared the common ratio of subjects of 1:1 to the ratio of 2:1. In the case of a normally distributed variable with known variance and a two-tailed significance level of 1%, a required power of 50% in the 1:1 situation would fall by 5.9% compared with the 2:1 situation. A loss of only 2.5% would occur if the two-tailed significance level were set at 5% and the required power at 95%, all other parameter values staying unchanged. All combinations in between these parameter values (significance levels between 1% and 5%, power levels between 50% and 95%, ratios between 1:1 and 1:2; all other values constant) would yield losses in power of between 5.9% and 2.5% Such small losses are ordinarily perfectly acceptable in the kind of research under consideration, unless one wants to detect very small differences.

Randomisation schemes

In what is called *simple or pure randomisation* the patients are entered one by one into the trial and assignment takes place by means of a list which specifies for each consecutive entry the treatment assigned. Which patient in the sequence is assigned which treatment is determined by means of a table of random numbers or a special computer program. Randomising in this way may have unwanted practical implications: there is no control on the tempo of influx of patients into one or the other treatment programme. One programme may purely by chance become 'favoured' for some time with, as an unwanted consequence, an overload of patients in this condition and underutilisation of the other programme.

An effective method to control for such a phenomenon is *blocked randomisation*. An example might clarify the method best. Take a trial into which 160 subjects are to be entered. The number of subjects in each block is set to, say, 16, which yields 10 blocks. Assume, for the sake of argument, equal assignment to two conditions, i.e. in each block 8 subjects placed into the control programme and 8 into the experimental one. For each block a randomisation list is prepared. In this example at most 16 (last 8 in block k, and first 8 in block $k + 1$) subjects in a row could be assigned to one and the same condition, which of course will hardly ever happen. In the same situation without blocking that theoretical number could be 80, which of course also will hardly ever happen. In order not to violate the assumptions of the statistical techniques to be applied the number of subjects in each block and the ratio of control to experimental subjects should remain fixed throughout the trial. With this method (correctable) statistical problems arise when there is a clear relation between the sequence of blocks and outcome (e.g. better outcome for blocks higher in the sequence). To adjust for this requires advice from a statistician.

If there is strong evidence that one or more patient factors (prognostic factors) might influence outcome *stratified randomisation*, i.e. randomisation within pre-chosen strata, is sometimes applied.

An example

An investigator, intending to run a RCT-P on day treatment versus psychiatric inpatient treatment, thinks he has firm reason to believe that female patients and depressive patients respond better to day treatment than others. He wants to make sure the percentage of females and the percentage of depressives in the study population are equal in both treatment conditions. This case implies the following four strata: depressive and female, depressive and male, not depressive and female, and not depressive and male. This method may prevent prognostic imbalance as sometimes might occur with unstratified randomisation, but only with regard to the chosen strata. Randomisation takes place within each stratum; either simple or blocked and equal-numbered or unequal-numbered randomisation can be applied. With limited numbers of patients available the number of strata should be kept low as otherwise many empty cells may be the result, which from an analytical point of view is highly undesirable. For example, 3 factors to be stratified, each of which has 2 classes, result in 8 strata. This will yield 16 cells if there are 2 treatment programmes to be compared.

A related scheme is *randomisation* after patients have been *matched* pairwise on one or more factors thought to be prognostic of outcome. Matching is a technique that quite often does not lead to satisfactory results, especially if matching is on three or more factors and with limited numbers of available patients. A distinct disadvantage of this kind of randomisation is that assignment of unequal numbers of subjects to the treatment programmes is impossible.

There is a real danger that stratified and matched randomisation make the trial less transparent and organisationally more difficult than one would wish. We agree with the stance taken by the *British Medical Journal* (Anonymous, 1977, p. 1239): 'Nowadays it is generally unnecessary to randomise patients within separate groups according to prognostic factors, since these are better allowed for retrospectively in the analysis.' The same position is taken by Peto *et al.* (1976). The latter authors see some room for stratification with small samples because of their susceptibility to imbalance. As noted before, the number of possible strata in small samples rapidly reaches its limit.

Blinding in RCT-P

Blinding aims at keeping information away from researchers and/or subjects that might elicit reactions producing false effects, i.e. effects that are not brought about by the interventions under investigation. Separation of false effects, as a result of bias or confounding, from true effects is the major methodological concern in experimentation. In RCT three categories of blinding should be distinguished: blinding to the combination 'patient–assignment to condition', blinding to the combination 'patient–administration of treatment' and blinding to the combination 'patient–measurement of outcome'. Double-blind trials (better described as treble-blind) comply with all three categories of blinding. This ideal is usually attained only in medication trials.

In RCT-P blinding to the assignment process is the only method of blinding possible. It can and must be accomplished in order to eliminate the all too human inclination to assign a given patient to the programme thought most appropriate for him or her, or to favour the experimental programme by assigning the less sick patients to it. The following procedure is fairly watertight. The randomisation list is converted into an ordered set of sealed envelopes containing the assignment decision; the order is exactly the same as on the list. When an eligible patient presents for treatment, his or her number in the sequence together with identification data and the time of presentation are filled in by an official. Another official having no contact with the patient is informed that patient no. X has arrived, upon which that official opens the top envelope and indicates to which treatment that patient is allotted. Promptly after that the official is also given the identification data. Variants are possible. In order to prevent predictability as to which condition is likely to come up next, as few people as possible should know about the blocks and in what ratio the patients are allotted to the conditions. In particular the official(s) to whom the patients present should be unaware of these matters. The tasks involved are not too difficult to accomplish. Adherence to explicit written instructions of when to do what in the assignment procedure is, however, an absolute requirement to avoid unintentional and intentional human interference.

As for the other two categories, the ideal of blinded therapeutic staff, blinded patients and blinded researchers is not feasible in the type of evaluation under consideration. Staff know which regimen they follow with which patients, and patients know what treatment they receive. There is hardly a way to blind the researchers. Only if all measurement occur without direct oral–verbal contact between researchers and patients can blinding be established. However, such a situation seldom occurs. Much of the measurement in the evaluation of psychiatric treatment programmes takes place by means of oral interviews and has to take place in that way because of the characteristics of the patients involved. In such interviews it is hardly possible for the patient not to speak about the kind of treatment he or she gets. Some interviews, such as those concerning satisfaction with the treatment received, would be virtually meaningless if no questions were asked about that specific treatment. The best one can achieve in RCT-P is to form research teams operating independently from the treatment teams and without vested interests in the programmes to be compared. Moreover, analyses of data and publication of results before the planned end of the trial should be avoided because they might provoke human reactions (Cook & Campbell, 1979) not compatible with the scientific standards being strived for. The latter statement does not apply, of course, if one of the programmes is evidently so inferior that the vital interests of the patients involved are at stake. It is therefore advisable to monitor during the experiment events such as suicides, deaths, and gross disruptions of the life of the patients and other people. It should be made explicit in the research protocol under what conditions the trial should be stopped.

Management trials and explanatory trials

In an influential article in the *New England Journal of Medicine* Sackett & Gent (1979) distinguished two basic types of trials in medicine: management trials and explanatory trials. They build on the work of Schwartz & Lellouch (1967) who pointed out the difference between a pragmatic and an explanation-directed attitude in therapeutic trials. Management trials are pragmatic by nature. Their aim is to simulate what happens in clinical practice if a new therapy or therapeutic programme is introduced in place of standard interventions. 'The management trial may . . . accept all comers, including patients with poor compliance, to obtain a better estimate of the usefulness of starting down a particular therapeutic path' (Sackett & Gent, 1979, p. 1411). By their nature RCT-P in psychiatry are management trials. The idea of comparing programmes is at odds with the experimental ideal of varying one or a few factors systematically in such a way that detected effects can be attributed only to the differences in those factors. Such strict control is for obvious reasons virtually impossible in RCT-P, especially in psychiatry.

An 'explanatory trial' is conducted in the laboratory or in circumstances as close to possible to laboratory conditions. 'Its main objective is to explain . . . by isolating the effects of specific variables and understanding the mechanisms of action' (Last, 1988, p. 45). Usually patients entered into such experiments are strictly selected with regard to their expected compliance and with regard to other characteristics conducive to completing the planned treatments. In general such trials are suited to identify which agents cause which effect, but not suited to provide the knowledge needed to work with the new treatment in realistic situations.

'Intention-to-treat' and 'as treated' groups: special problems in analysing management trials

Intricately connected with the concept of management trials is the concept of 'intention to treat' (Newcombe, 1988; Lee *et al.*, 1991; Newell, 1992). The treatment programme intended for a patient, given his or her assignment, may never have begun or not been completed. In clinical practice such occurrences are not uncommon, and neither are they in management trials as these try to simulate common practice in which all comers are accepted for the trial. Several reasons may account for this: the patient is non-compliant, the patient is not fit to undergo the treatment he or she is allocated to (e.g. surgery for patients with advanced cancer), the condition of the patient deteriorates during the trial to such a degree that the alternative treatment programme is tried in an attempt to stop the deterioration.

An example

A trial aims at assessing the efficacy of day treatment versus inpatient psychiatric care in clinical practice. In order to obtain a realistic estimate of what happens if hospitals adopt the attitude of attempting day treatment with all patients presenting for admission, no patients are excluded from the trial. The patients are randomly assigned to the condition 'day treatment' or the condition 'inpatient treatment'. It is known for certain that an (unknown) proportion of the patients presenting never will receive day treatment within a reasonable period because their condition forbids it. It is not known for certain which characteristics typify such patients. A management trial starting with the intention to treat patients according to their assigned treatment programme would be the trial of choice. The essential contrast is: the success (feasibility and outcomes) of the policy to attempt day treatment versus the success of the policy to apply inpatient treatment in all cases.

In management trials the statistical-analytical approach called for is the 'intention-to-treat analysis'. This says nothing other than that all patients assigned to the experimental condition should be contrasted with all patients assigned to the control condition, irrespective of whether they actually received the treatment implied by the condition of allocation or not. It aims at comparing clinical policies rather than specific treatments.

There is considerable argument over whether an 'intention-to-treat analysis' should be followed by comparisons between patient groups on the basis of the treatment they actually received (Lee *et al.*, 1991). The main counter-argument is that an analysis on the patients-as-treated would violate the good statistical conditions brought about by randomisation. However valid that argument is, 'as treated' analysis may produce important information and should in our view always be done. Otherwise important clues as to the impact of the treatments might be overlooked. One should contrast the patients in the experimental condition actually receiving the prescribed treatment with those who were switched to the control programme, to make sure, for example, that certain favourable outcomes are not mainly attributable to the latter patients. 'As treated' analysis should always be accompanied by a very careful analysis and description of the characteristics of the subgroups involved in the comparisons. Such analysis may lead to the detection of important distinguishing characteristics between compliers and non-compliers or may suggest clinically impressive differences in outcome. In 'as treated' analysis statistical tests need to be handled with great caution. Power is reduced because of smaller sample sizes: the patients in both the control and the experimental group are split into at least two subgroups, i.e. those receiving the treatment according to protocol and those not receiving that treatment. The p values may be wrongly estimated as the 'as treated' groups are not randomised groups.

Internal validity

Are observed differences in outcome between the control and experimental group accounted for by the differences between the control and experimental programme, or by alternative factors not related to the differences between the programmes, i.e. confounding variables? This question is the crux of the concept of internal validity.

Randomisation aims at ruling out differences in entry characteristics between the control and experimental group as causes for differences in outcome. Randomisation does not, however, always generate fully balanced groups; the degree to which it was successful should be checked and described. Special attention should be given to the consequences of consent. Consent may lead to (self-)selection bias if one of the conditions is viewed as more attractive, more beneficial, less restrictive, less dangerous, etc. It is also conceivable that patients with certain (e.g. social) characteristics tend to prefer one treatment and patients with different characteristics favour the other. Such (self-) selection, resulting in unequal numbers of patients per condition failing to consent, jeopardises internal validity. Special randomisation procedures have been proposed to tackle selection problems generated by the consent procedure (e.g. Zelen, 1979). For RCT-P in psychiatry such solutions as yet do not seem to be practicable as they probably will only add to the complexity these trials are already beset with. Stratified randomisation, with well-chosen stratifying (prognostic) factors, could be helpful in reducing to some extent imbalance caused by selection processes; it is certainly not a sufficient remedy. If (self-)selection as a consequence of the consent procedure occurs there is really no adequate way out. All one can hope for is to be able to show that the imbalance does not affect outcome, or if it does affect outcome that techniques that aim to correct for unbalanced prognostic factors, such as analysis of covariance, are applicable. The dangers of failure to consent should not be exaggerated however; for example, in no major RCT on day treatment and home treatment as (radical) alternatives to inpatient treatment were such problems reported.

Randomisation is a powerful tool; it does not, however, exercise any control over what happens afterwards. Several factors may then threaten internal validity. A very serious threat occurs if the loss to follow-up differs between the control and the experimental groups, thus creating imbalanced groups after all. 'Compensatory equalisation of treatments' may occur when 'the experimental treatment provides goods or services believed to be desirable, [and] there may emerge administrative and constituency reluctance to tolerate the focused inequality that results' (Cook & Campbell, 1979, p. 54). Treatment staff might be particularly susceptible to three processes:

- overreaction of staff administering the experimental treatment, manifesting itself in, amongst other things, a degree of attention given to the patients that is not repeatable in a normal, non-research situation;
- compensatory rivalry on the part of staff administering the less desirable treatment;
- resentful demoralisation of staff administering the less desirable treatment.

We refer to Cook & Campbell (1979) for an extensive list of potential threats to internal validity.

RCT-P in psychiatry are especially susceptible to threats to validity. It is seldom that two programmes differ only in one or two aspects; moreover, psychiatric patients are usually in need of an individualised approach. If, for example, day treatment is compared with inpatient treatment one would not know to which factor the differences in outcome should be attributed if one group were to get on average twice as much occupational therapy as the other or half the daily dose of neuroleptics. This point stresses the importance of recording of what is administered to the patients. Such records ought to show in what specific aspects the programmes being compared differed, and as such generate arguments for or against the internal validity of the outcomes of the trial.

The concept of internal validity was developed in connection with explanatory trials. Not much thought has as yet been given to its applicability to management trials with 'intention-to-treat' and 'as treated' groups. The assessment of the internal validity of such trials becomes seemingly very complicated. Perhaps Newcombe's proposal offers a way out. He suggests that the essential comparison to be made is that between two treatment *policies* rather than between two *specific* treatments: 'The term policy here is used in a particular sense: this is not as in, "The policy of hospital X is . . ." but rather something like, "Use A; if the patient responds, very well, otherwise try B, etc." Such a treatment plan is usually informally determined in clinical practice, but can usually be formalised to a great extent in the design of a therapeutic trial' (Newcombe, 1988, p. 696).

Generalisability

In order to substantiate his or her claims as to the generalisability of the results of the trial, the investigator has to demonstrate that the study sample accurately reflects the characteristics of the study population, and that the study population is representative of the target population. The hard part is showing the latter. The target population should be defined and data on its core characteristics should be available. The best one can hope for are national census data, such as the characteristics of a population admitted for inpatient treatment in some year. International census data are virtually non-existent. It is, however, hardly customary in psychiatric RCT-P to provide data on both the study population and the target population that allow the extent to which the former is representative of the latter to be judged. An analysis of ours of RCT-P on day treatment or home treatment versus inpatient treatment identified only one trial that adhered to this essential methodological requirement.

A judgement regarding the generalisability of results requires an unequivocal formulation of the inclusion and exclusion criteria. This requirement is seemingly obvious. In nearly all the RCT on day treatment versus inpatient treatment that we analysed such criteria were either absent or vague.

Conclusion

RCT-P in psychiatry are difficult – we believe more difficult than in most medical specialties. At least two factors contribute to this situation. Too little is still known about which psychopathological processes, inherent to the major psychiatric illnesses, might respond to which treatment or to which aspects of treatment. The way out is to try a given programme on broad, globally defined categories of patients and see what happens to whom. Mental illness produces, more often than not, behavioural disorders not conducive to the role of a passive, compliant subject. Both factors are in conflict with the ideal of the classic scientific experiment: the explanatory trial. Given these factors management trials might remain dominant in psychiatry for a long time to come. As management trials simulate clinical practice they are certainly in no way inferior to explanatory trials. Results from management trials might indicate detailed testing that should be carried out in explanatory trials. The applicability of results of such explanatory trials should, ideally, in their turn be tested in management trials.

In our opinion methodology has concentrated too much on analytically relatively easy, explanatory trials; management trials deserve a more thorough methodological elaboration than the collection of disparate papers available so far.

Randomised controlled trials in psychiatry are demanding enterprises. Psychiatry should not, however, avoid rigorous tests of new (and as yet untested conventional) treatment practices, by means of either explanatory or management trials. Our stance is that psychiatry should adhere to the current standards of somatic medicine, which imply rigorous experimental proof before a new drug or other kind of intervention is made generally available. Psychiatry has excepted itself too much and too long from the ethical and scientific obligation to demonstrate the efficacy of its intervention repertoire. It is all too easy to question the appropriateness of randomised controlled trials in psychiatry, by introducing objections of either a practical or fundamental nature into the argument. A detailed consideration of the arguments in such debates more often than not reveals their invalidity or futility. This does not alter the fact that experimentation in psychiatry is exacting. In the long run, however, the interests of patients are best served by tests as outlined in this chapter.

Appendix. A checklist of variables that might be important for RCT-P in psychiatry

As most RCT-P in psychiatry will pursue multiple objectives several *outcome variables* should be considered for inclusion in the design.

A checklist of *patient variables*:

- Diagnosis
- Other indicators of the nature and severity of the psychopathology
- Indicators concerning the capability for self-care
- Indicators concerning the capability to do work
- Indicators concerning the level of social functioning. 'Social role' is an effective concept for operationalising social functioning. Some examples of social roles are: partner in a (sexual) relationship, member of a family, parent, child, sibling, friend, housekeeper, employee, member of society at large
- Indicators concerning the structure of daily activities, including leisure activities
- Indicators of psychological (dys)functioning as to consciousness, sleep, concentration, memory, speech and thought, reality testing, volition, emotion and affect, psychomotor behaviour
- Satisfaction with treatment
- Satisfaction with life and quality of life
- Relapses
- Re(admissions)
- Costs of treatment and indirect costs
- Compliance with the programmes
- Time spent in the community (with and without attachment to an institution)
- Aggressive incidents, including homicide
- Suicide attempts
- Suicides
- Death

In each RCT-P the variables in this list that can be measured at baseline should be measured then. Those pretest measures are also part of the set of entry characteristics and should, together with other entry characteristics, be used to check whether the randomisation generated balanced groups.

Other *entry characteristics* to be assessed are: gender, age, living situation, marital status, educational status, employment career and status, career in psychiatry (especially the number and duration of previous admissions).

As psychiatric interventions might affect the *partner and family* of the patient in one way or another, serious consideration should be given to including the outcome measures:

- Burden on partner and/or family
- Satisfaction of partner and/or family with the treatment provided

Together with these the appropriate entry characteristics of the partner/family should be assessed.

All RCT-P on day treatment or home treatment versus inpatient treatment which we studied lacked an adequate *description of the programmes* as applied. This is highly unsatisfactory as it hinders a proper evaluation of the outcomes and obstructs further dissemination of the tested programmes. Together with its governing principles and its general content each programme should be described in terms of the type of care and how much of it each patient (and, if appropriate, the patient's partner and/or relatives) receives. Wherever possible the variables for the control and experimental condition should be the same. The organisation and execution of such a recording programme may be highly demanding: usually many professionals will provide care to each patient and all these efforts need to be recorded by each professional or by some central person who needs to be informed by each professional. Not much can be said about the specific contents of the variables as they depend on the nature of the programmes tested. Variables that might be important in most programmes are:

- Whereabouts of the patient by day and by night (e.g. hospital, outpatient department, day centre, home)
- Medication prescribed (daily dose, trade name, generic name, equivalence of daily dose to a reference medication)
- Number, duration and location of contacts with psychiatrist(s), (community psychiatric) nurses, occupational therapists, other therapists and other professionals

References

Anonymous (1977). Randomized clinical trials (leader). *British Medical Journal*, i, 1238-9.

Braun, P., Kochansky, G., Shapiro, R., Greenberg, S., Gudeman, J., Johnson, S. & Shore, M. (1981). Overview. Deinstitutionalization of psychiatric patients: a critical review of outcome studies. *American Journal of Psychiatry*, **138**, 736-49.

Campbell, D. & Stanley, J. (1963). *Experimental and Quasi-experimental Designs for Research*. Chicago: Rand McNally.

Cohen, J. (1969). *Statistical Power Analysis for the Behavioral Sciences*, 1st edn. San Diego, CA: Academic Press.

Cohen, J. (1988). *Statistical Power Analysis for the Behavioral Sciences*, 2nd edn. Hillsdale, NJ: Erlbaum.

Cohen, J. (1992). A power primer. *Psychological Bulletin*, **112**, 155-9.

Cook, D. & Campbell, D. (1979). *Quasi-Experimentation: Design and Analysis for Field Settings*. Chicago: Rand McNally.

Fletcher, R. & Fletcher, S. (1979). Clinical research in general medical journals: a 30-year perspective. *New England Journal of Medicine*, **301**, 180-3.

Hays, W. (1973). *Statistics for the Social Sciences*. London: Holt, Rinehart and Winston.

Kluiter, H., Giel, R., Nienhuis, F., Rüphan, M. & Wiersma, D. (1992). Predicting feasibility of day treatment for unselected patients referred for inpatient psychiatric treatment: results of a randomized trial. *American Journal of Psychiatry*, **149**, 1199-205.

Last, J. (1988). *A Dictionary of Epidemiology*. New York: Oxford University Press.

Lee, Y., Ellenberg, J., Hirtz, D. & Nelson, K. (1991). Analysis of clinical trials by treatment actually received: is it really an option? *Statistics in Medicine*, **10**, 1595–605.

McKhann, G. (1989). The trials of clinical trials. *Archives of Neurology*, **46**, 611–14.

Mendel, W. (1986). Psychiatric treatment outcome research. *International Journal of Partial Hospitalization*, **3**, 151–7.

Neter, J., Wasserman,W. & Kutner M.H. (1985). *Applied Linear Statistical Models: Regression, Analysis of Variance and Experimental Designs*, 2nd edn. Homewood, IL: R.D. Irwin.

Newcombe, R. (1988). Evaluation of treatment effectiveness in psychiatric research. *British Journal of Psychiatry*, **152**, 696–7.

Newell, D.J. (1992). Intention-to-treat analysis: implications for quantitative and qualitative research. *International Journal of Epidemiology*, **21**, 837–41.

Peto, R., Pike, M., Armitage, P., Breslow, N., Cox, D., Howard, S., Mantel, N., McPherson, K., Peto, J. & Smith, P. (1976). Design and analysis of randomized clinical trials requiring prolonged observation of each patient. I. Introduction and design. *British Journal of Cancer*, **34**, 585–612.

Pocock, S. (1979). Allocation of patients to treatment in clinical trials. *Biometrics*, **35**, 183–97.

Pocock, S. (1987). *Clinical Trials: A Practical Approach*. Chichester: Wiley.

Sackett, D. & Gent, M. (1979). Controversy in counting and attributing events in clinical trials. *New England Journal of Medicine*, **300**, 1410–12.

Schwartz, D. & Lellouch, J. (1967). Explanatory and pragmatic attitudes in therapeutic trials. *Journal of Chronic Diseases*, **20**, 637–48.

Wiersma, D., Kluiter, H., Nienhuis, F., Rüphan, M. & Giel, R. (1991). Costs and benefits of day treatment with community care as an alternative to standard hospitalization for schizophrenic patients: a randomized controlled trial in the Netherlands. *Schizophrenia Bulletin*, **17**, 411–19.

Zelen, M. (1979). A new design for randomized clinical trials. *New England Journal of Medicine*, **300**, 1242–5.

17

Individual patient outcomes

MIRELLA RUGGERI AND MICHELE TANSELLA

Introduction

Already in 1958 the World Health Organization (WHO), in a declaration extended recently, stated that:

> Health is a state of complete physical, mental and social wellbeing and not merely the absence of disease and infirmity. (WHO, 1958, 1985)

In fact, an individual's illness is usually dramatically characterised by feelings of discomfort, or perceptions of change in usual functioning, which are not necessarily correlated with clinical signs and symptoms. A correct evaluation of health should be based on how the patient feels, on his or her individual judgement, in addition to clinical signs or symptoms. Moreover, in chronic illnesses treatments should be evaluated mainly in terms of whether they are more or less likely to lead to an outcome of a life worth living in social and psychological, as well as physical, terms.

The WHO concept of health implicitly defines the efficacy of an intervention as its ability to bring an individual to a condition of complete or partial wellbeing, and clearly emphasises: (1) *social functioning* as a complement of the clinical signs; (2) the *comprehensiveness* and the *multidimensionality* of the enquiry; (3) the *subjectivity* of the evaluation. The model for outcome evaluation proposed by the WHO is a complex one, far from the simple, symptom-based model that clinicians frequently have in mind when evaluating outcome. If such a complex approach seems to provide extremely important information in all medical disciplines, it becomes absolutely necessary in psychiatry. Among others, Schulberg & Bromet in 1981 individuated issues and strategies for the measurement of outcome which raise problems currently unsolved and stated that:

Outcome studies should be sophisticated if they are to be valid and useful to programme planning.

(Schulberg & Bromet, 1981)

Referring to, and extending, their statements, outcome studies should aim to answer the following questions: Which intervention is efficacious? On what parameters? According to whom? In which subjects? Under which conditions?

Evaluation of outcome has been neglected in psychiatry. The lack of knowledge on the efficacy of psychiatric interventions has been outlined recently by various authors (Wright *et al.*, 1989; Jenkins, 1990; Mirin & Namerow, 1991; Attkisson *et al.*, 1992). The task force instituted by the National Institute of Mental Health (NIMH) on the topic 'Caring for people with severe mental disorders: a national plan of research to improve services' affirms:

> The first major problem is that little is known about which treatments work and which severely mentally ill patients benefit in various outcomes and circumstances. Even when the efficacy of individual clinical modalities is known, empirical information is usually lacking about how to combine and sequence them to achieve optimal outcomes. This picture is further complicated by the heterogeneity of the population, of potential providers and settings for treatment delivery, and of relevant outcomes.

(Attkisson et al., 1992)

Various and contrasting resistances have been offered to the evaluation of outcome in psychiatry. Clinicians, on the one hand, have been dominated by the fear that the measurement of their interventions' outcome would inevitably be accompanied by reductionism and by the feeling that only the therapist who is directly involved in caring for the patient can fully comprehend the complexity of the patient's problems and be the judge of the care provided. Researchers, on the other hand, have tended to apply simple, quantitative measures, which often produced not only reductive, but sometimes also misleading, outcome evaluations. Clinical and epidemiological knowledge should, instead, be integrated in order to formulate guidelines for the measurement of outcome and develop appropriate instruments for such a measurement. As Michael Shepherd stated:

> In so doing it would bring *Epidemiological Psychiatry* alongside *Psychiatric Epidemiology* to help advance its prospects in the next, potentially most exciting phase of its development.

(Shepherd, 1985)

This chapter, though not providing an exhaustive review of work in the field, will try, on the basis of available knowledge, to define guidelines and areas of research in order appropriately to measure outcome of psychiatric interventions.

The efficacy of psychiatric interventions

Among the major problems that psychiatric epidemiology must face there is the difficulty in describing and quantifying the variety of approaches used (biological, psychological, rehabilitative, etc.), the variety of contexts (hospital, sheltered hostel, outpatient facility, community service, etc.) where these approaches can take place, and the modifications that theoretical approaches can undergo when applied in different contexts. Complex and integrated interventions, such as those which take place in community-based services, are very difficult both to quantify and to evaluate. Moreover, in psychiatry decisions on which intervention is more effective in a specific situation seem to be influenced more by the ideology of the professional and by the sociodemographic characteristics of the patient than by proved efficacy and shared knowledge (Katz *et al.*, 1969).

Evidence on the efficacy of the vast majority of psychiatric interventions is insufficient. This evidence will not be considered in detail here; for a review of such findings see Jenkins (1990), Attkisson *et al.* (1992) and Burti & Yastrebov (1993).

The indicators of outcome

Dissatisfaction with the information provided in long-term psychiatric illnesses by traditional indicators of outcome, such as mortality and morbidity rates, facilitated the use of data on the *structure* (physical lay-out, economic resources, personnel available) and, mainly, on the *process* (service utilisation) of care as indicators of outcome. The rationale for this idea was, on one hand, that illness severity is linearly correlated with service utilisation and, on the other hand, that service utilisation is linearly correlated with outcome. Nowadays it is clear that outcome and service utilisation are *not* linearly correlated and that service utilisation may depend on many variables other than outcome, such as patients' sociodemographic characteristics, relationship with professionals, resources available, and 'intrinsic' characteristics of the service itself (Bergner *et al.*, 1979; Goldberg & Huxley, 1980).

What are the variables that better represent the outcome of psychiatric care and what are the main principles for their measurement? As already stressed, the measurement of outcome should be multidimensional, should consider both clinical and social variables, and should represent the individual patient's experience.

Change over time in *psychiatric symptoms* has for a long time been the main criterion for the evaluation of outcome. The measurement of psychopathology (the severity and course of symptoms, and their aggregation into syndromes) and the formulation of diagnostic criteria have been the main areas of work for psychiatric epidemiology in recent decades (Thompson, 1989). The study of co-morbidity, and the efficacy of the interventions not only on the main disorder but also on the co-morbid one, is a newer area of study which has increasing interest in the field of outcome evaluation.

Increasing attention has been paid by researchers to the relationship between psychopathology and social functioning (Dohrenwend & Dohrenwend, 1974; de Jong *et al.*, 1985, 1986). Initially, the level of social dysfunctioning was believed to be merely an epiphenomenon of psychopathology, conveying no additional information to that derived from measurement of psychopathology alone. Research in this field has disproved this belief, by showing that psychopathology and social functioning are not necessarily correlated and may be relatively independent manifestations of a mental disorder, on both a cross-sectional and a longitudinal basis. Cross-sectional correlations range from weak (Blumental & Dielman, 1975;Dohrenwend *et al.*, 1981; de Jong *et al.*, 1986) to moderate (Weissman *et al.*, 1978; Paykel *et al.*, 1978; Serban & Gidynski, 1979; Pai & Kapur, 1982), and differ according to diagnostic category (Hecht & Wittchen, 1988). In a longitudinal perspective, social dysfunctioning tends to have a less favourable and more protracted course than psychopathology (Paykel & Weissman, 1973; Bothwell & Weissman, 1977; Platt *et al.*, 1981; Waryszak, 1982; de Jong *et al.*, 1986).

Social functioning appears to react to different types of interventions from those designed for the treatment of psychopathological symptoms (Bothwell & Weissman, 1977; Platt *et al.*, 1981); community-based treatments, in contrast to hospital-based treatments, seem to determine a more marked improvement in social functioning than in psychopathology (Mignolli *et al.*, 1991; Anderson *et al.*, 1993).

Among indicators of social outcome, *social support* seems to have a relevant role. Having good social support seems to be positively correlated with improvement in social functioning and recovery from illness, and negatively correlated with mortality, incidence of mental disorders and low morale (Berkman & Syme, 1979; Lin *et al.*, 1979; Cohen *et al.*, 1987; Maes *et al.*, 1987; Zimmermann-Tansella & Siciliani, 1990; Brugha, 1990; Zimmermann-Tansella *et al.*, 1993).

Increasing importance is being accorded to the *quality of life* as a social indicator of outcome (Lehman & Burns, 1990; Oliver, 1991). High priority should be given in the near future to studying the relationship between quality of life and psychopathology, social functioning and self-perceived wellbeing. *Burden* on relatives (Fadden *et al.*, 1987), and patients' and relatives' *needs* (Wing, 1990; Thornicroft *et al.*, 1992) are other areas which should be taken into account when studying outcome.

Another variable that is receiving increasing attention by researchers is *satisfaction with services*. As early as 1966 Donabedian stated that:

> ... the effectiveness of care in achieving and producing health and satisfaction, as defined for its individual members by a particular society or subculture, is the ultimate validator of the quality of care.
>
> *(Donabedian, 1966)*

Patients' satisfaction with services represents 'a general sense in which the clients, overall, felt positive or negative about interventions' (Sheppard, 1993) and 'is defined differently by individuals as a result of varying backgrounds and experiences' (Ware *et al.*, 1983). Satisfaction with services may be viewed as a desirable outcome of care. Further, satisfaction may illuminate results obtained when measuring other outcome variables (such as psychopathology, social functioning, quality of life and burden on relatives).

A significant association between the level of patient satisfaction and treatment outcome was found in a few studies (Lebow, 1983). Various findings point to a strong relationship between client assessment of satisfaction and client global reports of outcome, but to a less strong relationship between reported satisfaction and client reports of more specific change. It seems that this correlation is time-dependent, change and satisfaction being likely to be perceived more independently during the engagement process than later in treatment. The correlations between patient satisfaction and therapist-rated change measures have tended to be lower than those between patient satisfaction and patient-rated change measures. These findings indicate that therapist ratings of change and client ratings of satisfaction probably tap different domains and further emphasise the need for a multidimensional measurement of outcome.

More reseach is needed to clarify the relationship between satisfaction and other outcome variables. In the light of current knowledge satisfaction should be considered one of the outcome variables but not a *substitute* for the information provided by research utilising these variables or for professional judgement. Moreover, one should be clear that increasing a service recipient's satisfaction is not necessarily the main goal of a service and psychiatrists should not feel, as they often do, threatened by the process of assessing clients' satisfaction or obliged to fulfil all patients' requests in order to be judged positively. It is obvious that there may be times when fulfilling clients' requests may prove too difficult or too costly, or may not be clinically indicated. As previously mentioned, the correlation of satisfaction with other outcome variables seems to be time-correlated. *Short-term dissatisfaction* may in some cases be considered a 'side effect' of a therapeutic intervention which changes the patient's perspective (such as, for example, putting into practice a shift from institutional to community care, or pursuing a change in the relationship of the patient with significant others): apart from the risk of early drop-out from treatment (which, in this case, may be considered an unfavourable outcome) dissatisfaction here is, probably, scarcely representative of outcome and may not be a worrying event. A certain relevance should, instead, be given to consumers' dissatisfaction in the long term. *Long-term dissatisfaction*, in fact, may provide important information on the view of patients regarding the outcome of a specific intervention and may indicate that the planned change did not contribute to an improvement in their life: in this case the suitability of such an intervention should be seriously reconsidered. It may also indicate that consumers do not have enough personal resources to appreciate the advantages of that intervention: in this case, if not a change in the therapeutic strategy, at least an improvement in communication between consumers and professionals is necessary.

The prejudice that mental illness can completely deprive an individual of the capacity to make considered and rational judgements, and the fact that patients' statements are often considered useful only as a basis for making and confirming a diagnosis, certainly played a major role in reservations about the practicality and measurability of satisfaction (Brandon, 1981). The reality is that the empirical data refute this prejudice. Various studies, in fact, have found that patients are sensitive to verbal and non-verbal elements of the health care process, fairly accurate in distinguishing the quality of provider behaviours, such as courtesy and competence, and that they base their satisfaction ratings on these discriminations. The satisfaction ratings of patients have also been found to correspond to criteria for physician excellence customarily used by health providers, such as more years of training, positive motivation of the physician towards patients and peer supervision of physicians (for a review of these data see Lebow, 1983).

Subjectivity certainly causes problems in the measurement of satisfaction; on the other hand, assessing subjective variables seems to be a unique opportunity in service evaluation to take account of and examine the perspective of consumers. Recently, studies conducted in South Verona within the framework of a quantitative and qualitative evaluation of this community-based psychiatric service (Tansella, 1991) found that, by using a newly developed instrument, the Verona Service Satisfaction Scale (VSSS) (Ruggeri & Dall'Agnola, 1993; Ruggeri & Greenfield, 1995; Ruggeri *et al.*, 1994, 1995), it was possible to measure satisfaction of patients and relatives in an acceptable, sensitive, valid and stable way. For a review of the literature on the state of the art of satisfaction measurement see Ruggeri (1994).

The subjective perspective on outcome

If health is not only 'the absence of illness' but also 'a sense of subjective wellbeing' (WHO, 1985), the measurement of outcome should give due relevance to the subjective perspective of the person receiving the psychiatric care.

A problem still partially to be solved is the content validity of the measurement of outcome according to differing perspectives, such as those of patients, relatives and professionals. Differences in patients' and professionals' views on service delivery have, in fact, been reported (Mayer & Rosenblatt, 1974; Dowds & Fontana, 1977; Sorensen *et al.*, 1979; Ruggeri & Dall'Agnola, 1993); if the user's perspective is not included, then there is a risk that outcome evaluation may be distorted within the narrow perception of the provider. However, instruments for the measurement of psychopathology and, to a certain extent, social functioning, rely heavily on

standards generated by professionals; their content validity according
to clients' views has seldom been studied. Moreover, differences in the
views of medical and paramedical personnel on patient outcome
should not be underestimated. Further, it is commonly believed that
relatives too may have requests, needs and views on the service which
markedly differ from those of patients (Solomon *et al.*, 1988; Grella &
Grusky, 1989).

Instruments for measuring outcome should, therefore, possibly
allow a *multiaxial evaluation*, so as to consider simultaneously the views
of all these groups. This seems to be a fundamental requisite in those
settings, such as community-based psychiatric services, where all
these groups interact continuously.

The importance of considering the subjective perspective further
outlines the role of parameters such as an individual's satisfaction,
needs, and burden on relatives in the measurement of outcome; it
should, however, be emphasised that differing perspectives among
these subjects is not only a requisite of 'softer' variables such as those
mentioned, but also of 'harder' variables such as severity of clinical
symptoms and impairment in social functioning (Brewin *et al.*, 1990;
Attkisson *et al.*, 1992).

The predictors of outcome

Epidemiological knowledge regarding predictors of outcome is clearly
needed. Of the research work done in this area, studies on predictors
of outcome are especially relevant; we will mention this body of work
only in passing in this chapter.

Diagnosis has been shown to predict the pattern of contact with
psychiatric services, and especially the type of treatment and its
length (Tansella *et al.*, 1986, 1995), but its relationship with outcome
seems to be a complex one. For example, if schizophrenia in some
studies has been shown to have a worse clinical and social outcome
than other disorders (such as schizoaffective disorder, major depression,
borderline personality disorder) (McGlashan 1984, 1986a), other
studies have shown that the outcome of schizophrenia is not necessarily
bad and depends on a variety of factors such as symptom severity at
onset, co-morbidity, relatives' expressed emotions, social support,
working conditions and stressful events (English *et al.*, 1986; McGlashan,
1986b, c, 1991; Avison & Speechley, 1987; Falloon *et al.*, 1987;

Harding *et al.*, 1987; Gabel & Pietzcher, 1987). *The International Pilot Study on Schizophrenia (IPSS)* and the *Study on the Determinants of Outcome of Severe Mental Disorders (DOSMED)* promoted by WHO showed a better outcome in developing than in developed countries (WHO, 1973, 1979; Jablensky *et al.*, 1992).

When evaluating the outcome of severe psychiatric illnesses, one should have clearly in mind that a complete clinical and social recovery is not always a realistic outcome and that the impact of treatments should be evaluated on the basis of this awareness. The possibility of defining the 'best possible outcome' in different subjects and different conditions goes together with obtaining knowledge on the *natural course* of mental disorders. This is an area it is extremely difficult to study due, on one hand, to the rarity of untreated severe diseases and, on the other, to the difficulty in following-up such conditions. A good example of this difficulty is the fact that long-term effects of institutionalisation have often been wrongly interpreted as signs of the natural course of schizophrenia (Abrahamson, 1993).

The lack of *specificity* and of *longitudinality* are among the main limitations of studies on outcome. Finally, the issue of treatment *drop-outs* should be raised when considering individual patients' outcomes from a wider point of view. Is dropping out from treatment an index of improvement or worsening of subjective wellbeing? Is it an index of dissatisfaction with service received? Is it an index of community stigma deriving from attending psychiatric services?

Conclusions

In the coming years an effort should be made to promote the habit of measuring outcome in a multidimensional, specific and longitudinal way. Specifically, a unique and challenging task faces researchers assessing the outcome of community-based care. In fact, despite the great number of studies published on community care, very little knowledge exists on the outcome of the integrated interventions which can take place in community-based psychiatric services. Here, a highly sophisticated multivariate research design is required: evaluation must become able to focus upon multiple components of care, consider heterogeneity of staff, patients and their families, and assess both subjective and objective variables. It is, however, unlikely that a large number of projects will be able to establish and maintain the complex protocols and methodological requirements needed for such designs. Different strategies should, therefore, be amalgamated and, through a sort of 'triangulation of findings', a better comprehension of outcome should be obtained by combining different types of studies.

Though not numerous, some controlled experimental studies on the outcome of specific interventions in community-based settings exist; instead, there is a lack of naturalistic studies. In the future, therefore, naturalistic studies should complement experimental studies. For this reason it is necessary to plan and produce survey studies in community settings that have as their main objective the multidimensional measure of outcome of mental health care interventions, possibly by using standardised instruments as part of the routine clinical activities within community-based psychiatric services.

A pilot study to test the feasibility of performing a standardised routine evaluation of the outcome in the South Verona community-based psychiatric service (a service operating since 1978 designed to be an alternative to, rather than to complement, hospital-based services and based on the principles of continuity and comprehensiveness of care; Tansella, 1991) and in the South Camberwell community-based psychiatric service (a service recently set-up, aiming at putting into practice a similar model to the Italian one), has been jointly promoted by the Department of Medical Psychology at the University of Verona, Italy, and by PRiSM at the Institute of Psychiatry of the University of London. The following indicators of outcome will be measured on a regular basis: psychopathology (Brief Psychiatric Rating Scale; Lukoff *et al.*,1986), social functioning (Disability Assessment Schedule; WHO, 1988), needs for care (Camberwell Assessment of Needs; Phelan & Slade, 1993), quality of life (Lancashire Quality of Life Profile; Oliver, 1991) and satisfaction with services (Verona Service Satisfaction Scale; Ruggeri & Dall'Agnola, 1993). Results obtained in this study will provide further evidence on theoretical and methodological problems in the multidimensional measurement of outcome and indicate areas where specific research is needed.

Developing and testing instruments for the measurement of outcome according to an approach which combines quantitative and qualitative, objective and subjective evaluation, and disseminating their use widely, will be one of the most important challenges of psychiatric epidemiology in the next decade.

Acknowledgements

This work was supported by the Consiglio Nazionale delle Ricerche (CNR, Roma), Progetto Finalizzato Fattori di Malattia (FATMA), Sottoprogetto 'Stress', Contracts no. 92.00186.PF41 and no. 93.00743.PF41 to Professor M. Tansella.

References

Abrahamson, D. (1993). Instituzionalization and the long-term course of schizophrenia. *British Journal of Psychiatry*, **162**, 533–8.

Anderson, J., Dayson, D., Wills, D., Gooch, C., *et al.* (1993). The TAPS project. XIII. Clinical and social outcomes of long-stay psychiatric patients after one year in the community. *British Journal of Psychiatry*, **162**, Suppl. 19, 45–56.

Attkisson, C., Cook, J., Karno, M., Lehman, A., *et al.* (1992). Clinical services research. *Schizophrenia Bulletin*, **18**, 627–68.

Avison, W.R. & Speechley, K.N. (1987). The discharged psychiatric patient: a review of social, social-psychological, and psychiatric correlates of outcome. *American Journal of Psychiatry*, **144**, 10–18.

Bergner, M., Bobbit, R.A., Kressel, S., *et al.* (1979). The sickness impact profile: conceptual formulation and methodology for the development of a health status measure. In *Sociomedical Health Indicators*, ed. J. Elinson & A.E. Siegmann. New York: Baywood.

Berkman, L.F. & Syme, S.L. (1979). Social networks, host resistance and mortality: a nine-year follow-up study of Alameda County residents. *American Journal of Epidemiology*, **109**, 186–204.

Blumenthal, M.D. & Dielman, T.E. (1975). Depressive symptomatology and role functioning in a general population. *Archives of General Psychiatry*, **32**, 985–91.

Bothwell, S. & Weissman, M.M. (1977). Social impairment four years after an acute depressive episode. *American Journal of Orthopsychiatry*, **47**, 231–7.

Brandon, D. (1981). *Voices of Experience: Consumer Perspectives of Psychiatric Treatment*. London: MIND.

Brewin, C.R., Veltro, F., Wing, J.K., McCarthy, B. & Brugha, T.S. (1990). The assessment of psychiatric disability in the community: a comparison of clinical, staff, and family interviews. *British Journal of Psychiatry*, **157**, 671–4.

Brugha, T.S. (1990). Social networks and support. *Current Opinion in Psychiatry*, **3**, 264–8.

Burti, L. & Yastrebov, V. (1993). Evaluation of procedures used in rehabilitation. In *Evaluation of Treatment Outcome in Psychiatry*. Geneva: World Health Organization.

Cohen, S., Mermelstein, R., Karmack, T., *et al.* (1987). Social network and mortality in an inner city elderly population. *International Journal of Ageing and Human Development*, **24**, 257–69.

Dohrenwend, B.P. & Dohrenwend, B.S. (1974). Social and cultural influences on psychopathology. *Annual Review of Psychology*, **25**, 417–52.

Dohrenwend, B.S., Cook, D. & Dohrenwend, B.P. (1981). Measurement of social functioning in community populations. In *What is a Case? The Problem of Definition in Psychiatric Community Surveys*, ed. J.K. Wing, P. Bebbington & L.N. Robins, pp. 183–201. London: Grant McIntyre.

Donabedian, A. (1966). Evaluating the quality of medical care. *Mildbank Memorial Fund Quarterly*, **44**, 166–203.

Dowds, B. & Fontana, A. (1977). Patients' and therapists' expectations and evaluations of hospital treatment. *Comprehensive Psychiatry*, **18**, 295–300.

English, J.T., Sharfstein, S.S., Scherl, D.J., *et al.* (1986). Diagnosis-related groups and general hospital psychiatry: the APA study. *American Journal of Psychiatry*, **143**, 131–9.

Fadden, G., Bebbington, F. & Kuipers, L. (1987). The burden of care: the impact of functional psychiatric illness on the patient's family. *British Journal of Psychiatry*, **150**, 285–93.

Falloon, I.R.H., McGill, C.W., Boyd, J.L., *et al.* (1987). Family management in the prevention of morbidity of schizophrenia: social outcome of a two year longitudinal study. *Psychological Medicine*, **17**, 59–66.

Gabel, W. & Pietzcher, A. (1987). Prospective study of course of illness in schizophrenia. III. Treatment and outcome. *Schizophrenia Bulletin*, **13**, 307–16.

Goldberg, D. & Huxley, P. (1980). *Mental Illness in the Community: The Pathway to Psychiatric Care*. London: Tavistock.

Grella, C.E. & Grusky, O. (1989). Families of the seriously mentally ill and their satisfaction with services. *Hospital and Community Psychiatry*, **40**, 831–5.

Harding, C.M., Brooks, G.W., Ashikaga, T., *et al.* (1987). The Vermont longitudinal study of persons with severe mental illness. II. Long-term outcome of subjects who retrospectively met DSM-III criteria for schizophrenia. *American Journal of Psychiatry*, **144**, 727–35.

Hecht, H. & Wittchen, H.U. (1988). The frequency of social dysfunction in a general population sample and in patients with mental disorders. *Social Psychiatry and Psychiatric Epidemiology*, **23**, 17–29.

Jablensky, A., Sartorius, N., Ernberg, G., *et al.* (1992). *Schizophrenia: Manifestations, Incidence and Course in Different Cultures. A World Health Organization Ten-Country Study*. Psychological Medicine Monograph Supplement 20. Cambridge: Cambridge University Press.

Jenkins, R. (1990). Toward a system of outcome indicators for mental health care. *British Journal of Psychiatry*, **157**, 500–14.

Jong, A.de, Giel, R., Soloff, C.J. & Wiersma, D. (1985). Social disabilities and outcome in schizophrenic patients. *British Journal of Psychiatry*, **147**, 621–36.

Jong, A.de, Giel, R., Soloff, C. & Wiersma, D. (1986). Relationship between symptomatology and social disability. *Social Psychiatry*, **21**, 200–14.

Katz, M.M., Cole, J.O. & Lowery, H.A. (1969). Studies of the diagnostic process: the influence of symptom perception, past experience, and ethnic background on diagnostic decisions. *American Journal of Psychiatry*, **125**, 937–46.

Lebow, J.L. (1983). Similarities and differences between mental health and health care evaluation studies assessing consumer satisfaction. *Evaluation and Program Planning*, **6**, 237–45.

Lehman, A.F. & Burns, B.J. (1990). Severe mental illness in the community: quality of life assessment. In *Quality of Life Assessments in Clinical Trials*, ed. B. Spilker. New York: Raven Press.

Lin, N., Simeone, R., Ensel, W., *et al.* (1979). Social support, stressful life events and illness: a model and an empirical test. *Journal of Health and Social Behaviour*, **20**, 108–19.

Lukoff, D., Nuechterlein, K. & Ventura, J. (1986). Appendix A. Manual for expanded Brief Psychiatric Rating Scale (BPRS). *Schizophrenia Bulletin*, **4**, 594–602.

Maes, S., Vingerhoets, A. & Van Heck, G. (1987). The study of stress and disease: some developments and requirements. *Social Science and Medicine*, **25**, 567–78.

Mayer, J. & Rosenblatt, A. (1974). Clash in perspective between mental patients and staff. *American Journal of Orthopsychiatry*, **44**, 432–41.

McGlashan, T.H. (1984). The Chestnut Lodge follow-up study. II. Long-term outcome of schizophrenia and the affective disorders. *Archives of General Psychiatry*, **41**, 586–601.

McGlashan, T.H. (1986a). The Chestnut Lodge follow-up study. III. Long-term outcome of borderline personalities. *Archives of General Psychiatry*, **43**, 20–30.

McGlashan, T.H. (1986b). The Chestnut Lodge follow-up study. IV. The prediction of outcome in chronic schizophrenia. *Archives of General Psychiatry*, **43**, 167–76.

McGlashan, T.H. (1986c). Predictors of shorter-, medium-, and longer-term outcome in schizophrenia. *American Journal of Psychiatry*, **143**, 50–5.

McGlashan, T.H. (1991). Selective review of recent North American long-term follow-up studies of schizophrenia. In *Psychiatric Treatment: Advances in Outcome Research*, ed. S.M. Mirin, J.T. Grosset & J.C. Grob. Washington, DC: American Psychiatric Press.

Mignolli, G., Faccincani, C. & Platt, S. (1991). Psychopathology and social performance in a cohort of patients with schizophrenic psychoses: a seven year follow-up study. In *Community-Based Psychiatry: Long Term Patterns of Care in South-Verona*, ed. M. Tansella. Psychological Medicine Monograph Supplement 19. Cambridge: Cambridge University Press.

Mirin, S.M. & Namerow, M.J. (1991). Why study treatment outcome? *Hospital and Community Psychiatry*, **42**, 1007–13.

Oliver, J.P. (1991). The social care directive: development of a quality of life profile for use in community services for the mentally ill. *Social Work and Social Science Review*, **3**, 4–45.

Pai, S. & Kapur, R.L. (1982). Impact of treatment intervention on the relationship between dimensions of clinical psychopathology, social disfunctioning and burden on the family of psychiatric inpatients. *Psychological Medicine*, **12**, 651–8.

Paykel, E.S. & Weissman, M.M. (1973). Social adjustment and depression. *Archives of General Psychiatry*, **28**, 659–63.

Paykel, E.S., Weissman, M.M. & Prusoff, B.A. (1978). Social maladjustment and severity of depression. *Comprehensive Psychiatry*, **19**, 121–8.

Phelan, M. & Slade, M. (1993). The development of the CAN (Camberwell Assessment of Needs). Paper presented at Community Care: Making It Work: the first PRISM Conference.

Platt, S., Hirsh, S.R. & Knights, A.C. (1981). Effects of brief hospitalization on psychiatric patients' behavior and social functioning. *Acta Psychiatrica Scandinavica*, **63**, 117–28.

Ruggeri, M. (1994). Patients' and relatives' satisfaction with psychiatric services: the state of the art of its measurement. In *Designing Instruments for Mental Health Service Research*, part 1, ed. G. Thornicroft & M. Tansella. *Social Psychiatry and Psychiatric Epidemiology*, **28**, 212–27.

Ruggeri, M. & Dall'Agnola, R. (1993). The development and use of the Verona Expectations for Care Scale (VECS) and the Verona Service Satisfaction Scale (VSSS) for measuring expectations and satisfaction with community-based psychiatric services in patients, relatives and professionals. *Psychological Medicine*, **23**, 511–23.

Ruggeri, M. & Greenfield, T. (1995). The Italian version of the Service Satisfaction Scale (SSS-30) adapted for community-based psychiatric services: development, factor analysis and application. *Evaluation and Program Planning*, **18**, 191–202.

Ruggeri, M., Dall'Agnola, R., Agostini, C. & Bisoffi, G. (1994). Acceptability, sensitivity and content validity of VECS and VSSS in measuring expectations and satisfaction in psychiatric patients and their relatives. *Social Psychiatry and Psychiatric Epidemiology*, **29**, 265–76.

Ruggeri, M., Dall'Agnola, R., Greenfield, T. & Bisoffi, G. (1995). Factor analysis of the Verona Service Satisfaction Scale-82 and development of reduced versions. *International Journal of Methods in Psychiatric Research*, **5**, 147.

Schulberg, H.C. & Bromet, E. (1981). Strategies for evaluating the outcome of community services for the chronically mentally ill. *American Journal of Psychiatry*, **138**, 930–5.

Serban, D. & Gidynski, C.B. (1979). Relationship between cognitive defect, affect response and community adjustment in chronic schizophrenics. *British Journal of Psychiatry*, **134**, 602–8.

Shepherd, M. (1985). Psychiatric epidemiology and epidemiological psychiatry. *American Journal of Public Health*, **75**, 275–6.

Shepherd, M. (1993). Client satisfaction, extended intervention and interpersonal skills in community mental health. *Journal of Advanced Nursing*, **18**, 246–59.

Solomon, P., Beck, S. & Gordon, B. (1988). Family members' perspective on psychiatric hospitalization and discharge. *Community Mental Health*

Journal, **24**, 108–17.

Sorensen, J., Kantor, L., Margolis, R. & Galano, J. (1979). The extent, nature and utility of evaluating consumer satisfaction in community mental health centers. *American Journal of Community Psychology*, **7**, 329–37.

Tansella, M. (ed.) (1991). *Community-Based Psychiatry: Long Term Patterns of Care in South-Verona*. Psychological Medicine Monograph Supplement 19. Cambridge: Cambridge University Press.

Tansella, M., Micciolo, R., Balestrieri, M. & Gavioli, I. (1986). High and long-term users of the mental health services: a case-register study in Italy. *Social Psychiatry*, **21**, 96–103.

Tansella, M., Micciolo, R., Biggeri, A., Bisoffi, G. & Balestrieri, M. (1995). Episodes of care in first-ever psychiatric patients: a long-term case-register evaluation in a mainly urban area. *British Journal of Psychiatry*, **167**, 220–7.

Thompson, C. (ed.) (1989). *The Instruments of Psychiatric Research*. New York: Wiley.

Thornicroft, G., Brewin, C. & Wing, J. (eds.) (1992). *Measuring Mental Health Needs*. London: Gaskell/Royal College of Psychiatrists.

Ware, J.E., Snyder, M.K., Wright, W.R. & Davies, A.R. (1983). Defining and measuring patient satisfaction with medical care. *Evaluation and Program Planning*, **6**, 247–63.

Waryszak, Z. (1982). Symptomatology and social functioning of psychiatric patients before and after hospitalization. *Social Psychiatry*, **17**, 149–54.

Weissman, M.M., Prusoff, B.A. & Thompson, W.D. (1978). Social adjustment by self report in a community sample and in psychiatric outpatients. *Journal of Nervous and Mental Disease*, **166**, 317–26.

WHO (1958). *The First Ten Years: The Health Organization*. Geneva: World Health Organization.

WHO (1973). *The International Pilot Study of Schizophrenia*, vol. I. Geneva: World Health Organization.

WHO (1979). *Schizophrenia: An International Follow-up Study*. Chichester: Wiley.

WHO (1985). *Targets for Health for All by the Year 2000*. Copenhagen: World Health Organization, Regional Office for Europe.

WHO (1988). *Disability Assessment Schedule (DAS-II)*. Geneva: World Health Organization.

Wing, J.K. (1990). Meeting the needs of people with psychiatric disorders. *Social Psychiatry and Psychiatric Epidemiology*, **25**, 2–8.

Wright, R.G., Heiman, J.R., Shupe, J. & Olvera, G. (1989). Defining and measuring stabilization of patients during 4 years of intensive community support. *American Journal of Psychiatry*, **146**, 1293–8.

Zimmermann-Tansella, C. & Siciliani, O. (1990). Social problems, social support and emotional distress in the community. In *The Public Health Impact of Mental Disorder*, ed. D. Goldberg & D. Tantam. Toronto: Hogrefe & Huber.

Zimmermann-Tansella, C., Donini, S., Galvan, U., *et al.* (1993). Social support, adversities and emotional distress in an Italian community sample. *Journal of Clinical Epidemiology*, **46**, 65–75.

18

Caregiving in severe mental illness: conceptualisation and measurement

AART H. SCHENE, RICHARD C. TESSLER AND
GAIL M. GAMACHE

Introduction

Severe mental disorders such as schizophrenia, bipolar and major depression, and personality disorders may represent obstacles to independent living and life satisfaction for those who suffer from them. Employment opportunities may be reduced, self-care may be impeded, and the capacity for social relationships may be severely diminished. In most cases these problems involve a serious disruption of the patient's expected life course, and may have profound caregiving consequences for family members. It is in this sense that family or caregiver burden is relevant to mental health service evaluation.

The purpose of this chapter is to assist mental health services researchers in conceptualising and measuring family burden. We elaborate the concept of caregiving and set it within the context of changing policies towards adult persons with severe mental disorders, provide a summary of studies of family burden and mental illness since the 1950s, and discuss methodological issues in conducting family burden research. A major point to be discussed is how caregiver burden may be incorporated as a measure in mental health service evaluation. The chapter concludes with implications for improving family outcomes and needs for future research.

Over the life cycle, caregiving can involve parents caring for a mentally ill adult child, adult children caring for a mentally ill parent, a well spouse caring for an ill spouse, or a sibling caring for a disabled brother or sister. Excluded from this chapter, although important, are caregiving to minor children with serious developmental disorders and to the elderly with dementias (see Biegel *et al.*, 1991).

The concept of caregiving

Caregiving needs to be distinguished from dependency relationships that are age appropriate and culturally expected. We begin and may end our lives with a period of dependency during which it is crucial to our own survival and that of our species that others provide care and support. The institution that typically provides this care is the family unit. Kinship ties are among the most enduring of all supports available, although expectations may vary from culture to culture, and from one historical era to another. In modern industrialised societies, adult persons are expected to be independent of their family of origin and to care for themselves from the moment they end their education until they retire from the (paid) labour force.

Caregiving is a relatively modern concept that has come to describe the relationship the exists between *adult* individuals who are related through kinship. One, the caregiver, assumes an unpaid and unanticipated responsibility for another. That second, the care recipient, is typically disabled and unable to fulfil the reciprocal obligations associated with normative adult relationships. Care becomes caregiving when it is out of synchrony with the appropriate stage in the life cycle. Caregivers are bound by kinship obligations that go beyond those normatively associated with a family role at a particular stage. It is the addition of the caregiving role to existing family roles which makes it burdensome, although caregiving may also be a source of satisfaction (Fisher *et al.*, 1990; Bulger *et al.*, 1993). In virtually all societies caregivers are disproportionately female (Ascher-Svanum & Sobel, 1989).

Changing policies towards persons with mental illness

Social policies towards persons with mental illness in the last three decades mandate an increasing emphasis on community care. This *deinstitutionalisation* movement brought age-old responsibilities back to family members, who saw themselves after a hundred years of a policy of institutionalisation confronted with *new obligations* towards their ill or handicapped members. This policy has often been blamed for increasing the burden on patients' relatives.

Although the situation differs from country to country, it is estimated that between one-third and one-half of patients live with family (Lamb & Oliphant, 1978; Fisher *et al.*, 1990; Schene & van Wijngaarden, 1993). If family relationships are more traditional, or if residential alternatives are scarce, the proportion living with family members may be substantially higher (Arey & Warheit, 1980; Thompson & Doll, 1982).

The family remains the safety net of last resort, and when this obligation is accepted, the family will surely find itself involved with the patient during crisis, whether or not they live in the same household (Tessler *et al.*, 1987). As informal providers, families worry about the lack of mental health care in the community, poor communication with professionals, strain between patient and family members, and in some cases the prospect that the patient might become homeless (Carpentier *et al.*, 1992).

Previous research on caregiver burden

Perspectives have changed on the meaning of mental illness for family members of persons with severe mental illness. We can distinguish three historical periods of research:

1940–1960

Although most family burden research is associated with deinstitutionalisation, Treudley (1946) studied family reactions to mental illness as early as the 1940s. Her descriptive study noted many aspects that were to become focal points in later burden research. She was especially concerned about the effects on children.

In the mid-1950s Clausen and Yarrow dedicated a special edition of the *Journal of Social Issues to* 'Mental Illness and the Family'. Their study of 33 families in which a husband with a mental disorder was hospitalised is the classic sociological study of the impact of mental illness on the family. Although the sample was small and limited to wives, the study was the first to examine systematically the family reaction to mental illness using such concepts as social perception, labelling, deviance, changing role structures and coping (Clausen & Yarrow, 1955).

During the 1950s, interest in attitudes towards the mentally ill steadily increased in conjunction with the emerging influences of the social sciences and community psychiatry. It now became essential to ascertain under which conditions persons with mental illness could live their own lives among 'normal people' in an acceptable way. The first studies on the effects of short-term hospital treatment were carried out in the United Kingdom by Brown *et al.* (1958) and in the United States by Freeman & Simmons (1958, 1959). Lystad (1958) was the first to study attitudes of family members towards day care. Rose (1959) investigated the attitudes of relatives of patients after long-term hospitalisation.

1960–1975

In the 1960s more data on attitudes, labelling (Scheff, 1966), stigma (Cumming & Cumming, 1965), and specific effects of different kinds of psychiatric treatments became available. Lewis & Zeichner (1960) studied the impact of admission to a mental hospital on the patient's family. Evans *et al.* (1961) and Deykin (1961) studied chronic schizophrenic patients returning home after hospitalisations of at least 5 years.

Mandelbrote & Folkard (1961), investigating mental health care in Gloucester, England, were among the first researchers to investigate the degree of burden resulting from community psychiatry. They concluded that community psychiatry may result in 'burden to the family', but that, as Freeman & Simmons (1959) had earlier observed, different families have 'differential tolerance of deviance'.

Dudgeon, Wing and Waters studied recently discharged patients in the United Kingdom. Dudgeon (1964) conducted structured interviews with 471 patients or their relatives, and found in 30% of cases a serious disturbance of family life. Wing *et al.* (1964) studied the correlation between family relations and the course of the patient's illness after discharge. Waters & Northover (1965) conducted a follow-up study of 42 long-stay patients with schizophrenia following discharge from a mental hospital rehabilitation unit. They observed that families needed a considerable amount of help to deal with severe types of burden.

Hoenig & Hamilton (1966a, b) were the first to distinguish objective and subjective burden. They defined objective burden as the effects on the household and subjective burden as the informant's own perception of whether the household had suffered some degree of burden.

In the 1960s, only two *controlled* studies were conducted in which family burden was one of the outcome measures. Grad & Sainsbury (1963, 1968) performed a non-randomised controlled trial comparing hospital-based service and community care, concluding that the latter resulted in more 'social cost'. Pasamanick *et al.* (1967) compared treatment in a state hospital versus home care with medication for admittable schizophrenic patients and found no significant difference in burden.

At the beginning of the 1970s, Kreisman & Joy (1974) reviewed family responses to mental illness of a relative. Their seminal review was to be the only synthesis of this literature for at least 15 years.

During this period improvements in the measures for assessing burden were made by a number of investigators, including an interview protocol developed by Spitzer *et al.* (1971). The focus of attention also became broader so as to include not only the negative impact of the patient on the family (burden), but also the negative influence of family members on patients (expressed emotion).

1975

From the mid-1970s onwards, three different scientific traditions relating to caregiver research can be distinguished. First there was theoretical and empirical interest in the burden concept and its measurement (Platt *et al.*, 1980; Schene, 1986; Tessler *et al.*, 1987). Although most earlier literature focused especially on schizophrenia, more recently Fadden (1984), Fadden *et al.* (1987), Jacob *et al.* (1987), Coyne *et al.* (1987) and Chakrabarti *et al.* (1992) have studied burden in relatives of patients with affective disorders.

Second, progress was made in developing more sophisticated instruments, and using burden as an outcome measure in mental health service evaluation (Stein *et al.*, 1975; Platt *et al.*, 1980), and in controlled studies (Washburn *et al.*, 1976; Herz *et al.*, 1977; Fenton *et al.*, 1979; Pai & Kaipur, 1982; Reynoulds & Hoult, 1984).

Third, theoretical findings on burden and expressed emotion (Brown *et al.*, 1972) were gradually incorporated into treatment programmes with a psycho-educational approach (Beels, 1978; Leff *et al.*, 1982; Kopeikon *et al.*, 1983; Falloon & Liberman, 1983; Anderson *et al.*, 1986). The last decade has witnessed a proliferation of studies of psychosocial intervention with families in which a member suffers from schizophrenia. The studies in the early 1980s were based on the assumption that high expressed emotion resulted from a lack of knowledge. Hence a gain in knowledge among family members was one of the outcome measures. A second generation of studies is evaluating the impact of educational programmes on the relatives' distress and objective burden (Lam, 1991).

The nature of the caregiver burden

The negative consequences of being related to someone suffering from severe mental illness can be roughly divided into the obligation to offer long-term extensive *care* and the emotional *distress* and *worries* related to the patient. The former requires close contact between patient and family member, while the latter may also exist when kinship ties have unravelled or the amount of contact is very small. Graham (1983) described this distinction as caring *for* and caring *about*.

Relationships

Either caring for or caring about the patient may have an impact on family and marital relationships, as well as on social relations outside the household. When reciprocal relationships are disrupted by illness, other family members may be forced to take on a greater proportion of formerly shared tasks. As a consequence the interpersonal relationships within the household can become strained. In cases of spouses, disruption of the marital relationship is not uncommon, and 'living together apart' and divorce are prevalent.

Just as the personality of the relative suffering from mental illness may change, so may the relationship with that person. Some family members experience a sense of loss with accompanying grief, comparable to the process of bereavement (Miller *et al.*, 1990). The great difference, however, is that with mental illness the 'lost' person stays alive and the relationship may need to be reconstructed.

Relationships outside the household may also be affected adversely, first by having less time to spend on social relations, and second by social stigma for both the patient and family members, leading primary kin in extreme cases to attempt to conceal their relative's mental illness. In addition, many caregivers have ambivalent relationships with mental health professionals. They often report feeling unsupported, uninformed, misinformed, and blamed and judged, which reinforces feelings of guilt. Any of the above may influence the amount of social contact outside the family and result in a profound sense of isolation. The loss of social network and accompanying loss of social support may have a further negative impact on the psychological wellbeing of family members.

Stages

Responses can be described in terms of stages, although the process of adaptation varies from family to family. In the first phase of the illness family members are uncertain about the disorder itself and the consequences of it. Once they know and accept the diagnosis, they want to have the best treatment available, but may not have the money to pay for mental health service, or do not know where to obtain help. In later stages they might be worried if the patient does not seek any treatment at all, if he or she is going in and out of hospitals without any progress, or in extreme cases is wandering through the streets, eating from dustbins, and using alcohol or drugs.

Some family members must live with uncertainty because they have lost all contact, and do not know where their mentally ill relative can be found. When family members are in contact with the patient, and particularly when the patient is dependent on them financially and in other ways, they worry about the future and what will happen to the patient when they are no longer there to help (Gubman *et al.*, 1987; Tessler *et al.*, 1987).

Caring and coping

Family members who choose to remain involved often provide a great deal of assistance in activities of daily living: provision of personal care, cooking, doing household chores and laundry, shopping, and helping with transportation. Some of them also have to learn to cope with frightening, troublesome, disruptive or annoying psychiatric symptoms such as delusions, hallucinations, attention seeking, stealing, inappropriate sexual behaviour, making unreasonable demands, being verbally abusive, being noisy at night, behaviours that are threatening or violent, talk or threats of suicide, and drug abuse. Coping with these symptoms and behaviours may often require lengthy, complex and distressing negotiations.

Finances

If the onset of mental illness comes after the attainment of gainful employment, there may be financial consequences when the patient is not able to work at all or when because of the illness he or she works fewer hours. Caregiving may also force relatives to work less or to give up their jobs. Ironically this may occur along with a rise in expenses related to psychiatric or health care, and medication. Other economic repercussions may flow from the patient's inability to manage money, or as a result of destructive behaviour.

Children

When the patient is also a parent, it may be necessary for other family members to help in caring for the minor child(ren). Although most of the more severely mentally ill do not have children, the negative effect of a psychiatric disabled parent on his or her children has been studied by burden researchers from the very beginning. There is also a separate scientific tradition in which the mental health of the child is the focus of attention. In these investigations, growing up with a parent with mental illness is studied as a risk factor for the healthy psychological development of the child (Doniger, 1962; Anthony, 1969; Beardslee *et al.*, 1983; Silverman, 1989; Dunn, 1993).

Health

Caring for or about a mentally ill relative may have consequences for the physical and mental health of the family members involved. These health consequences are typically the result of chronic stress. While rare, there are also reported cases of injuries resulting from physical abuse by the patient.

Thus, caregiver burden is a general concept, referring to a broad range of difficulties experienced by family members in caring for and dealing with their mentally ill relatives. It does not lend itself to a single measure but rather invites a multidimensional approach (Hatfield, 1978; Platt, 1985; Tessler *et al.*, 1987; Wahl & Harman, 1989; Schene, 1990).

Methodological issues

The preceding discussion of the nature of burden clearly shows the range of problems, and the variety of family relationships that are affected. It is evident that the study of family burden hinges on how it is defined and measured, who in the family is interviewed, and the theory that underlies the analysis of the collected data. How researchers resolve such issues will have much to do with the results and interpretations, as well as the generalisability and applicability, of the research.

Sampling and design

Most recent studies of family burden are actually studies of primary caregivers. In a typical study, patients are asked to identify the family member with whom they are most involved on a daily basis, or who provides them with the most support or care. Some studies further limit the sample to carers who are living with the patient. This also implies that in most cases *family burden* is a misnomer, in as much as all family members are rarely, if ever, interviewed. The term *caregiver burden* better describes most recent studies.

Research indicates that substantially higher levels of burden will be detected if the sample is limited to those primary caregivers who are currently living with the patient. However, co-residence does not necessarily determine involvement with the patient, since even family members who live apart may sustain high levels of personal involvement, while people living under the same roof may interact negatively or not at all.

Sampling issues are clearly linked to the research questions. For instance without interviewing multiple kin, examination of the distribution of burden in families is possible in only the most limited ways. If only primary caregivers are investigated, no information is available about family members not presently involved with the patient, such as siblings, who may be asked to 'take up the slack' when parental caregivers age and die. If, however, the aim is to evaluate whether burden is reduced by a programme designed for carers, then selecting for primary caregivers may be more appropriate.

In designing studies of family burden, it is important to build into the research design one or more meaningful bases for comparison.

Various alternatives exist. One is to study large samples, and to compare diagnostic groups, different types of family members, and different living conditions. Another possibility, rarely pursued, is to use a comparison group of families without a member with mental illness, as Clark & Drake (1993) recently did in analysing economic burden. Other solutions to the *compared to what* problem are to investigate the same population over time, treating each individual family member as his or her own control, or to incorporate experimental and control groups into the research design.

To increase the generalisability of descriptive research, it is necessary that characteristics of the patient and caregiver, their relationships and residential arrangements be carefully described. Such information gives other researchers and policy makers the opportunity to judge the relevance and generalisability of research findings. Ultimately, meta-analysis combining results from different studies may provide the most comprehensive picture of family and caregiver burden.

Measurement issues

Recently we collected and studied 21 distinct burden instruments currently available in English (Schene *et al.*, 1994). Many of these instruments use a recall period of approximately 1 month. The advantages of a limited time frame for asking about burden are that it aids in accurate recall, increases reliability of measurement, makes a comparison with other instruments possible, and allows for a more sensitive measure of change. The main disadvantages are that the past month may not be representative, and that some very burdensome experiences may be missed because they occurred months or years ago. The choice of a time frame depends on the aims of the investigation. For a descriptive study, a longer time frame than 4 weeks may be worthwhile. For the measurement of change, however, one needs a short time frame focusing on relatively common aspects of burden.

Reliability is also influenced by the method of data collection. The available methods are in-person interviewing, questionnaires and telephone interviewing. Which one to choose depends on the aims of the study. For a descriptive study in-person interviewing is certainly the method of choice. When resources are a constraining factor in large sample studies, questionnaires can provide a viable alternative.

The same is true in clinical trials in which one has control over the conditions in which the questionnaires are administered. Telephone interviews are possible with only minimal attrition once a respondent has completed an in-person interview. More than half of the reviewed instruments offer the option of either a structured or a semi-structured personal interview (Schene et al., 1994).

The response categories used in measuring severity also need to be carefully considered. To indicate the *severity* of burden on a particular item, two approaches have been used. First, one can ask family members in very objective terms how many days a week or how many hours a day they spent in varying types of caregiving. However, some respondents may have difficulty responding in such specific terms. A more commonly used approach is to use questions pertaining to specific behaviours with ordinal response categories such as 'never', 'sometimes', 'regularly', 'often', or '(almost) always' to produce scales with Likert-like qualities (Likert, 1932).

Although family burden researchers view the distinction between *objective* and *subjective* burden as important, there exists considerable uncertainty about how the subjective component should be measured. Different approaches have been used (Schene, 1990). In the first, subjective burden is directly related to particular symptoms or behaviours, as in the Social Behavior Assessment Schedule in which researchers ask family members how difficult or stressful they experience each of these behaviours (Platt et al., 1980). In the second approach an assessment is made of the subjective response to such caregiving tasks as helping, activating, supervising and paying money. Here family members are asked how difficult or distressing they experience each of these domains (Creer et al., 1982). In the third approach subjective burden can be considered as a distinct entity related to the caregiver's overall life situation (Maurin & Barmann Boyd, 1990). These three approaches to measuring subjective burden also differ in their relatedness to the relationship with the patient.

The subjective side of burden has also proved to be difficult to measure empirically because it is unclear how best to differentiate burden and resignation. Resignation may indicate that one has given up and simply endures without complaint or that one has become used to carrying the burden. On the other hand, if one measures subjective burden in terms of distress one may be picking up not how badly the respondent feels, but how urgently he or she would like to be rid of the burden.

There is disagreement among researchers as to whether or not burden can be reduced to a single (total) score. Most researchers take a multidimensional approach. In some cases the scales are derived empirically on the basis of factor analysis. In other cases, they are constituted *a priori* by combining items with high face validity (Schene *et al.*, 1994). For a given area one can sum all items within that area. To get a total cumulative burden score one can sum all burden measures, but one should not necessarily expect a high degree of internal consistency. In some cases individual items may provide the most insight into the family experience.

Our recent review of 21 instruments that have been used or developed during the last 10 years (including several which have not yet been published) enumerates the many choices available. However, the final choice of an instrument depends on a variety of considerations including the purpose(s) for which the study is being conducted and the population under study. For specific guidelines for choosing a family burden instrument most appropriate to particular research and clinical aims, the reader is referred to our review article (Schene *et al.*, 1994).

When the aim is to assess burden as an outcome measure in mental health service evaluation, there may be no obvious reason to expand the scope of the interview beyond the measurement of burden. When, however, the investigator wishes to examine the burden concept or models of caregiving (Biegel *et al.*, 1991), it becomes necessary to measure other relevant constructs, such as patterns of residence and contact, services to patient and family, and social support.

Models of analysis

As in other areas of research, analysis of the collected data will benefit from a well-defined theory. While theories of family burden may be framed at the level of either the family as a whole or the individual caregiver, until now caregiving models have concentrated on the individual level (Maurin & Barmann Boyd, 1990; Gallop *et al.*, 1991; Biegel *et al.*, 1991). Most of these models include care recipient or patient variables, caregiver or family member variables, objective burden, subjective burden or distress measures, and mediating or intervening variables. Cultural, subgroup or religious ideas and expectations about caregiving and personal characteristics of the caregiver such as beliefs, attitudes, attributions, stress management and his or her own physical and mental health are quite difficult to disentangle, but together they have a strong influence on how the caregiver may experience the caregiving task. Symptomatology and functional status are the most important clinical variables influencing what patients do and what they do not do, which forms the basis of the objective burden (Schene, 1990).

Objective burden itself covers all those things that the caregiver and/or his or her family has to do (helping, supervising, controlling, paying, etc.), experiences (disturbed family and/or social relations), or is not allowed to do any longer (hobbies, clubs, career, work) as a consequence of the caregiving task. How a family member cognitively experiences this objective burden, reacts and responds to it, and adapts and copes, are assumed to be determinants of subjective burden.

Caregiving is a process that takes place within a social context which is influenced by social networks, the organisation and delivery of mental health care, and the community at large. Thus there are a host of variables possibly associated with levels of objective and subjective burden. These include the composition of the family, the way roles are divided among its members, and the amount of contact between patient and caregiver. Socioeconomic status is also important, because it is strongly related to the prevalence of mental disorders and it can determine the availability of mental health care. Greater income can also lessen the impact of the financial burden of caregiving, for example by providing access to larger living quarters which offer the space for patient and caregiver to withdraw.

The large number of variables involved invite multivariate approaches to data analysis. Contradictions in results from studies conducted in the 1960s and 1970s may stem in part from the limitations of univariate and bivariate analyses (Schene, 1990).

Improving family outcomes

Family burden research strives to learn about the relationship between the mentally ill patient and his or her family members, and how that relationship may be best supported (Kuipers & Bebbington, 1985; Francell *et al.*, 1988). Positive outcomes include preventing the breakdown of kinship relationships, keeping intact the patient's natural support network, relieving subjective burden, educating family members about mental illness, and enhancing partnerships between patients, family members and professionals (Mintz *et al.*, 1987). Future initiatives should consider the accumulating evidence of the beneficial effects of services that are intended specifically for families (Pfeiffer & Mostek, 1991). Among the possible approaches that have been highlighted are respite care (Geiser *et al.*, 1988), family education (Strachan, 1992), including family members in treatment planning (Hatfield, 1979), and developing mobile teams that are responsive to families when the client is in crisis (Francell *et al.*, 1988).

In addition, professionals should be aware of the consequences of mental illness for family members. This may mean helping them to accept and grieve, educating them about the disorder and the treatment, and teaching them to solve problems and cope with symptoms and behaviours. Because most caregivers are very responsible in helping the patient, professionals should help them to acknowledge their own needs. Professionals may need special skills and perhaps specific training to be helpful in these ways (Bernheim & Lehman, 1985; Bernheim & Switalski, 1987; Berkowitz *et al.*, 1990).

Activities by non-professionals may be just as important in improving family and carer outcomes as activities within psychiatry (Katschnig & Konieczna, 1989). For instance, self-help groups sponsored by family organisations provide information about psychiatric disorders, encourage adaptive coping strategies, offer support and mutual help, and advocate in a political way (Lamb *et al.*, 1986; Schene & van Wijngaarden, 1993).

Directions for future research

After an era in which the institutionalisation of persons with serious mental illness was the predominant philosophy, the contemporary emphasis is on providing opportunities to the patient for leading as normal a life as possible. One consequence of this changing social policy is the impact on family members, which under certain conditions may prove to be quite burdensome. We need to continue to study family burden as part of the social costs of community care so as to enable family members also to lead as normal a life as possible.

There are a variety of issues in need of further study (see also Schene, 1990). As in other areas of chronic illness, it is important to describe how social roles are affected by the onset and progression of the disorder. There is a need to refine and standardise the measurement of burden and the underlying structure of the concept. Our recent review of family burden instruments (Schene *et al.*, 1994) showed that researchers more or less agree about the dimensions that comprise the burden concept, but there is less agreement with regard to the definition of burden and how best to measure objective and subjective burden. We believe that some standardisation is needed. Otherwise we can end up in a situation comparable to that of social support and social functioning research where there are many instruments and none that is really accepted as a standard measure.

Until now burden research has concentrated on the negative effects of caregiving. This needs to be redressed by research on the positive side of the ledger by looking at such things as patient contributions to the family and reciprocal emotional support. The emphasis has also been on the family of origin, particularly parents, rather than on the patient's family of procreation. The increase in the fertility rate of women with severe mental illness suggests the need to pay attention to the care of minor children which may represent a hidden aspect of burden (Gamache *et al.*, 1995).

Most of our present knowledge of family burden comes from studies carried out in urban and suburban areas. However, rural areas are unique in a variety of ways that are likely to affect the family experience. Rural areas exhibit relative physical isolation from formal sources of care, and possibly more stigma associated with psychiatric help-seeking. The rural family, though, is also thought to be more inclusive and may be more accepting of the patient and the disability.

Although we have not dealt with caregiving to the elderly with dementias, there is much research available. The same is not true for the burden of caring for a child with a serious emotional disturbance. This is an important future area of study because the burden of caring for such a child may be a significant factor in understanding placement decisions, which have major consequences for the child, the family and the society.

Most research on adult patients has been done on the major mental illnesses, namely schizophrenia and affective disorders. Little is known about the burden to a family caused by patients suffering from addictive, somatisation, anxiety, obsessive–compulsive and personality disorders.

Finally, much of the burden literature has been conducted with middle and upper middle class samples. More research is needed to represent better the experiences and coping strategies of poor and minority families. We also need to know much more about the prevalence of burden cross-culturally and about the factors that might reduce it.

It is important to remember that families will vary in the rate at which they cope and adapt (Tessler *et al.*, 1987). Some family members may be overwhelmed by the onset of the illness, and never really come to terms with the loss of the pre-morbid relationship. Others adapt more successfully and are able to lower their expectations of their relative's social and vocational achievements and accept the loss of reciprocal support. These are matters which are best studied over various stages that define the life cycle of the family. In so doing, we can expect to learn more about the complicated relationship between caregiver burden, expressed emotion, coping behaviour, social support and stressful life events (Kuipers & Bebbington, 1988; Jackson *et al.*, 1990; Mueser *et al.*, 1993). We join with others in recommending the integration of these historically distinct constructs (McFarlane, 1990), and the need to examine them from a developmental point of view (Birchwood & Smith, 1992).

References

Anderson, C.M., Reiss, D.J. & Hogarty, G.E. (1986). *Schizophrenia in the Family: A Practitioner's Guide to Psychoeducation and Management.* New York: Guilford Press.

Anthony, E.J. (1969). A clinical evaluation of children with psychotic parents. *American Journal of Psychiatry*, **126**, 177–84.

Arey, S. & Warheit, G.J. (1980). Psychosocial costs of living with psychologically disturbed family members. In *The Social Consequences of Psychiatric Illness*, ed. L. Robins & J.K. Wing. New York: Brunner/Mazel.

Ascher-Svanum, H. & Sobel, T.S. (1989). Caregivers of mentally ill adults: a women's agenda. *Hospital and Community Psychiatry*, **40**, 843–5.

Beardslee, W.R., Bemporad, J., Keller, M.B. & Klerman, G.L. (1983). Children of parents with major affective disorder: a review. *American Journal of Psychiatry*, **140**, 825–32.

Beels, C.C. (1978). Social networks, the family and the schizophrenic patient. *Schizophrenia Bulletin*, **4**, 512–20.

Berkowitz, R., Shavitt, N. & Leff, J.P. (1990). Educating relatives of schizophrenic patients. *Social Psychiatry and Psychiatric Epidemiology*, **25**, 216–20.

Bernheim, K.F. & Lehman, A.F. (1985). Teaching mental health trainees to work with families of the mentally ill. *Hospital and Community Psychiatry*, **36**, 1109–11.

Bernheim, K.F. & Switalski, T. (1988). Mental health staff and patient's relatives: how they view each other. *Hospital and Community Psychiatry*, **39**, 63–8.

Biegel, D.E., Sales, E. & Schulz, R. (1991). *Family Caregiving in Chronic Illness*. London: Sage Publications.

Birchwood, M. & Smith, J. (1992). Specific and non-specific effects of educational intervention for families living with schizophrenia. *British Journal of Psychiatry*, **160**, 645–52.

Brown, G.W., Carstairs, G.M. & Topping, G. (1958). Post-hospital adjustment of chronic mental patients. *Lancet*, **2**, 685–9.

Brown, G.W., Birley, J.L.T. & Wing, J.K. (1972). Influence of family life on the course of schizophrenic disorder: a replication. *British Journal of Psychiatry*, **121**, 241–58.

Bulger, M.W., Wandersman, A. & Goldman, C.R. (1993). Burdens and gratifications of caregiving: appraisal of parental care of adults with schizophrenia. *American Journal of Orthopsychiatry*, **63**, 255–65.

Carpentier, N., Lesage, A., Goulet, J., Lalonde, P. & Renaud M. (1992). Burden of care of families not living with young schizophrenic relatives. *Hospital and Community Psychiatry*, **43**, 38–43.

Chakrabarti, S., Kulhara, P. & Verma, S.K. (1992). Extent and determinants of burden among families of patients with affective disorders. *Acta Psychiatrica Scandinavica*, **86**, 247–52.

Clark, R.E. & Drake, R.E. (1993). Family costs associated with severe mental illness and substance abuse: a comparison of families with and without dual disorders. Presented at the Annual Meeting of the Association for Health Services Research.

Clausen, J.A. & Yarrow, M.R. (1955). Paths to the mental hospital. *Journal of Social Issues*, **11**, 25–32.

Coyne, J.C., Kessler, R.C., Tal, M., Turnbull, J., Wortman, C.B. & Greden, J.F. (1987). Living with a depressed person. *Journal of Consulting and Clinical Psychology*, **55**, 347–52.

Creer, C., Sturt, E. & Wykes, T. (1982). The role of the relatives. In *Longterm Community Care Experience in a London Borough. Psychological Medicine Monograph Supplement*, **2**, 29–39.

Cumming, J. & Cumming, E. (1965). On the stigma of mental illness. *Community Mental Health Journal*, **1**, 135–43.

Deykin, E. (1961). The reintegration of the chronic schizophrenic patient discharged to his family and community as perceived by the family. *Mental Hygiene*, **45**, 235–46.

Doniger, C.B. (1962). Children whose mothers are in a mental hospital. *Journal of Child Psychology and Psychiatry and Allied Disciplines*, **3**, 165–73.

Dudgeon, M.Y. (1964). The social needs of the discharged mental hospital patient. *International Journal of Social Psychiatry*, **10**, 45–56.

Dunn, B. (1993). Growing up with a psychotic mother: a retrospective study. *American Journal of Orthopsychiatry*, **63**, 177–89.

Evans, A., Bullard, D. & Solomon, M. (1961). The family as a potential resource in the rehabilitation of the chronic schizophrenic patient: a study of 60 patients and their families. *American Journal of Psychiatry*, **117**, 1075–83.

Fadden, G.B. (1984). The relatives of patients with depressive disorders: a typology of burden and strategies of coping. MPhil thesis, Institute of Psychiatry, University of London.

Fadden, G., Bebbington, P. & Kuipers, L. (1987). Caring and its burdens: a study of the spouses of depressed patients. *British Journal of Psychiatry*, **151**, 660–7.

Falloon, I.R.H. & Liberman, R.P. (1983). Behavioral family interventions in the management of chronic schizophrenia. In *Family Therapy in Schizophrenia*, ed. W.R. McFarlane. New York: Guilford Press.

Fenton, F.R., Tessier, L. & Struening, E.L. (1979). A comparative trial of home and hospital psychiatric care: one year follow-up. *Archives of General Psychiatry*, **36**, 1973–9.

Fisher, G.A., Benson, P.R. & Tessler, R.C. (1990). Family response to mental illness: developments since deinstitutionalization. *Research in Community and Mental Health*, **6**, 203–36.

Francell, C.G., Conn, V.S. & Gray, D.P. (1988). Families' perceptions of burden of care for chronic mentally ill relatives. *Hospital and Community Psychiatry*, **12**, 1296–1300.

Freeman, H.E. & Simmons, O.G. (1958). Mental patients in the community: family settings and performance level. *American Sociological Review*, **22**, 147–54.

Freeman, H.E. & Simmons, O.G. (1959). Social class and posthospital performance levels. *American Sociological Review*, **24**, 345–451.

Gallop, R., McKeever, P., Mohide, E.A. & Wells, D. (1991). *Family Care and Chronic Illness: The Caregiving Experience. A Review of the Literature.* Toronto: Faculty of Nursing.

Gamache, G., Tessler, R. & Nicholson, J. (1995). Childcare as a neglected dimension of family burden research. *Research in Community and Mental Health*, **8**, 63–80.

Geiser, R., Hoche, L. & King, J. (1988). Respite care for mentally ill patients and their families. *Hospital and Community Psychiatry*, **39**, 291–5.

Grad, J. & Sainsbury, P. (1963). Mental illness and the family. *Lancet*, **i**, 544–7.

Grad, J. & Sainsbury, P. (1968). The effects that patients have on their families in a community care and a control psychiatric service. *British Journal of Psychiatry*, **114**, 265–78.

Graham, R.W. (1983). Adult day care: how families of the dementia patient respond. *Journal of Gerontological Nursing*, **15**, 27–31.

Gubman, G.D., Tessler, R.C. & Willis, G. (1987). Living with the mentally ill: factors affecting household complaints. *Schizophrenia Bulletin*, **13**, 727–36.

Hatfield, A. (1978). Psychological costs of schizophrenia to the family. *Social Work*, **23**, 355–9.

Hatfield, A. (1979). The family as partner in the treatment of mental illness. *Hospital and Community Psychiatry*, **30**, 338–40.

Herz, M.I., Endicott, J. & Spitzer, R.L. (1977). Brief hospitalization: a two-year follow-up. *American Journal of Psychiatry*, **134**, 502–7.

Hoenig, J. & Hamilton, M.W. (1966a). The schizophrenic patient in the community and the effect on the household. *International Journal of Social Psychiatry*, **26**, 165–76.

Hoenig, J. & Hamilton, M.W. (1966b). The burden on the household in an extramural psychiatric service. In *New Aspects of the Mental Health Services*, ed. H.L. Freeman & W.A.J. Farndale. Oxford: Pergamon Press.

Jackson, H.J., Smith, N. & McGorry, P. (1990). Relationship between expressed emotion and family burden in psychotic disorders: an exploratory study. *Acta Psychiatrica Scandinavica*, **82**, 243–9.

Jacob, M., Frank, E., Kupfer, D.J. & Carpenter, L.L. (1987). Recurrent depression: an assessment of family burden and family attitudes. *Journal of Clinical Psychiatry*, **44**, 395–400.

Katschnig, H. & Konieczna, T. (1989). What works in work with families? A hypothesis. *British Journal of Psychiatry*, **155**, 144–50.

Kopeikon, H.S., Marshall, V. & Goldstein, M.J. (1983). Stages and impact of crisis oriented family therapy in the aftercare of acute schizophrenia. In *Family Therapy in Schizophrenia*, ed. W.R. McFarlane. New York: Guilford Press.

Kreisman, D. & Joy, V. (1974). Family response to the illness of a relative: a review of the literature. *Schizophrenia Bulletin*, **1**, 34–57.

Kuipers, L. & Bebbington, P. (1985). Relatives as a resource in the management of functional illness. *British Journal of Psychiatry*, **147**, 465–70.

Kuipers, L. & Bebbington, P. (1988). Expressed emotion research in schizophrenia: theoretical and clinical implications. *Psychological Medicine*, **18**, 893–909.

Lam, D.H. (1991). Psychosocial family intervention in schizophrenia: a review of empirical studies. *Psychological Medicine*, **21**, 423–41.

Lamb, R. & Oliphant, E. (1978). Schizophrenia through the eyes of families. *Hospital and Community Psychiatry*, **29**, 803–6.

Lamb, H.R., Hoffman, A., Hoffman, F. & Oliphant, E. (1986). Families of schizophrenics: a movement in jeopardy. *Hospital and Community Psychiatry*, **37**, 353–7.

Leff, J.P., Kuipers, L., Berkowitz, R., Eberlein-Fries, R. & Sturgeon, D. (1982). A controlled trial of social intervention in schizophrenia families. *British Journal of Psychiatry*, **141**, 121–34.

Lewis, V. & Zeichner, A. (1960). Impact of admission to a mental hospital on the patient's family. *Mental Hygiene*, **44**, 121–34.

Likert, R. (1932). A technique for the measurement of attitudes. *Archives of Psychology*, **22**, 140.

Lystad, M.H. (1958). Day hospital care and changing family attitudes toward the mentally ill. *Journal of Nervous and Mental Disorders*, **127**, 145–52.

Mandelbrote, B. & Folkard, S. (1961). Some factors related to outcome and social adjustment in schizophrenia. *Acta Psychiatrica Scandinavica*, **37**, 223–35.

Maurin, J.T. & Barmann Boyd, C. (1990). Burden of mental illness on the family: a critical review. *Archives of Psychiatric Nursing*, **4**, 99–107.

McFarlane, W.R. (1990). Can the family literature be integrated? In *Families as Allies in Treatment of the Mentally Ill*, ed. H.P. Lefley & D.L. Johnson. Washington, DC: American Psychiatric Association.

Miller, F., Dworkin, J., Ward, M. & Barone D. (1990). A preliminary study of unresolved grief in families of seriously mentally ill patients. *Hospital and Community Psychiatry*, **41**, 1321–5.

Mintz, L.I., Liberman, R.P., Miklowitz, D.J. & Mintz J. (1987). Expressed emotion: a call for partnership among relatives, patients and professionals. *Schizophrenia Bulletin*, **13**, 227–35.

Mueser, K.T., Gingerich, S.L. & Rosenthal, C.K. (1993). Familial factors in psychiatry. *Current Opinion in Psychiatry*, **6**, 251–7.

Pai, S. & Kaipur, R.L. (1982). Impact of treatment intervention on the relationship between dimensions of clinical psychopathology, social dysfunction and burden on the family. *Psychological Medicine*, **12**, 651–8.

Pasamanick, B., Scarpitti, F.R. & Dinitz, S. (1967). *Schizophrenics in the Community: An Experimental Study in the Prevention of Hospitalization.* New York: Appleton Century Crofts.

Pfeiffer, E.J. & Mostek, M. (1991). Services for families of people with mental illness. *Hospital and Community Psychiatry*, **42**, 262–4.

Platt, S. (1985). Measuring the burden of psychiatric illness on the family: an evaluation of some rating scales. *Psychological Medicine*, **15**, 383–93.

Platt, S., Weyman, A., Hirsch, S. & Hewett, S. (1980). The Social Behaviour Assessment Schedule (SBAS): rationale, contents, scoring and reliability of a new interview schedule. *Social Psychiatry*, **15**, 43–55.

Reynoulds, I. & Hoult, J.E. (1984). The relatives of the mentally ill: a comparative trial of community oriented psychiatric care. *Journal of Nervous and Mental Disease*, **172**, 480–9.

Rose, C. (1959). Relatives' attitudes and mental hospitalization. *Mental Hygiene*, **43**, 194–203.

Scheff, T.J. (1966). *Being Mentally Ill: A Sociological Theory.* Chicago: Aldine.

Schene, A.H. (1986). Thuis bezorgd: een literatuurstudie naar het verschijnsel 'Burden on the family'. (*Worried at Home: A Monograph on Burden on the Family in Psychiatry.*) Utrecht: NcGv.

Schene, A.H. (1990). Objective and subjective dimensions of family burden: towards an integrative framework for research. *Social Psychiatry and Psychiatric Epidemiology*, **25**, 289–97.

Schene, A.H. & van Wijngaarden, B. (1993). Familieleden van mensen met een psychotische stoornis; een onderzoek onder Ypsilonleden (*Family Members of People with a Psychotic Disorder: A Study among Members of Ypsilon*). Amsterdam: Department of Psychiatry, University of Amsterdam.

Schene, A.H., Tessler, R.C. & Gamache, G.M. (1994). Instruments measuring family or caregiver burden in severe mental illness. *Social Psychiatry and Psychiatric Epidemiology*, **29**, 228–40.

Silverman, M.M. (1989). Children of psychiatrically ill parents: a prevention perspective. *Hospital and Community Psychiatry*, **40**, 1257–65.

Spitzer, R.L., Gibbon, M. & Endicott, J. (1971). *Family Evaluation Form.* New York: New York State Department of Mental Hygiene.

Stein, L.I., Test, M.A. & Marx, A.J. (1975). Alternative to the hospital: a controlled study. *American Journal of Psychiatry*, **132**, 517–22.

Strachan, A. (1992). Family management. In *Handbook of Psychiatric Rehabilitation*, ed. R.B. Lieberman, pp. 182–212. New York: Macmillan.

Tessler, R.C., Killian, L.M. & Gubman, G.D. (1987). Stages in family response to mental illness; an ideal type. *Psychosocial Rehabilitation Journal*, **10**, 3–16.

Thompson, E.H. & Doll, W. (1982). The burden of families coping with the mentally ill: an invisible crisis. *Family Relations*, **31**, 379–88.

Treudley, M.B. (1946). Mental illness and family routines. *Mental Hygiene*, **15**, 407–18.

Wahl, O.F. & Harman, C.R. (1989). Family views of stigma. *Schizophrenia Bulletin*, **15**, 131–9.

Washburn, S., Vanicelli, M., Longabaugh, R. & Scheff, B.J. (1976). A controlled comparison of psychiatric daytreatment and inpatient hospitalization. *Journal of Consulting and Clinical Psychology*, **44**, 665–75.

Waters, M. & Northover, J. (1965). Rehabilitated longstay schizophrenics in the community. *British Journal of Psychiatry*, **111**, 258–67.

Wing, J.K., Monck, E., Brown, G.W. & Carstairs, G.M. (1964). Morbidity in the community of schizophrenic patients discharged from London Mental Hospitals in 1959. *British Journal of Psychiatry*, **110**, 10–21.

19

Needs assessment

GRAHAM THORNICROFT, MICHAEL PHELAN AND GERALDINE
STRATHDEE

Introduction

In recent years a consensus has emerged between clinicians and
planners in many countries that mental health services should be
provided in relation to needs, but often are not. If such services aim to
meet needs, at the levels both of the individual patient and of the
whole population, then three key issues emerge: how can needs be
defined, who should assess them and how can this information be best
used? This chapter addresses these issues in three stages: by presenting
definitions of need, by reviewing methods of assessing individual
needs for treatment, and by discussing how needs for services at the
population level can be measured.

Defining needs

There is at present no consensus on how needs should be defined
(Holloway, 1994), and who should define them (Ellis, 1993; Slade,
1994). The *Oxford English Dictionary* offers 'necessity, requirement and
essential'; and in a different sense 'destitution, distress, indigence,
poverty or want'. These clusters of meanings overlap in so far as they
define 'need' as a vital element which is lacking, and this chapter will
use this sense as its point of departure. 'Need' will therefore be used
here to refer to significant essentials of life which are insufficient. The
fact that a need is defined does not mean that it can be met. For
example, some needs may remain unmet because other problems take
priority, because an effective method is not available locally, or
because the person in need refuses treatment.

In psychological terms, Maslow (1968) has set out a hierarchy of four levels reflecting, in sequence, needs for physiological functioning, safety, love and self-actualisation. Similarly, from a philosophical analysis of the field, Liss (1990) has distinguished four elements of need. First is the 'ill health' approach which equates need with a deficiency in health that requires medical care. In this model the required intervention is simply the provision of the absent treatment. For Mallman & Marcus (1980), for example, need is 'an objective requirement to avoid a state of illness' (p. 165). Second, Liss describes the 'supply notion', where the existence of a need presumes that an acceptable and effective treatment exists to offer remedy, and this is referred to by Stevens & Gabbay (1992) as 'the ability to benefit in some way from health care'. Third, the 'normative notion' of need proposes that need is a matter of opinion, and therefore a needs assessment has to be put in the context of the beliefs of those involved, often referred to as 'felt' or 'perceived' needs to distinguish them from needs that are considered to have a more objective basis. The view that 'need is seen as a shortfall compared with a state of being which is generally acceptable' exemplifies this approach (Davies & Challis, 1986, p. 562). Fourth, the 'instrumental view' of need is that health is required to reach a certain state or defined goal. The accuracy of the needs assessment and the effectiveness of the treatment intervention can therefore be gauged by the extent to which the instrumental goal is achieved. Tracy (1986) expressed this as 'a need of a living system is a lack of a specific resource which is useful for or required by the purposes of that system' (p. 212).

In an alternative formulation to the definition of need, it can be distinguished from demand (expressed wish) and supply (utilisation) (Table 19.1).

Need, demand and supply are related to each other as shown in Fig. 19.1, A demand for care exists when an individual expresses a wish to receive it. In an alternative formulation, demand is what people would be willing to pay for in a market or might wish to use in a system of free health care (Stevens & Raftery, 1994). Supply includes interventions, agents and settings, whether or not they are used in any particular case. Care coordination entails providing such a pattern of service after initial assessment and then updating the assessment regularly to assess outcomes and to modify the care if needs remain unmet. In this scheme, overprovision is provision in excess of need, while underprovision is need in excess of provision

Table 19.1. *Definitions of need, demand and supply*

Need = What people benefit from
Demand = What people ask for
Supply = What is provided

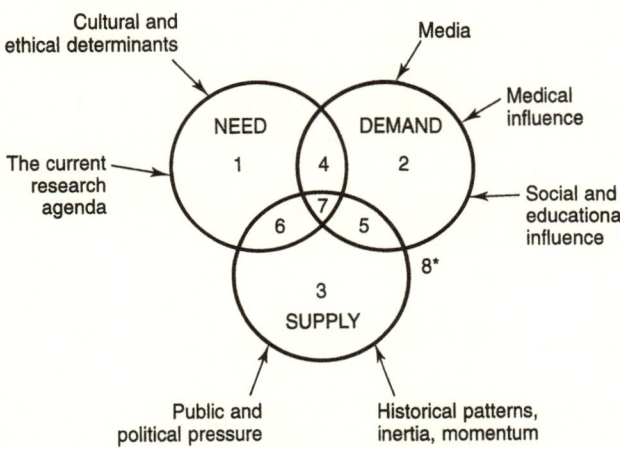

*Fig. 19.1. Need, demand and supply: influences and overlaps. * The external field where a potential service is not needed, demanded or supplied. NEED, what people benefit from; DEMAND, what people ask for; SUPPLY, what is provided. (From Stevens & Galway, 1991.)*

(unmet need). As Fig. 19.1 shows, need, demand and supply are usually not coterminous. Need may not match demand; and demand is not necessarily followed by provision or supply (utilisation).

A need may exist, as defined by a professional, even if the intervention is refused by a patient. At the same time, a proper needs assessment process should not lead to the imposition of expert solutions upon patients. A professionally defined need may remain unmet, and have to be replaced by one acceptable to the patients. Another approach to defining need has been suggested by health economists. Their contributions include first the proposal that need refers both to the capacity to benefit from an intervention and the amount of expenditure required to reduce the capacity to benefit to zero – it is therefore a product of benefit and cost-effectiveness (Culyer & Wagstaff, 1992). Second, health economists have proposed that diagnosis-related groups are notably irrelevant for mental health services (McCrone & Strathdee, 1994), and thirdly that empirical data should guide operational needs definitions (Beecham *et al.*, 1993).

In terms of mental health services specifically, needs have been described by the difference between service needs of a patient population and actual service provision. Lehtinen *et al.* (1990), for example, interpret needs as reflecting an inadequate level of service for the severity of the problem, and so patients with severe disorders receiving primary rather than specialised psychiatric care would be rated as having unmet need. Similarly, for Shapiro *et al.* (1985), unmet needs are defined as the combination of definite morbidity and lack of mental health service utilisation. A third view is that needs represent an insufficient supply of particular treatment interventions, and this approach is embodied in the three individual needs assessment instruments now described.

Measuring individual needs

In an ideal planning framework, a comprehensive needs assessment would be undertaken on all patients and the aggregated data would be used to plan the overall service. In practice this is seldom possible, but systematic assessment, review, and evaluation over months and years of contact should allow services to work with their users to evolve services more appropriate to their needs (Brewin *et al.*, 1987). Patients who suffer from severe mental illness have a range of needs which goes far beyond the purely medical, such as those described in the National Institute of Mental Health's document *Toward a Model Plan for a Comprehensive Community-Based Mental Health System* (1987).

The issue of how best to make an individual assessment of need has taxed both researchers and clinicians, not least because their requirements differ. An ideal assessment tool for use in a routine clinical setting would be one which is brief, easily learned, takes little time to administer, does not require the use of personnel additional to the usual clinical team, is valid and reliable in different settings and, above all, can be used as an integral part of routine clinical work. Macdonald (1991) suggests that in addition such a scale should be sensitive to change, the potential inter-rater and test-retest reliability should be high, and it should logically inform clinical management (Hillier *et al.*, 1991; Thornicroft & Bebbington, 1995). The decision about which scale to use will depend on whether the approach is to

Table 19.2. *Areas of potential need included in the CAN (Camberwell Assessment of Need)*

Accommodation
Occupation
Specific psychotic symptoms
Psychological distress
Information about condition and treatment
Non-prescribed drugs
Food and meals
Household skills
Self-care and presentation
Safety to self
Safety to others
Money
Childcare
Physical health
Alcohol
Basic education
Telephone
Public transport
Welfare benefits

focus on particular diagnostic or care groups, and on the balance to be struck between economy of time and inclusiveness of the ratings, and should include a range of areas of clinical and social functioning.

The Camberwell Assessment of Need

A clinically orientated and relatively brief instrument is the CAN (Camberwell Assessment of Need; see Table 19.2), which has been recently published by the PRiSM team at the Institute of Psychiatry in London. It is intended for both research and clinical use, especially in relation to the requirements of the National Health Service and Community Care Act (House of Commons, 1990) to undertake needs assessments of people with severe mental health problems, and it includes both patient and staff views, considers a comprehensive range of health and social needs, and assesses need separately from interventions. The areas assessed by the CAN are described by Thornicroft (1994).

The principles which have guided the development of the CAN are that needs are universal, that many psychiatric patients have

Table 19.3. *Camberwell Assessment of Needs:*
summary of reliability scores

		r	Significance level
Inter-rater	Staff	0.99	$p < 0.001$
	Patient	0.98	$p < 0.001$
Test–retest	Staff	0.78	$p < 0.001$
	Patient	0.71	$p < 0.001$

multiple needs, that needs assessment should be an integral part of clinical practice, and that this should allow ratings by both staff and by patents. In the construction of the scale we attempted to establish that it had adequate psychometric properties, could be completed within 30 minutes, was comprehensive, was usable by wide range of staff, could record help from informal carers and staff, and would be suitable for both research and clinical use. The areas of assessment included refer to basic needs (accommodation, food and occupation), health needs (physical health, psychotic and neurotic symptoms, drugs and alcohol, safety to self and others), social needs (company, intimate relationship and sexual expression), everyday functioning (household skills, self-care and childcare, basic education, budgeting) and service receipt (information, telephone, transport and welfare benefits).

The psychometric properties of the CAN have now been established both in terms of validity (face, consensual, content, criterion and construct) and reliability (Phelan *et al.*, 1995) and the results are acceptable (Table 19.3). It was striking that in a survey of severely disabled psychiatric patients in south London, the mean number of problems identified by staff was 7.5 (95% CI, 6.7–8.4), and by patients was 7.9 (6.8–8.9). When examined in detail, however, the degree of agreement by staff and patients for individual items was rather poor, rejecting the hypothesis that staff and patients would rate problems similarly (Slade, 1994). The CAN is now being introduced to field trials in routine clinical settings, is being translated into 12 European languages, and is being published in an electronic PC version (called PELiCAN).

The MRC Needs for Care Assessment

The MRC Needs for Care schedule (Brewin, 1992) is based on the following formal definition of need for care: (1) a need is present when (a) a patient's functioning (social disablement) falls below or threatens to fall below some minimum specified level, and (b) this is due to a remediable, or potentially remediable, cause; (2) a need (as defined above) is met when it has attracted some at least partly effective item of care, and when no other items of care of greater potential effectiveness exist; (3) a need is unmet when it has attracted only a partly effective or no item of care and when other items of care of greater potential effectiveness exist.

In this schedule 'needs for care' have been defined as requirements for specific activities or interventions that have the potential to ameliorate disabling symptoms or reactions. In contrast, 'needs for services' reflect institutional requirements and are defined as needs for specific agents or agencies to deliver those interventions (Brewin *et al.*, 1987). Mangen & Brewin (1991) outline a procedure for deriving estimates of needs for services from individuals' needs for specific items of care. Substantial data have now been presented on individual needs assessments using this instrument (Brewin *et al.*, 1988, 1990; MacCarthy *et al.*, 1988; Lesage *et al.*, 1991; Pryce *et al.*, 1993; van Haaster *et al.*, 1994) along with a detailed critique of this approach (Hogg & Marshall, 1992; Brewin & Wing, 1993).

Cardinal Needs Schedule

A third formal approach to individual needs assessment is that of Marshall (1994), who is developing the Cardinal Needs Schedule. This is a modification of the MRC Needs for Care approach, and identifies cardinal problems as those which satisfy three criteria:

1 the 'cooperation criterion' (the patient is willing to accept help for the problem);
2 the 'carer stress criterion' (the problem causes considerable anxiety, frustration or inconvenience to people caring for the patient);
3 the 'severity criterion' (the problem endangers the health or safety of the patient, or the safety of other people.

To rate this schedule, data are collected using the Manchester Scale for mental state assessment, the REHAB scale and a specially developed additional information questionnaire. A computerised version (Autoneed) has also been developed. Patients' views are rated using the Client Opinion Interview and the Carer Stress Interview which includes carers' ratings, and the author is undertaking both inter-rater and test–retest reliability studies.

Population-based needs assessment

A comprehensive method for the development of appropriate local services would be based on a systematic assessment of the needs of the population of individuals identified as mentally ill within the service's catchment area. Levels of need detected in individuals would then be aggregated on the basis of a case register, and services developed in relation to the identified unmet population needs (Wing, 1989).

Often direct data on service needs are absent or of very poor quality, and indicators or proxy variables may need to be used. A number of methods may be used as proxies in assessing local needs for services, each with its own limitations (Shapiro et al., 1985). First, estimates of need may be based on epidemiological work which estimates the national prevalence of mental disorders that may bring individuals into contact with the psychiatric services. Secondly, calculations of services needed locally may be derived from data on service utilisation rates found nationally (Goldberg & Huxley, 1980, 1992; Goldman, 1981). Third, a deprivation weighted approach may be used, adjusting estimates of service need according to current knowledge of the relationships of mental health disorders to age, sex, ethnic group, marital status, economic status and other social variables (Thornicroft, 1991). Fourthly, levels of provision locally may simply be compared with levels of provision nationally, a method which is not strictly based on needs but which allows a rough comparison to be made between the development of local services and the national picture. Finally, the degree of fit between services and local needs should be assessed not only in terms of numbers of places provided in a variety of services, but also from a geographical perspective: location of services should make them as accessible as possible to all, and should particularly take into account demographic variations in catchment areas which may produce particularly high levels of need in certain areas.

Table 19.4. *Estimated prevalence of psychiatric disorders in England*

	Estimated prevalence per 500 000 population
Schizophrenia	1 000–2 500
Affective psychosis	500–2 500
Depression	10 000–25 000
Anxiety	8000–30 000

Source: Department of Health (1994).

Estimated levels of psychiatric morbidity in the general population

Taking the first of the above approaches, a simple estimate of local morbidity may be derived from epidemiological studies of levels of morbidity nationally. Table 19.4 shows estimated levels of community morbidity in England per 500 000 population (Department of Health, 1994). Epidemiological data of this form have the strength of providing an overall estimate of needs to be met in the community. However, they do not give any indication of which particular forms of service are likely to be needed: most people with depression or anxiety will not require referral to specialist services. As far as schizophrenia and other psychoses are concerned data of this form are rather more useful, in that it may be assumed that most patients with severe mental illness of these types are likely to need provision for some form of long-term contact with psychiatric services.

Estimates of service need based on national patterns of service utilisation

The work of Goldberg & Huxley (1980, 1992) may be used as the basis of an approach which takes data on service utilisation as well as findings from epidemiological population surveys into account (Table 19.5). It has been established that in any year, one quarter (25%) of the adult population will suffer from a mental illness of at least moderate severity. Of this number, very few are referred to mental health services (1.7%) and less than half are admitted (0.6% of the population at risk).

Table 19.5. *Expected psychiatric morbidity and service use*

Measure	Annual prevalence (%)
Number of adults suffering from mental illness/distress	25
Number of consulting primary care	23
Number identified as having mental illness/distress	14
Number referred to mental health services	1.7
Number admitted to psychiatric hospital	0.6

Source: Goldberg & Huxley (1992).

Table 19.6. *Estimates for psychiatric service use by type of service*

Type of contact	No. per 250 000 total population
No. of patients attending GP per annum	64 250
No. of patients attending outpatients per annum	2858
Total no. of outpatient attendances per annum	8586
No. of inpatients on one day, stay < 1 year	135
No. of acute admission per annum	1095
No. of inpatients on one day, stay 1–5 years	93
No. of inpatients on one day, stay > 5 years	70
No. in Local Authority residential care on one day	18
No. in Local Authority long-term day place on one day	63

Source: Wing (1992).

Table 19.7. *Use of Local Government Authority (Municipality) Social Services (number of places per 10 000 population)*

	Municipal residential places	Other residential care places	Day centre places
England	0.4	0.3	4
Rural counties	0.2	0.2	3
Outer London	0.5	0.9	4
Inner London	1.2	2.2	8

Data for people in contact with psychiatric services are cited by Wing (1992) on the basis of the Local Authority Profile of Social Services for 1989/90 (Tables 19.6, 19.7). National figures, such as those used in Tables 19.6 and 19.7, do, however, have the disadvantage of frequently being based on relatively unreliable data: returns may

Table 19.8. *Outpatient and domiciliary visit contact rates in case register areas*

Type of contact	Contact rates in case register areas
Persons per 100 000 who attend outpatients during 1 year	798–1355 per 100 000 population
No. of visits per person	2.9–3.9
Persons per 100 000 who receive a domiciliary visit during 1 year	89–208 per 100 000 population
Domiciliary visits per person	1.0–1.1

Source: Gibbons *et al.* (1984).

often be incomplete or inaccurate, and this is likely to apply particularly to information on more community-based services (Glover, 1991). More reliable data on service utilisation may be found in studies based on case registers, where data collection is likely to be considerably more complete and accurate than in national surveys. For utilisation rates for specific services based on data from case registers in five areas, Gibbons *et al.* (1984) give the figures for use of outpatient and domiciliary services shown in Table 19.8.

The deprivation-weighted population approach to needs assessment

There is strong evidence that social and demographic factors are closely associated with the measured rates of psychiatric disorder. The association between psychiatric disorders and social class (particularly for schizophrenia and depression) is one of the most consistent findings in psychiatric epidemiology. The Jarman combined index of social deprivation, for example, has been shown to be highly correlated with psychiatric admission rates for Health Districts in the South East Thames Region, and may be used to estimate the degree of excess morbidity (Jarman, 1983, 1984; Hirsch, 1988; Thornicroft, 1991; Thornicroft *et al.*, 1993; Jarman & Hirsch, 1992). It seems reasonable, therefore, to use a deprivation-weighted population score to estimate morbidity within psychiatric sectors or provider units. Apart from overall deprivation, a number of specific factors are relevant in planning mental health services. These are discussed in turn below.

Homelessness

The homeless is a group whose specific needs for mental health care have received considerable attention in the United States in the past 10 years and who have now begun also to be the focus of research in the United Kingdom. Most studies have focused particularly on the homeless in hostels, but work has also begun on the evaluation of the psychiatric status of the street homeless. This body of research suggests that the homeless in hostels and night shelters and on the street probably have a rate of mental illness of between 30% and 50%, and that functional psychoses predominate (Marshall, 1989; Timms & Fry, 1989; Marshall & Reed, 1992; Scott, 1993). Conventional psychiatric services often fail to contact or engage consistently the homeless mentally ill, so that specific services for this group are needed. For example, clinics may be provided in places where the homeless tend to congregate or assertive outreach work can be carried out on the street. The extent of the local homeless population thus needs to be known in order to plan a comprehensive service for the long-term mentally ill.

The first step towards planning adequate provision for this group, which needs urgently to be taken, is to carry out some form of enumeration, and to attempt to assess their needs and levels of mental illness among them, as organisations working with the homeless suggest that the characteristics of local populations of the street homeless vary widely, and need to be assessed locally in each area. The capture–recapture technique recently described by Fisher et al. (1994) is likely to be one of the most accurate means of estimating the extent of this group.

Population requirements for services

There is considerable debate about the numbers of psychiatric treatment and care places that are necessary (Wing, 1971, 1989; Thornicroft & Strathdee, 1994). The 1975 British White Paper suggests targets of 50 District General Hospital beds per 100 000 of the population, together with 35 for the elderly severely mentally infirm and 17 for the 'new' long-stay patients. More recently, the House of Commons Social Services Committee Report on Community Care (1985) noted that 'a smaller number of in-patients beds is now thought necessary for general psychiatric services', and a Royal

Table 19.9. *Estimated numbers of places required in residential settings for an 'ideal' mental health service*

Type of provision	Range of places
24-hour staffed residences	40–150
Day staffed residences	30–120
Acute psychiatric care	50–150
Unstaffed group homes	48–80
Adult placement schemes	0–15
Local secure places	5–10
Respite facilities	0–5
Regional secure unit	1–10

Source: Strathdee & Thornicroft (1992).

College of Psychiatrists working party has specified this as 44 acute beds for a population of 100 000 (Hirsch, 1988).

Strathdee & Thornicroft (1992) have set out targets for service provision based on likely prevalences of mental illness nationally (Table 19.9). These targets assume that services should as far as possible be community based, with community-based residential places and day care taking the place of institutional care. Wing (1992) provides some figures for targets for day provision by mental health services, which again take account of the prevalence of severe mental illness in the community. These figures exclude patients in residential mental health services, many of whom will of course also require day services.

Service needs from a local perspective

To meet needs across the catchment area, services need not only to provide adequate numbers of places in a range of forms of care, but also to locate these services so that they are as accessible as possible to their users. Two principles are important in this respect: sectorisation, and the development of services which are highly accessible to those parts of the catchment area where particularly high levels of need are likely to be found.

Sectorisation, as in many European countries, is now generally regarded in the United Kingdom as an essential prerequisite to the development of effective community services. The term 'sector' now generally refers to a delineated geographic area, with a defined catchment population. Internationally the concept of the sector permeates community service development. The first sectors were formed in France in 1947, and by 1961 the country had over 300. In America the Kennedy Community Mental Health Centres Act of 1963 introduced the principle of a catchment area for each CMHC, and by 1975, 40% of the population had services based on the notion. In Europe throughout the 1970s sector development grew but with sector sizes varying between countries (Lindholm, 1983). A recent study (Johnson & Thornicroft, 1993) indicates that 81% of districts in England have divided their catchment area into sectors.

There is evidence that sectorisation may facilitate the development of community alternatives to inpatient hospital treatment. In Nottingham (UK), Tyrer *et al.* (1989) found the following reductions: number of admissions (5%), duration of admissions (4%), use of inpatient beds (38%). One Swedish study (Hansson, 1989) found a decrease in: number of admissions (20%), beds-days used (40%) and compulsory admissions (25%). In addition, sectorisation allows for effective assessment of need at a local level, liaison with primary care teams and local social services, greater opportunities for home treatment, and the possibility of establishing local bases for provision of a range of services which are highly accessible to the local population.

General practitioners play a major role in the care of those with both acute and chronic psychological disorders (Shepherd *et al.*, 1966; Goldberg & Blackwell, 1970; Sharp & Morrell, 1989; Kendrick *et al.*, 1991). For many patients with severe, long-term disorders the general practitioner is indeed the only source of continuing care (Pantellis *et al.*, 1988). Given the nature of the involvement of health, social and the range of non-statutory agencies, the organisation of services is therefore fundamental to their ability to fulfil the principles of delivery.

Between one-fifth and one-quarter of all consultations in the average general practitioner's daily surgeries are undertaken by individuals who have a mental health component as either the sole or a major component of their problems (Shepherd *et al.*, 1966). In the average consultation time of 6 minutes, just under half of these problems are recognised by the doctors (Goldberg & Bridges, 1988). While the majority of mental health disorders fall within the less severe or 'neurotic' areas, of those individuals identified as having a mental health disorder, one-tenth have a chronic disorder defined as continually present for 1 year or requiring prophylactic treatment. The primary care team has always dealt with the majority of mental health morbidity within the community. Only about 1 in 20 patients is referred on for specialist care. General practice consultations are in a ratio of 10:1 with psychiatric outpatient attendances and 100:1 with psychiatric admissions.

The development of registers of vulnerable individuals can form a practical focused first step to the development of good liaison between primary and secondary care services to establish local need. Such initiatives are facilitated by general practices having computerised age/sex registers with repeat prescribing lists and by local mental health services having care programme approach or other comprehensive registers. Without registers of the most vulnerable individuals general practitioners are at risk of being unaware of the needs or existence of this client group until they present in crisis. Having identified such individuals, the joint development of practice policies in optimal care offers a useful strategy for the organisation of practices to maximise care of this client group (Strathdee & Phelan, 1993).

Service utilisation as a proxy for need

Traditionally service-level needs have been approximated from service utilisation data, especially hospital bed use. This is now increasingly inaccurate for several reasons. First, inpatient care is a small and diminishing part of mental health care. Second, in many respects inpatient care actually represents an alternative model of care to that practised (i.e. community based) for certain patients. Third, the chronicity and episodic nature of mental illness means that episodes are often part of a longer sequence and are very varied in length and intensity. Fourth, there is a greater diversity of health professional contacts, i.e. psychiatrists, psychologists, community psychiatric nurses and occupational therapists.

In terms of the needs for general adult mental health services for a defined population, Table 19.9 presents data from a British consensus survey of expert opinion and suggests that (1) the emphasis should be upon the number of places available rather than upon the number of beds, (2) a range of provisions should exist, (3) the number of places needed in each category depends upon the extent of provision in the other categories, and (4) the overall requirement for services will

Table 19.10. *Guidelines to distinguish high, medium and low support patient groups for specialist mental health services*

Group	Patient characteristics
High support group	Individuals with severe social dysfunction (e.g. social isolation, unemployment and/or difficulty with skills of daily living) as a consequence of severe or persistent mental illness or disorder. In particular, individuals with the following difficulties will be identified for high levels of support: • current or recent serious risk to self or to others or of self-neglect • severe behavioural difficulties • high risk of relapse • history of poor engagement with mental health services • little contact with other providers of care • precarious housing (e.g. bed and breakfast) • carers who experience particular difficulty in coping with a relative suffering from mental illness Such patients often require a staff:patient ratio of about 1:15
Medium support group	Individuals with a moderate degree of social disability arising from mental illness or disorder, e.g. those able to work at least part-time and/or to maintain at least one enduring relationship. This group will also include the following individuals: • those likely to recognise, and to seek help when early in relapse • those receiving appropriate services from other agencies
Low support group	Individuals who, following assessment, have been found to have specific and limited mental-health-related needs which do not require extensive, multidisciplinary input. In general, such individuals are likely to respond to brief or low-intensity intervention. For example, patients with: • psychosis in remission (with or without medication) • moderately severe personality disorder

Source: Strathdee and Thornicroft (1995).

correlate closely with the degree of socio-economic deprivation experienced by that particular population, and therefore a range of places is given for each category.

Within groups of patients in contact with a clinical service there may remain a requirement to differentiate degrees of relative need, for example for setting case loads for staff members. Table 19.10 shows one approach to this triage function.

Table 19.11. *Principles to guide services to meet unmet needs*

Services should meet the range of special needs of psychiatric patients, with particular attention being paid to those with physical disabilities, mental retardation, the homeless or imprisoned

Services should be local and accessible and to the greatest extent possible delivered in the individual's usual environment

Services should be comprehensive and address a wide range of needs

Services should be flexible by being available whenever and for whatever duration needed

Services should be consumer-oriented, that is, based on the needs of the user rather than those of providers

Services should empower clients by using and adapting treatment techniques which enable clients to enhance their self-help and retain the fullest possible control over their own lives

Services should be racially and culturally appropriate

Services should focus on strengths, and should be built on the skills and strengths of clients to help them maintain a sense of identity, dignity and self-esteem

Services should incorporate natural supports by being in the least restrictive, most natural setting possible. The usual work, education, leisure and support facilities in the community should be used in preference to specialised developments

Services should be accountable to the consumers and informal carers and evaluated to ensure their continuing appropriateness, acceptability and effectiveness on agreed parameters

Conclusion

Although there exists among many research and clinical staff reasonable agreement about which principles should guide the development and provision of services (Table 19.11), very often clinical practice falls far short of the implementation of these principles. More specifically, it is now commonplace to state that services should be needs-led, yet four vital issues currently prevent the realisation of this intent. First, as this chapter shows, there is no widespread agreement on how to define needs for services for individuals or for populations. Second, leading on from this, the measurement of need is still in its early development. Third, we still have only limited information on the cost-effectiveness of specific interventions for specific mental-health-related needs. Finally, if these three prior steps were complete, the results of mental health service evaluative studies would more precisely indicate the extent to which such services are underfunded.

References

Beecham, J., Knapp, M. & Fenyo, A. (1993). Costs, needs and outcomes in community mental health care. In *Costing Community Care*, ed. A. Netten & J. Beecham. Aldershot: Ashgate.

Brewin, C. (1992). Measuring individual needs for care and services. In *Measuring Mental Health Needs*, ed. G. Thornicroft, C.R. Brewin & J. Wing. London: Gaskell/Royal College of Psychiatrists.

Brewin, C. & Wing, J. (1993). The MRC Needs for Care Assessment: progress and controversies. *Psychological Medicine*, **23**, 837–41.

Brewin, C., Wing, J.K., Mangen, S.P., Brugha, T.S. & MacCarthy, B. (1987). Principles and practice of measuring needs in the long-term mentally ill: the MRC Needs for Care Assessment. *Psychological Medicine*, **17**, 971–82.

Brewin, C., Wing, J., Mangen, S., *et al.* (1988). Needs for care among the long-term mentally ill: a report from the Camberwell High Contact Survey. *Psychological Medicine*, **18**, 457–68.

Brewin, C., Veltro, F., Wing, J., *et al.* (1990). The assessment of psychiatric disability in the community: a comparison of clinical, staff, and family interviews. *British Journal of Psychiatry*, **157**, 671–4.

Burton, P. (1993). Community Profiling: *A Guide to Identifying Local Needs*. Bristol: School for Advanced Urban Studies, University of Bristol.

Culyer, A. & Wagstaff, A. (1992). *Need, Equity and Equality in Health and Health Care*. York: Centre for Health Economics, Health Economics Consortium, University of York.

Davies, B. & Challis, D. (1986). *Matching Resources to Needs in Community Care*. London: Gower.

Department of Health (1994). The Health of the Nation, 2nd edn. London: HMSO.

Ellis, K. (1993). *Squaring the Circle: User and Carer Participation in Needs Assessment*. York: Joseph Rowntree Foundation.

Fisher, N., Turner, S.W., Pugh, R. & Taylor, C. (1994). Estimating numbers of homeless and homeless mentally ill in North East Westminster by using capture–recapture analysis. *British Medical Journal*, **308**, 27–30.

Gibbons, J.L., Jennings, C. & Wing, J.K. (1984). *Psychiatric Care in Eight Register Areas*. Southampton: University Department of Psychiatry.

Glover, G. (1991). The official data available on mental health. In *Indicators for Mental Health in the Population*, ed. R. Jenkins & S. Griffiths. London: HMSO.

Goldberg D.P. & Blackwell, B. (1970). Psychiatric illness in general practice: a detailed study using a new method of case identification.

British Medical Journal, **ii**, 439–43.

Goldberg, D. & Bridges K. (1988). Somatic presentation of psychiatric illness in primary care settings. *Journal of Psychosomatic Research*, **32**, 137–44.

Goldberg, D. & Huxley, P. (1980). *Mental Illness in the Community*. London: Tavistock.

Goldberg, D. & Huxley, P. (1992). *Common Mental Disorders: A Bio-Social Model*. London: Routledge.

Goldman, H. (1981). Defining and counting the chronically mentally ill. *Hospital and Community Psychiatry*, **32**, 21–7.

Hansson, L. (1989). Utilisation of psychiatric in-patient care. *Acta Psychiatrica Scandinavica*, **79**, 571–8.

Hillier, W., Zaudig, M. & Mobour, W. (1991). Development of diagnostic checklists for use in routine clinical care. *Archives of General Psychiatry*, **47**, 782–4.

Hirsch, S. (1988). *Psychiatric Beds and Resources: Factors Influencing Bed Use and Service Planning*. London: Gaskell/Royal College of Psychiatrists.

Hogg, L. & Marshall, M. (1992). Can we measure need in the homeless mentally ill? Using the MRC Needs for Care Assessment in hostels for the homeless. *Psychological Medicine*, **22**, 1027–34.

Holloway, F. (1994). Need in community psychiatry: a consensus is required. *Psychiatric Bulletin*, **18**, 321–3.

House of Commons (1985). *Second Report from the Social Services Committee, Session 1984–85*, Community Care. London: HMSO.

House of Commons (1990). *The National Health Service and Community Care Act*. London: HMSO.

Jarman, B. (1983). Identification of underprivileged areas. *British Medical Journal*, **286**, 1705–9.

Jarman, B. (1984). Underprivileged areas: validation and distribution of scores. *British Medical Journal*, **289**, 1587–92.

Jarman, B. & Hirsch, S. (1992). Statistical models to predict district psychiatric morbidity. In *Measuring Mental Health Needs*, ed. G. Thornicroft, C. Brewin & J.K. Wing, chapter 4. London: Gaskell/Royal College of Psychiatrists.

Johnson, S. & Thornicroft, G. (1993). The sectorisation of psychiatric services in England and Wales. *Social Psychiatry and Psychiatric Epidemiology*, **28**, 45–7.

Kendrick, A., Sibbald, B., Burns, T. & Freeling, P. (1991). Role of general practitioners in care of long term mentally ill patients. *British Medical Journal*, **302**, 508–11.

Lehtinen, V., Joukamaa, M., Jyrkinen, E., *et al.* (1990). Need or mental health services of the adult population in Finland: results from the Mini Finland Health Survey. *Acta Psychiatrica Scandinavica*, **81**, 426–31.

Lesage, A.D., Mignolli, G., Faccincani, C., *et al.* (1991). Standardised assessment of the needs for care in a cohort of patients with schizophrenic psychoses. In *Community-Based Psychiatry: Long-Term Patterns of Care in South Verona*, ed. M. Tansella, pp. 27–33. *Psychological Medicine Monograph*, Supplement 19.

Lindholm, H. (1983). Sectorised psychiatry. *Acta Psychiatrica Scandinavica*, **67**, Supplement 304.

Liss, P. (1990). *Health Care Need: Meaning and Measurement*. Studies in Arts and Science. Linkoping.

MacCarthy, B., *et al*. (1988). The role of relatives. In *Community Care in Practice: Services for the Continuing Care Client*, ed. A. Lavender & F. Holloway, pp. 207–27. Chichester: Wiley.

Macdonald, A. (1991). How can we measure mental health? In *Indicators for Mental Health in the Population*, ed. R. Jenkins & S. Griffiths. London: HMSO.

Mallman, C.A. & Marcus, S. (1980). Logical clarifications in the study of needs. In *Human Needs*, ed. K. Lederer, pp. 163–85. Cambridge, MA: Oelgeschlager, Gunn & Hain.

Mangen, S. & Brewin, C.R. (1991). The measurement of need. In *Social Psychiatry: Theory, Methodology and Practice*, ed. P.E. Bebbington, pp. 163–81. Transaction Press.

Marshall, M. (1989). Collected and neglected: are Oxford hostels filling up with disabled psychiatric patients? *British Medical Journal*, **299**, 706–9.

Marshall, M. (1994). How should we measure need? *Philosophy, Psychiatry and Psychology*, **1**, 27–36.

Marshall, M. & Reed, A. (1992). Psychiatric morbidity in homeless women. *British Journal of Psychiatry*, **160**, 761–8.

Maslow, A. (1968). *Towards a Psychology of Being*, 2nd edn. New York: van Nostrand.

McCrone, P. & Strathdee, G. (1994). Needs not diagnosis: towards a more rational approach to community mental health resourcing in Great Britain. *International Journal of Social Psychiatry*, **2**, 79–86.

National Institute of Mental Health (1987). *Toward a Model Plan for a Comprehensive Community-Based Mental Health System*. Washington, DC: National Institute of Mental Health.

Pantellis, C., Taylor, J. & Campbell, P. (1988). The South Camden schizophrenia survey. *Psychiatric Bulletin*, **12**, 98–101.

Phelan, M., Slade, M., Thornicroft, G., *et al*. (1995). The Camberwell Assessment of Need (CAN): the validity and reliability of an instrument to assess the needs of the seriously mentally ill. *British Journal of Psychiatry*, in press.

Pryce, I., Griffiths, R., Gentry, R., Hughes, I., Montaguss, L., Watkins, S., Champney-Smith, J. & McLackland, B. (1993). How important is the assessment of social skills in a long-stay psychiatric in-patients? *British Journal of Psychiatry*, **163**, 498–502.

Scott, J. (1993). Homelessness and mental illness. *British Journal of Psychiatry*, **162**, 314–24.

Shapiro, S., Skinner, E.A., Kramer, M., *et al*. (1985). Measuring need for mental health services in a general population. *Medical Care*, **23**, 1033–43.

Sharp, D. & Morrell, D. (1989). The psychiatry of general practice. In *Scientific Approaches on Epidemiological and Social Psychiatry. Essays in Honour of Michael Shepherd*, ed. P. Williams, G. Wilkinson & K. Rawnsley.

London: Routledge.

Shepherd, M., Cooper, B., Brown, A., *et al.* (1966). *Psychiatric Illness in General Practice*. London: Oxford University Press.

Slade, M. (1994). Needs assessment: who needs to assess? *British Journal of Psychiatry*, **165**, 287–92.

Stevens, A. & Gabbay, J. (1991). Needs assessment, needs assessment. *Health Trends*, **23**, 20–3.

Stevens, A. & Gabbay, J. (1992). The purchaser's information requirements on mental health needs and controlling for mental health services. In *Measuring Mental Health Needs*, ed. G. Thornicroft, C. Brewin & J.K. Wing, chapter 3. London: Gaskell/Royal College of Psychiatrists.

Stevens, A. & Raftery, J. (1994). Introduction. In *Health Care Needs Assessment*, ed. A. Stevens & J. Raftery, pp. 11–30. Oxford: Radcliffe Medical Press.

Strathdee, G. & Phelan, M. (eds.) (1993). *The Maudsley Practical Clinical Handbook Series for General Practitioners*. (i) Crisis Intervention (in press), (ii) Making Use of the Consultation (in preparation), (iii) Suicide (Health of the Nation), (iv) Depression, (v) Anxiety, (vi) Organic Disorder, (vii) Drugs and Alcohol, (viii) Eating Disorders. Nottingham: Boots.

Strathdee, G. & Thornicroft, G. (1992). Community sectors for needs-led mental health services. In *Measuring Mental Health Needs*, ed. G. Thornicroft, C. Brewin & J.K. Wing, chapter 8. London: Gaskell/Royal College of Psychiatrists.

Strathdee, G. & Thornicroft, G. (1995). Community psychiatry and service evaluation. In *Essentials of Psychiatry*, ed. R. Murray, P. Hill & P. McGuffin. Cambridge: Cambridge University Press (in press).

Strathdee, G. & Williams, G. (1984). A survey of psychiatrists in primary care: the silent growth of a new service. *Journal of the Royal College of General Practitioners*, **34**, 615–8.

Thornicroft, G. (1991). Social deprivation and rates of treated mental disorder: developing statistical models to predict psychiatric service utilisation. *British Journal of Psychiatry*, **158**, 475–84.

Thornicroft, G. (1994). The NHS and Community Care Act, 1990. *Psychiatric Bulletin of the Royal College of Psychiatrists*, **18**, 13–7.

Thornicroft, G. & Bebbington, P. (1995). Quantitative methods in the evaluation of community mental health services. *Modern Community Psychiatry* (in press).

Thornicroft, G. & Strathdee, G. (1994). How many psychiatric beds? *British Medical Journal*, **309**, 970–1.

Thornicroft, G., Brewin, C. & Wing, J. (1992). *Measuring Mental Health Needs*. London: Royal College of Psychiatrists.

Thornicroft, G., De Salvia, G. & Tansella, M. (1993). Urban–rural differences in the associations between social deprivation and psychiatric service utilization in schizophrenia and all diagnoses: a case-register study in Northern Italy. *Psychological Medicine*, **23**, 487–496.

Timms, P. & Fry, A. (1989). Homelessness and mental illness. *Health Trends*,

21, 70–1.

Tracy, L. (1986). Toward an improved need theory: in response to legitimate criticism. *Behavioral Science*, **31**, 205–18.

Tyrer P., Turner, R. & Johnson, A. (1989). Integrated hospital and community psychiatric services and use of inpatient beds. *British Medical Journal*, **299**, 298–300.

van Haaster, I., Lesage, A., Cyr, M. & Toupin, J. (1994). Problems and needs for care of patients suffering from severe mental illness. *Social Psychiatry and Psychiatric Epidemiology*, **29**, 141–8.

Wing, J. (1971). How many psychiatric beds? *Psychological Medicine*, **1**, 189–90.

Wing, J. (ed.) (1989). *Health Services Planning and Research: Contributions from Psychiatric Case Registers*. London: Gaskell.

Wing, J.K. (1992). *Epidemiologically Based Needs Assessments: Review of Research on Psychiatric Disorders*. London: Department of Health.

PART VI

HEALTH ECONOMICS IN MENTAL HEALTH

20

Programme-level and system-level health economics

M A R T I N K N A P P A N D J E N N I F E R B E E C H A M

Costs and health economics

Cost-effectiveness is in vogue. The search for cost-effectiveness (or 'value for money' or 'efficiency') is being conducted at all levels of government, in most health care systems, and from a number of perspectives. All such searches are examples or special cases of economic evaluation. The search for cost-effectiveness is not confined to national health care strategies and systems' reorganisations, but is actively under way at both the programme level and systems level. Creating the right incentives and the right micro- and macro-systems for effective and cost-effective delivery of mental health care must be a fundamental objective.

By repute, cost-effectiveness analysis – or economic evaluation more generally – is neither simple nor uncontroversial. In fact, it is merely 'an effort to bridge the gap between a conceptual model – theoretic welfare economics – and actual social policy' (Weisbrod & Helming, 1980). Welfare economics is that branch of economics concerned with the relationship between an economic system and the wellbeing of individuals. It has developed the techniques of economic evaluation as means of appraising efficiency in contexts where markets either do not exist or cannot be relied on to generate efficiency automatically. Where economic evaluation differs from other evaluative techniques is in its examination of a fuller range of causes and effects. The common theme of all evaluative research is to enquire whether a particular project or course of action is worthwhile. The difference between economic and other evaluations is the meaning attached to the term 'worthwhile': economic evaluations add the cost dimension.

Economic evaluation does not seek to replace the sound or educated judgement of the decision maker. Final decisions will be made by politicians (at the systems level) or clinicians (at the programme level), advised by administrators and interpreted by managers, in the light of available information. It is the principal aim of all evaluative research, and economic evaluation is certainly no exception, to provide a more considered and sound information base for policy decisions. Some years ago, Weisbrod (1979) made the important point that this technique will never 'make decisions', but if it is vigorously pursued it will 'make decisions better informed'.

Economic evaluations are not restricted to answering questions about efficiency, for increasingly they have sought to examine *distributional* implications. They can provide answers to a wide variety of questions (Williams, 1974): *What* treatment or support service is more or most appropriate in given circumstances? *When* should treatment be provided? *Where* should it be provided? *To whom* should treatment be delivered, and *how*? Answers to these five generic questions should obviously aid the decision-making tasks of mental health care purchasers and providers at both local and central levels, as well as managers and politicians. We return to these evaluative questions later in the chapter.

The aims of this chapter are to introduce the methods of economic evaluation as they are applied to mental health services at the programme (micro) and systems (macro) levels, to illustrate these methods with examples from recent evaluations, and to discuss their relevance. The aims of an economic evaluation as we interpret them are usually the following:

- to collect data on service utilisation, accommodation, medication, employment and 'informal care' in order to calculate the costs associated with each of a number of interventions;
- to describe the total and component costs, over time and by funding agency or individual, for each intervention; and then to examine variations in total and component costs and their associations with characteristics of individuals and by reference to the nature of alternative treatments or interventions;
- to collect and analyse data on the outcomes of treatment for individuals; and
- to analyse, at both aggregate and individual levels, the links between costs, needs (and other individual characteristics) and outcomes.

Methodologically, economic evaluations of systems or programmes are little different. It is the scale of the enterprise and the magnitude of measures that will vary, rather than the framework. At the systems level we might measure costs in thousands of pounds per year and outcomes as, say, a reduction in suicide rate. By contrast, at the programme level we might measure cost in pounds per week and outcomes as changes in clinical symptoms or behaviour for individual people with mental health problems.

The stages of economic evaluation

It is helpful to distinguish six stages for an economic evaluation:

1 identify or define the alternatives to be evaluated;
2 list the costs and outcomes (or effects);
3 quantify and value the costs and outcomes;
4 compare the costs and outcomes, reaching a tentative conclusion or recommendation;
5 examine that conclusion or recommendation in the light of risk, uncertainty and sensitivity; and
6 examine the distributional implications of the alternatives.

Stage one: Identify the alternatives

The exact nature of the range of mental health treatment or care options to be evaluated needs to be made explicit at the outset. The research question must be clear. For example, are we concerned with whether or not to provide treatment A, or are we choosing between treatments A and B? Policy or practice constraints may narrow the range of options, perhaps to a single intervention type. We might then use the evaluative framework to provide information on 'How much of this intervention is optimal?' Clearly, in this first stage there is no difference between an economic evaluation and any other evaluation: both need careful explication of the objectives and hypotheses.

Stage two: List the costs and outcomes

At the second stage, all the likely costs and outcomes need to be listed, although no attempt is made to measure them just yet. Even if a cost or outcome is considered to be immeasurable it should still be listed so as not to be forgotten in the final discussion and interpretation. Costs and outcomes are not always distinct. Consider, for example, the comparison of hospital and community care for elderly people with dementia. One important cost of community care may be the burden and strain borne by relatives. But the removal of this burden is also an outcome of hospital care, and so an evaluation of the two options must be careful not to double count it.

Costs fall on the agency directly responsible for providing and/or purchasing care (such as the psychiatric unit or a residential facility). Costs also fall indirectly on other agencies such as a public sector housing department, primary health care service or the criminal justice system, and there are often costs for users (patients), relatives and neighbours. The direct costs are those immediately and readily attributable to service users through agency accounts: the average weekly cost of inpatient hospital treatment or residential care or nursing home for elderly people. Indirect costs are associated with services such as social work teams and primary health care, and are also incurred by families and others. Financial costs to families can be high. McGuire (1991) reports the work of Franks' unpublished PhD dissertation (1987), who estimated both the out-of-pocket expenses related to their relative's illness and the time implications of their caregiving role. More recently, Weinberger *et al.* (1993) found primary caregivers spent 105 hours per week on care activities. Netten (1993) provides a useful framework for valuing the opportunity cost of informal care. Indirect costs, depending on the scope of the research question, may also include the value of lost output due to the reduced productivity caused by illness. This could be measured using the average loss of net earnings as a result of time taken off work (Ratcliffe, 1993).

A classificatory schema is detailed in Table 20.1, where examples of the different types of cost are drawn from the range of services for elderly people with mental health problems in the United Kingdom. (All of these cost dimensions – and many of the outcome dimensions described below – were addressed in our own evaluation of two community care alternatives to long-stay hospital residence. See Knapp *et al.* (1994b). In their path-breaking evaluation of community care with care management for elderly people, Davies & Challis (1986) covered all these dimensions.) Costs included in the table are of three kinds:

- *living costs* (expenditure on provisions, clothing, personal needs and so on);

Table 20.1. *A costs classification with illustrations from the support of elderly people with dementia*

| | Examples of costs incurred by: | | |
	Direct care agency	Other agencies	Users and others
Direct costs	Inpatient hospital; residential or nursing homes; home help	Public sector housing; voluntary organisation homes	Elderly people's own housing and food expenditures; user charges for residential care
Indirst costs	Community nursing; speech or occupational therapy	Local authority care management; field social work; voluntary sector day care	Families' caring 'burden' – lost work or leisure opportunities

- *labour costs* (staff costs in hospitals and residential homes, and costs incurred by relatives providing family care); and
- *capital costs* (durable resource inputs such as the residential home, the client's own home and so on).

Many mental health evaluations and commentaries have concerned themselves only with the direct costs or resource implications for the main providing agency. Häfner and an der Heiden (1989, 1990) take this approach in their evaluation of community care in Mannheim, Germany, and all the studies of diagnostic-related groups appear to have focused solely on inpatient hospital admissions. This narrow measurement of costs is becoming increasingly inappropriate with the growing practice of providing community-based and comprehensive alternatives to inpatient treatment. Evaluations which concentrate on the cost burdens or savings to the traditional mental health system (see, for example, Wiersma *et al.*, 1991) will not only underestimate the costs of community care but also forgo the opportunity to examine the distributional impact of service innovation.

Health service managers might argue that requirements for greater financial acuity make it hard for them to be concerned with costs incurred by other organisations or by users. This is short-sighted though understandable. Many of the non-health service costs fall directly to the taxpayer or impose unwanted or heavy burdens on families, and a decrease in the expenditure or costs included in the left-hand column of Table 20.1 will be quite likely to produce an *increase* in the costs included in the other two columns. In fact, in our experience few managers or practitioners argue against the *principle* of including these other costs, but budgetary constraints mean they often have to take decisions which reduce their own costs to the disadvantage of others. There is a need for changes in *incentives* in order to avoid actions which are clearly not in the broader social interest. In the United Kingdom, introducing these uncertainties is one of the aims of the community care reforms.

On the outcome or effectiveness side we can similarly distinguish outcomes or effects enjoyed by or relating to users, by people directly associated with users (mainly family members), and by other members of society. We could further make the distinction between 'observed' and 'concealed' effects. The former are readily identified in research or provision by observation of users and others. In the case of services for elderly people with dementia these observed effects might range over mobility, incontinence, self-care capacity and wandering behaviour. In contrast, changes in some mental health symptoms such as affect or anxiety, morale or subjective quality of life are less easily assessed; they can only really be measured by asking or assessing users themselves. This two-way classification of outcomes – benefits to whom, and how assessed – is detailed in Table 20.2 and illustrated again with examples taken from services for elderly people. Historically, most evaluations of mental health services focus only on the easily observed user outcomes in the top left-hand cell of Table 20.2. Other chapters in this book address outcome measurement principles in mental health evaluations.

The classification of costs and outcomes in this way has the signal advantage of ensuring that the full range of factors or dimensions is considered even if it later proves impossible to obtain measures for all of them. This is particularly important where international comparisons are undertaken, such as that attempted by Moscarelli *et al.* (1991), as not only may the scope of the evaluation or mental health system *per se* be different across countries but the medical purchasing power in each country may be different. However, there is still one more task to undertake at this second stage in an economic evaluation. This is to ensure that the listing of the costs and outcomes is consistent and sensible. There are four main issues to address.

The first is to exclude *transfer payments*, that is any transfers of money from one person to another which are not payment for goods or services

Table 20.2. *An outcome classification with illustrations from the support of elderly people with dementia*

	Example of the outcomes experienced by:		
	Users	Families	Wider society
Observed	Self-care capacity, mobility, incontinence	Employment opportunities for carers; increased leisure time	Availability of housing if elderly people in long-stay hospital or residential care
Concealed	Morale, loneliness	Psychological burden and joys of informal care	Benefits of seeing elderly people with proper care and support

received. Prime examples are taxation, unemployment and social security benefits. Second, we should be wary of *double counting*, particularly if we want to measure the costs and outcomes of alternative services over as wide a range as possible. Third, we should take care when including *secondary effects*, i.e. outcomes and costs accruing to people other than the immediate beneficiaries or sufferers. They should be included only if they have not already been taken into account by the market-determined valuations of the immediate or primary effects. Of course, transfer payments, some forms of double counting and secondary effects may well be important in examinations of the distributional consequences of different treatment or care options.

A fourth difficulty is to decide the length of time over which to measure costs and outcomes. The outputs of some mental health services could be argued to accrue over the full lifespan of people with mental health problems, but clearly we cannot wait that long before completing an evaluation. The cut-off point is thus sometimes arbitrary and usually determined by balancing the wish to measure outcomes and costs over as long a period as possible with the contrary pressure to produce a result.

Stage three: Quantify and value the costs and outcomes

There are actually two steps here: the quantification or measurement of the costs and outcomes listed at the second stage, and their subsequent valuation in monetary terms.

Cost measures are generally based on service utilisation data obtained from or for each individual user during a period of care or treatment. In our programme-level research, service utilisation data are collected using variants of the Client Service Receipt Interview or CSRI (Beecham & Knapp, 1992; Beecham, 1994). To date, the CSRI has been employed in more than 36 separate studies. Some service use data may also come from case notes, hospital records, depot clinic statistics and other sources. Costs can then be attached to each service or element of support in turn, using the best available estimates of long-run marginal opportunity cost, where 'marginal' refers to the addition of total cost attributable to the inclusion of one more patient, and 'opportunity cost' refers to the opportunities forgone by not using a resource in its best alternative use (Knapp, 1993). The short-run average revenue cost (obtained from a complete set of agency accounts), plus appropriately measured capital and overhead elements, is usually assumed to be close to the long-run marginal cost for many services, and there is now an excellent compendium of service costings for the United Kingdom, updated annually, which greatly assists this stage of the research (Netten & Smart, 1993; Netten, 1994). Costs for individual facilities are ideally based on local data, and ward-level costings often need to be calculated for inpatient hospital treatment.

Data collected from an interview instrument such as the CSRI can be cross-checked. For expensive items of a total 'care package', such as hospital inpatient admissions, information can be sought from hospital records. For specific service interventions such as cognitive-behavioural therapy, a particular drug regime or a psycho-educational package, further independent data can be gleaned from providers, although this obviously adds to the research task. Accommodation and living expenses comprise another large cost element, and the information needed can usually come from non-patient sources.

The most common economic evaluations are cost-effectiveness, cost-benefit and cost-utility analyses; CEA, CBA and CUA, respectively. Each sets out to measure costs comprehensively in accordance with the principles just outlined, but they treat outcome measurement differently. CEAs compare the costs of different policies in achieving an identical outcome, such as a uniform reduction in hospital readmission rates or different degrees of success, such as cost per readmission avoided. A multivariate CEA admits more than one outcome, examining the cost–outcome links *statistically* (see below).

The measures of outcome to be enjoyed in such an analysis will be driven by the broader needs of evaluation, and earlier chapters in this book have addressed their measurement.

A CBA values outcomes in monetary terms, making it possible to compare treatment costs with benefits using the same measure of value. The disadvantage is that a CBA might sometimes squeeze multifarious, complex effects into a monetary straitjacket. The simple comparison of 'costs incurred' with 'costs saved' may be a worthwhile exercise, but it is *not* a CBA for it neglects the impacts of services or treatments on users. A CUA compares cost with a global measure of quality-adjusted life year or QALY, allowing treatments to be compared in terms of cost per QALY. There has, as yet, been little development towards a usable QALY measure for mental health care applications (Wilkinson *et al.*, 1990, 1992).

Thus a CUA compares the costs of securing more quality-adjusted life years across different clinical interventions, a CBA indicates whether the outcomes of an intervention exceed the resources expended, and a (simple) CEA compares the costs of achieving a single consistent outcome. More complex cost-effectiveness analyses – using what economists would identify as cost function analyses based upon multivariate statistical methods – offer the opportunity to analyse more than one outcome simultaneously.

Cost-of-illness studies form a significant part of the applied health economics literature. They aim to calculate, at a national or systems level, the direct and indirect costs resulting from an illness. Grey & Fenn (1993), for example, calculate the cost of Alzheimer's disease in England to be £1039 million per year. Rice *et al.* (1992) estimated that the total cost of mental illness in the United States was $103.7 billion in 1985. This total includes both direct costs associated with detection, treatment and response to the consequences of ill-health and indirect costs such as the loss of productive output (Croft-Jeffreys & Wilkinson, 1989).

Debate arises over the use of such data. One strand of argument suggests that these data assist in the appropriate allocation of resources – those illnesses with the greatest resource consequences should be the focus of intervention programmes. The problem with this argument is that it assumes the benefits of an intervention can be equated with the financial savings, ignoring the outcomes of intervention. To make allocative decisions, policy-makers require information about the health gain of an intervention as well as the resource implications.

Stage four: Compare the costs and outcomes

By the start of this fourth stage, the evaluator will have obtained measures of costs and outcomes for each alternative treatment or service configuration. These costs and outcomes will often be spread over a period of some years. Typically a new project requiring substantial capital investment will have high costs in the first one or two years followed by a period of low costs, whilst there may be no user outcomes at all until the service is in operation. We therefore need to be able to compare costs incurred today with outcomes enjoyed tomorrow. As individuals, we generally prefer, say, $200 today rather than $200 tomorrow, because we have a whole day between now and then in which to use the money – a set of options which is not available tomorrow. This is what the economist calls time preference and, in an evaluation, may require the weighting of future costs and outcomes so as to render them comparable with present costs and outcomes.

In an evaluation the researcher must select a suitable value for these weights, called the *discount rate*, which is assumed to measure society's rate of time preference. A typical discount rate used in UK evaluations today is 5% or 6%. Weisbrod (1983) allowed 8% on the estimated value of the land and replacement cost of the buildings and fittings. The choice of discount rate is crucial and most economic evaluations will examine the implications of more than one numerical value (see Stage Five). The larger the discount rate the smaller the present value of a future cost or outcome. Therefore, if the major costs of a new policy or mode of treatment are incurred early and the outcomes are realised later, a discount rate which is 'too high' will tend to undervalue the present value of the outcomes relative to the costs.

The decision rules at the comparison stage were described earlier for the three main variants of economic evaluation: CEA, CBA and CUA. The simplest decision rule is to compare the costs and summary outcomes for each group of people or treatment option, and to conclude that the option with the lowest cost per given level of outcome is the more efficient. Obviously, this may not be easy to apply in practice, particularly with multidimensional outcome measures which do not move in concert. If some outcome dimensions register improvements and others deteriorate, or if the cost and outcome comparisons point to different preferred solutions, the simple decision rule may be difficult to implement. One option is to leave the weighting of costs and outcomes to the clinician, manager or other decision-maker, but to help them by providing accurate and informative summary results.

Another and not mutually exclusive option is to estimate supplementary cost functions. In its fully specified form, the cost function is the estimated relationship between the cost of providing an intervention on the one hand, and, on the other, the user outcomes, input prices and other factors with a hypothesised influence on cost. The precise form of a cost function is determined by the interaction of theoretical considerations and statistical findings (see, for example, Beecham *et al.*, 1991). It can be interpreted as a multivariate version of cost-effectiveness analysis. The cost function helps to tease out and statistically 'explain' inter-individual variations, and will usually illuminate cost–outcome and cost–need linkages.

Stage five: Take account of risk, uncertainty and sensitivity

The costs and outcomes calculated for the treatments or care practices being evaluated are often estimated, expected or predicted values. Their measurement will be subject to some error. It is important to qualify the decision rules and their recommendations by taking account of these errors. We can distinguish between risk, when we do not know the exact value of a cost or outcome variable but we do know its probability distribution, and *uncertainty*, when neither the variable nor its probability distribution is known. Uncertainty is more common than risk. Other errors are possible; for example, we may set the discount rate too high, compute a mistaken unit cost or allow too short a time lapse for follow-up. The evaluator should therefore conduct sensitivity analyses, examining the implications of alternative key assumptions. McGuire (1991), for example, showed that using a discount rate of 4% rather than 8% on Weisbrod's cost data considerably reduced the cost advantage of the community programme relative to standard hospital-based treatment. McGuire also reports the wide cost variations found by Cannon *et al.* (1985) during the examination of the capital cost implications of the Massachusetts Mental Health Centre.

Stage six: Examine the distributional implications

The three main types of economic evaluation are mainly prompted by, and concerned with, *efficiency* considerations. How does this new treatment or that new care policy influence the cost of achieving specified outcomes, or how does it improve the outcomes obtained from a specified level of expenditure? But it is often important to examine the equity implications.

One course of action is to include a different set of weights at the third stage so as to take account of the fact that the outcomes may be falling mainly to the more or less affluent (or less or more needy) members of society. The evaluator would probably want to examine the implications of a number of different sets of distributional weights via a sensitivity analysis. In practical circumstances, weights have been based on relative incomes, marginal rates of gross taxation, marginal rates of net taxation (benefit–burden ratios) and the weights implicit in other governmental decisions. An alternative course of action would be to assume equal weights but comment at the end of the analysis on their distributional or equity implications. A danger of including other distributional weights before aggregation 'is that this becomes just another part of the "tool kit", another issue that [economic evaluation] "solves" for the decision maker' (Drummond, 1981, p. 141). There is also the danger that equity might get subsumed under efficiency and that the evaluation merely becomes a vehicle for the evaluator's own prejudices. However, it would be wrong for the analyst not to make clear the implications of alternative treatments or policies for individuals in different socio-economic groups or different areas of the country. In some cases, of course, the distributional implications may be too small to be of consequence, although this ought to be checked carefully.

Questions addressed by economic evaluations

Economic evaluations can provide valuable information of the kind needed for a variety of treatment or policy discussions and decisions. Earlier we identified five main types of evaluation question which we can now use to structure a discussion of some of the central issues which economic evaluations can address, illustrated with evidence from recent research. Not all the studies cited below conform to the standard structure for economic evaluation, nor do all of these succeed in adhering fully to the methodological recommendations described above, but we summarise the results as indicative of research activities at the programme and systems levels.

What care service or treatment mode is more or most appropriate in given circumstances?

As an example of how economic evaluation addresses the 'what' question we can draw on the recent UK discussion of clozapine for the treatment of schizophrenia. Davies & Drummond (1993) offer some interesting evidence of clozapine's comparative cost-effectiveness over conventional neuroleptic therapy. This UK study was not typical or standard, for it was retrospective, based on US data not obtained from randomisation, and used Delphi judgements rather than actual placements and outcomes. Nevertheless, it usefully raised important economic questions about drug therapies. After sensitivity analysis (allowing key assumptions to vary), Davies and Drummond concluded that clozapine was cost-saving or cost-neutral under the conditions of psychiatric practice in the United Kingdom, and was cost-effective for people with severe, chronic schizophrenia.

Prospective, controlled studies, embodying economic evaluations, are obviously needed for other drugs treating schizophrenia (such as risperidone) and for other psychiatric problems. The same is true for other forms of treatment such as psychological therapies, including cognitive-behavioural therapy (Tarrier *et al.*, 1993; Kingdon & Turkington, 1993). Crits-Christoph (1992) found that brief dynamic psychotherapy is about as effective as other forms of psychotherapy and medication. Although cost issues were not addressed in this article we might assume that the reduction in duration of treatment brings with it a cost advantage. However, there may be financial incentives not to provide this form of treatment. Mechanic (1991) suggests that payment on a fee-for-service basis creates incentives to provide therapy beyond the point at which it could be cost-effective. Another example of an economic evaluation addressing the 'what' question is the study of experimental home-based treatment in South London by Burns *et al.* (1993). People receiving this new service fared better than those receiving conventional care; in particular a substantial reduction in inpatient stays was found for people with schizophrenia when compared with those with other diagnoses.

When should care or treatment be provided?

It is common for health economists to examine the efficacy and efficiency of preventive measures, but not – it would seem – in relation to mental health problems. Backhouse *et al.* (1992) listed more than 300 English language health economics studies of prevention, but only one in psychiatry, and this was a modest evaluation of case registers published in 1980.

It is in the field of child psychiatry that the 'when' question can be most usefully illustrated. Two short articles have recently summarised the key aspects of the debate (Cottrell, 1993; Light & Bailey, 1993). An important question is whether child psychiatry services can muster good arguments for additional resources to meet need or produce health gain. Light and Bailey suggest that expenditure on child psychiatry services for disturbed and abused children reduces costs to education, health, social care and criminal justice services in the short term. Moreover, 'as untreated cases show a high probability of pathology in later childhood, adolescence and adulthood' (p. 17), the health gain can be measured not only in terms of the child's wellbeing (reduction in pain, shame and the private horrors of abuse) but also in the prevention of poverty, crimes, injuries and self-induced illnesses. While the cost of meeting needs for child psychiatry services is much higher than the current resource allocation, the cost of not meeting them is arguably even higher: 'child mental health services are a prime example of the kind of service that can provide long-term benefits in exchange for relatively cheap early intervention' (Cottrell, 1993).

In the field of adult mental health the timing of treatment has generally not been the focus of much evaluative attention from health economists. In the United Kingdom, Burns *et al.* (1993) and Merson *et al.* (1992) examined prompt or early intervention services. An evaluation of community psychiatric nursing services in Greenwich showed that the introduction of care management practices was a cost-effective alternative to standard care, but only in the first 6 months after referral to the service. In the longer term differences were not significant (McCrone *et al.*, 1994).

Where should care or treatment be provided?

Policy debates about mental health provision in the United Kingdom have been dominated by the balance between inpatient and community care. As far as the *long-term* care of people with chronic mental health problems is concerned, UK evidence should encourage the further move away from hospital inpatient treatment. A North London study of the closure of two hospitals found evidence of lower community care costs for most former long-stay inpatients, except those with more challenging symptoms and behavioural problems (Knapp *et al.*, 1993; Hallam *et al.*, 1994), whilst outcomes after 1 year of community residence were as good as or better than outcomes for matched stayers in hospital (Anderson *et al.*, 1993).

Health economics evidence also points to the potential for cost-effective diversion away from inpatient admission. The Maudsley Hospital Daily Living Programme (DLP) provided problem-oriented, home-based care for people with severe mental illness facing emergency admission, modelled on earlier experiments with intensive community support teams, particularly in Madison, Wisconsin (Stein & Test, 1980). A randomised, controlled evaluation compared the DLP with standard inpatient hospital-based care, and found that the new service improved symptoms and social adjustment slightly more, and enhanced patients' and relatives' satisfaction over a period of 20 months after admission (Marks *et al.*, 1994). Using a methodology for the economic evaluation similar to that described earlier, the DLP was also found to be significantly less costly than standard treatment over this period (Knapp *et al.*, 1994a).

The move away from inpatient care is apparent in other countries. Häfner & an der Heiden's work in Mannheim, Germany (1990) examines the impact of outpatient appointments on length of stay in the hospital and in the community. In the United States, Dickey *et al.* (1989) compare a traditional inpatient-based system with a new day hospital-inn programme which showed significant cost advantages, though the authors suggest that financial incentives alone are not enough to encourage such relocation of care.

Some studies address the question of where, within the range of community provision, care should be provided. Wiersma *et al.* (1991), for example, examine the feasibility of day treatment with community care. Service location within the developing mixed economy is also an issue. In North London services provided by the independent sectors for former hospital residents were found to be more cost-effective than those managed by the public sector after standardising for needs and outcomes. Health-authority-managed services in particular were shown to be more costly than expected (Beecham *et al.*, 1991). Sectoral efficiency has long been a research issue in the United States. McCue & Clement (1993), for example, found patients had longer admissions in private (for-profit) psychiatric hospitals and that public general hospitals played a more significant role than private hospitals in treating mental illness among indigent persons. Looking particularly at nursing home facilities, Weisbrod & Schlesinger (1986) found differences in quality of care and frequency of resident complaints between non-profit and for-profit providers.

Kavanagh *et al.* (1993, 1994) describe two systems-level balance of care studies. Each of the studies describes the current balance of provision for people with a particular condition (dementia in one case; schizophrenia in the other), the services received, their associated cost and the projected cost-effectiveness improvements that might be secured by altering the balance. Both studies build on a number of programme-level economic and other evaluations.

To whom should care or treatment be provided?

Economic evaluations in psychiatry have rarely addressed this 'to whom' question, although the controversy over the efficacy of clozapine relates in part to its targeting during the US trial on particular groups of people with schizophrenia (Healy, 1993). Similarly, a study of inpatient hospital stays for risperidone treatment related only to patients with schizophrenia who completed a year of treatment and who thus tolerated the drug well (Addington *et al.*, 1993). However, the factors which limit the generalisability of trial results might simultaneously assist in the targeting of comparatively expensive treatments.

Surgery for epilepsy is another treatment mode which is known to be most effective for a small proportion of people with the condition: where the patient's condition is resistant to drug therapy, where the pattern and severity of seizures is unacceptable, and where the origin of the condition is from an organic brain lesion (Rossi, 1990). In the same article Rossi asserts that 'the results that surgery can offer to epileptics, not helped sufficiently by pharmacological treatment, can be very good' (p. 61), with a range of outcomes from the disappearance of seizures to the very rare case of deterioration. Silfvenius (1988), when calculating the economic costs of epilepsy, was more optimistic, suggesting that surgery will lead to functioning at a normal level for 20% of patients and that 50% of those operated on will become seizure-free. The economic gain can be calculated in *indirect costs*, for example due to patients returning to or starting work thereby reducing the costs to unemployment benefit and increasing productivity.

The direct costs would also be reduced as there is a lower need for supervised care.

Indications are filtering through from research evidence that this 'to whom' question might be an important consideration in the implementation of care management. Intagliata (1982) defined case management as a process 'to enhance the continuity of care and its accessibility, accountability and efficiency'. By 1986, nineteen US states had Medicaid-supported case management programmes. Two years later the Griffiths Report, a highly influential review of British community care, identified the need for case management (Thornicroft, 1991), although experimental projects have existed in the United Kingdom since the early 1980s. There is evidence to suggest that people who are unwilling to attend hospital-based services, who show poor medication compliance and poor ability to monitor themselves, and who have frequent crises are most likely to benefit from 'assertive case-management' (Skeer & Diamond, 1985, quoted in Thornicroft, 1991).

More generally, disaggregated data are needed to tease out the *individual* characteristics of patients associated with different outcomes and costs. For example, the disaggregation of costs in the North London psychiatric reprovision study described earlier had considerable predictive power, showing how community care costs responded to patients' pre-discharge symptoms and needs. Disaggregated cost analyses were also conducted for the DLP study, revealing associations between the downstream costs of treatment and the characteristics of people at admission (Knapp, 1995). Neither of these studies attempted to direct purchasers or providers to concentrate available treatment on particular groups of patients, but they demonstrated the cost consequences of doing so. Under conditions of resource scarcity, such inter-personal comparisons are inevitable and the people who must decide on the allocations of treatment resources at both systems and programme levels should ordinarily benefit from having health economics and other evidence to assist their decisions.

How should treatment be provided?

This final evaluative question is closely linked to the others, for the organisation of treatment usually cannot be separated from its location or targeting. At the systems evaluation level we can identify a number of North American studies which explore the implications of insurance and other funding mechanisms. Bigelow & McFarland (1989), for example, show how attempts to contain costs can push up administrative overheads, resulting in fewer people being seen by mental health services, fewer illnesses treated and fewer treatment procedures covered by insurance. Frank & Jackson (1989) examined the impact of different payment and budgetary arrangements on psychiatric admissions. Pre-set budgets, rather than reimbursement after the event, were associated with a fall in admission rates and substitution of outpatient services for inpatient treatment. Similar results were found in a two-group case–control study, which also found no significant differences between the groups in patient satisfaction or clinical outcome (Sederer *et al.*, 1992). Capitated budgets, such as those used within the US Preferred Provider Organizations and Health Maintenance Organizations, create incentives to provide as little care as necessary (Mechanic, 1991). Mental health provision shifted from psychiatrists and psychologists to general physicians and social workers, resulting in lower intensity of service use by patients and lower costs.

This fifth evaluation question can be distinguished from the other generic questions at the programme evaluation level by its emphasis on improved *coordination* of support and treatment, whether through care programmes (North & Ritchie, 1993; Schneider, 1995), care management (Huxley, 1992) or other case-level coordinating activities aiming for better and multi-agency assessments and closer links between needs and services.

In providing care management services for elderly people in the United Kingdom, evaluations of the early experimental projects found budgetary devolution to staff with smaller caseloads and comprehensive information could produce less costly packages which were also better for elderly people and their informal carers (Challis & Davies, 1986). There have, as yet, been few such in-depth studies of care management for people with mental health problems in Europe. In the United States, an experiment which gave vouchers to clients to 'buy' services through budget-holding case management programmes promoted choice and flexibility for clients but also required new organisational and administrative mechanisms which would permit users to make choices (Bertsch, 1992). The results of evaluations of case management provide conflicting evidence on cost-effectiveness, although the consequences of not having such arrangements could be dire (Melzer *et al.*, 1991).

Is economic evaluation suitable for mental health care?

This chapter has considered evaluation at both systems level and programme level. Indeed, from the perspective which we have adopted it is often difficult to separate the two, for the level at which one addresses economic questions generally need not change the methodology. The questions we posed in the previous section are as applicable to systems-level data as to programme-level data, as evidenced by the research used to illustrate them. Moreover, one might generalise from programme results to the systems implications, as tended to happen in UK mental health policy documents of the early 1980s exhorting the replacement of hospital care with community care, and as we have ourselves done in making national cost extrapolations for hospital closure (Knapp *et al.*, 1992a).

What does change from level to level is the means of undertaking the evaluation. At the programme level one might set up a controlled design, perhaps randomly allocating people to experimental and standard services. This design is not always possible in the real world of mental health care, and before-and-after studies, matched designs or quasi-experimental studies can all be undertaken within the over-arching methodological approach described here. This is particularly important at the systems level where an RCT (randomised controlled trail) would be almost inconceivable.

This discussion of the stages of economic evaluation has highlighted two things: first, the mode of analysis is probably less straightforward than it may at first appear, harbouring, as it does, a number of difficulties of both theory and application, but – second – it can also be very informative (Knapp, 1995). There are other features of economic evaluations which need to be appreciated, as well as some misconceptions to lay to rest.

Economic evaluations will be of limited help in the choice between, say, the expansion of nursing home facilities for elderly people and the provision of more child and adolescent psychiatry sessions, nor do they claim to do more than give indicative results. Two other misconceptions are that economic evaluations only consider monetary items and that they attempt to place monetary values on items that are 'priceless' or 'beyond money'. The first thing to notice is that some items are only without prices by historical accident. Blood, for example, was not marketed in Britain until 1983, when the National Health Service introduced charges for private hospitals (and then the 'market' was very limited), while it is marketed in many other countries. Just because an item is not marketed in one society does not mean that it can *never be marketed*, and we must not confuse positive and normative views on these issues. Second, decision makers are usually attaching *implicit* valuations to many items or eventualities. Whenever a clinician, nurse, care manager or government minister allocates resources between services or users, a decision has been made as to the relative costs and outcomes of competing claims on those resources. Whether the values underlying these allocations are 'correct' is obviously a value judgement. One aim of an evaluation, therefore, should be to make these values explicit so that decisions might be more consistent and better informed.

Cost-effectiveness and other modes of economic evaluation are more art that science. They are ways of organising thought rather than mechanistic rules for allocating resources. Evaluations cannot replace the judgements of decision-makers but they can supplement and inform them. They can help the decision-maker formulate policy questions sensibly and logically, and then (generally) provide a range of *answers* from which the decision-maker might choose. If the decision-maker misinterprets these answers it is the evaluator's responsibility to point this out. It is not, however, the evaluator's responsibility to determine policies. The interplay of economic appraisal and clinical and political priorities is the sensible way to proceed.

References

Addington, D.E., Jones, B., Bloom, D., *et al.* (1993). Reduction of hospital days in chronic schizophrenia patients treated with risperidone: a retrospective study. *Clinical Therapeutics*, **15**, 917–26.

Anderson, J., Dayson, D., Wills, W., *et al.* (1993). The TAPS Project 13: clinical and social outcomes of long-stay psychiatric patients after one year in the community. *British Journal of Psychiatry*, **162** (Supplement 19), 45–56.

Backhouse, M.E., Backhouse, R.J. & Edey, S.A. (1992). Economic evaluation bibliography. *Health Economics*, **1** (Supplement), 1–236.

Beecham, J.K. (1994). Collecting and estimating costs. In *The Economic Evaluation of Mental Health Care*, ed. M. R. J. Knapp. Aldershot: Ashgate.

Beecham, J.K. & Knapp, M.R.J. (1992). Costing psychiatric interventions. In *Measuring Mental Health Needs*, ed. G. Thornicroft, G. Brewin & J. Wing, pp. 163–83. Oxford: Oxford University Press.

Beecham, J.K., Knapp, M.R.J. & Fenyo, A.J. (1991). Costs, needs and outcomes. *Schizophrenia Bulletin*, **17**, 427–39.

Bertsch, E.F. (1992). A voucher system that enables persons with severe mental illness to purchase community support services. *Hospital and Community Psychiatry*, **43**, 1109–13.

Bigelow, D.A. & McFarland, B.H. (1989). Comparative costs and impacts of Canadian and American payment systems for mental health services. *Hospital and Community Psychiatry*, **40**, 805–8.

Burns, T., Raftery, J., Beadsmoore, A., *et al.* (1993). A controlled trial of home-based acute psychiatric services. II. Treatment patterns and costs. *British Journal of Psychiatry*, **163**, 55–61.

Cannon, N.L., McGuire, T.G. & Dickey, B. (1985). Capital cost in economic program evaluation: the case of mental health services. In *Economic Evaluation of Public Programs, New Directions for Program Evaluation*, vol. 26, ed. J. Cotterall, pp. 69–82. San Francisco: Jossey-Bass.

Challis, D. & Davies, B. (1986). *Case Management in Community Care*: Aldershot: Gower.

Cottrell, D. (1993). Pound foolish: a review. *Psychiatric Bulletin*, **17**, 480.

Crits-Christoph, P. (1992). The efficacy of brief dynamic psychotherapy: a meta-analysis. *American Journal of Psychiatry*, **149**, 151–8.

Croft-Jeffreys, C. & Wilkinson, G. (1989). Estimated costs of neurotic disorder in UK general practice 1985. *Psychological Bulletin*, **19**, 549–58.

Davies, B.P. & Challis, D.J. (1986). *Matching Resources to Needs in Community Care*. Aldershot: Gower.

Davies, L.M. & Drummond, M.F. (1993). Assessment of costs and benefits of drug therapy for treatment-resistant schizophrenia in the United Kingdom. *British Journal of Psychiatry*, **162**, 38–42.

Dickey, B., Binner, P.A., Leff, S., Vydea, M.K., Schlesinger, M.J. & Gudeman, J.E. (1989). Containing mental health treatment costs through program design: a Massachusetts study. *American Journal of Public Health*, **79**, 863–7.

Drummond, M.F. (1981). Welfare economics and cost benefit analysis in health care. *Scottish Journal of Political Economy*, **28**, 125–45.

Frank, R.G. & Jackson, C.A. (1989). The impact of prospectively set hospital budgets on psychiatric admissions. *Social Science and Medicine*, **28**, 861–7.

Grey, A. & Fenn, P. (1993). Alzheimer's disease: the burden of the illness in England. *Health Trends*, **25**, 31–7.

Häfner, H. & an der Heiden, W. (1989). The evaluation of mental health care systems. *British Journal of Psychiatry*, **155**, 12–17.

Häfner, H. & an der Heiden, W. (1990). Effectiveness and cost of community care for schizophrenic patients. *Hospital and Community Psychiatry*, **40**, 59–63.

Hallam, A., Beecham, J.K., Knapp, M.R.J. & Fenyo, A. (1994). The costs of accommodation and care: community provision for former long-stay psychiatric hospital patients. *European Archives of Psychiatry and Clinical Neuroscience*, **243**, 304–10.

Healy, D. (1993). Psychopharmacology and the ethics of resource allocation. *British Journal of Psychiatry*, **162**, 23–9.

Huxley, P. (1992). Social services assessment and care management: getting it right. *Journal of Mental Health*, **1**, 285–94.

Intagliata, J. (1982). Improving the quality of community care for the chronically mentally disabled: the role of case management. *Schizophrenia Bulletin*, **8**, 655–74.

Kavanagh, S., Schneider, J., Knapp, M.R.J., Beecham, J.K., *et al.* (1993). Elderly people with cognitive impairment: costing possible changes in the balance of care. *Health and Social Care in the Community*, **1**, 69–80.

Kavanagh, S., Opit, L., Knapp, M.R.J. & Beecham, J.K. (1994). *Schizophrenia: Costs and Balance of Care in England*. Discussion paper 954. University of Kent at Canterbury: Personal Social Services Research Unit.

Kingdon, D.F. & Turkington, D. (1993). *Cognitive Therapy in Schizophrenia*: New York: Guilford Press.

Knapp, M.R.J. (1993). Background theory. In *Costing Community Care*, ed. A. Netten & J. K. Beecham, pp. 9–24. Aldershot: Ashgate.

Knapp, M.R.J. (1994a). The health economics of schizophrenia treatment. *The Clinician*, **12**, 39–52.

Knapp, M.R.J. (1994b). In *The Economic Evaluation of Mental Health Care*, ed. M.R.J. Knapp. Aldershot: Ashgate.

Knapp, M.R.J. (1995). Community mental health services: towards an understanding of cost-effectiveness. In *Evaluation of Community Psychiatric Services*, ed. F. J. Creed & P. Tyrer. Cambridge: Cambridge University Press.

Knapp, M.R.J., Beecham, J.K. & Gordon, K. (1992a). Predicting the community cost of closing psychiatric hospitals: national extrapolations. *Journal of Mental Health*, **1**, 315–25.

Knapp, M.R.J., Cambridge, P., Thomason, C., *et al.* (1992b). *Care in the Community: Challenge and Demonstration*. Aldershot: Ashgate.

Knapp, M.R.J., Beecham, J.K., Hallam, A. & Fenyo, A. (1993). The costs of community care for people with long-term mental health problems. *Health and Social Care in the Community*, **1**, 193–201.

Knapp, M.R.J., Beecham, J.K., Koutsogeorgopoulou, V., *et al.* (1994a). Service use and costs of home-based care versus hospital-based care for people with serious mental illness: service use and costs. *British Journal of Psychiatry*, **165**, 195–203.

Knapp, M.R.J., Cambridge, P., Thomason, C., *et al.* (1994b). Residential care as an alternative to long-stay hospital: a cost-effectiveness evaluation. *International Journal of Geriatric Psychiatry*, **9**, 297–304.

Light, D. & Bailey, V. (1993). Pound foolish. *Health Service Journal*, 11 February.

Marks, I.M., Connolly, J. & Muijen, M. (1994). Home-based versus hospital-based care for people with serious mental illness. *British Journal of Psychiatry*, **165**, 179–94.

McCrone, P., Beecham. J., & Knapp, M.R.J. (1994). Community psychiatric nurse teams: cost-effectiveness of intensive support versus generic care. *British Journal of Psychiatry*, **165**, 218–21.

McCue, M.J. & Clement, J.P. (1993). Relative performance of for-profit psychiatric hospitals in investor-owned systems and nonprofit psychiatric hospitals. *American Journal of Psychiatry*, **150**, 77–82.

McGuire, T. (1991). Measuring the economic costs of schizophrenia. *Schizophrenia Bulletin*, **17**, 375–88.

Mechanic, D. (1991). The social dimension. In *Psychiatric Ethics*, ed. S. Bloch & P. Chadoff, pp. 47–64. Milton Keynes: Open University Press.

Melzer, D., Hale, A.S. & Malik, S.J. (1991). Community care for patients with schizophrenia one year after hospital discharge. *British Medical Journal*, **303**, 1023–6.

Merson, S., Tyrer, P., Onyett, S., *et al.* (1992). Early intervention in psychiatric emergencies: a controlled trial. *Lancet*, **339**, 1311–13.

Moscarelli, M., Capri, S. & Neri, I. (1991). Cost evaluation of chronic schizophrenia patients during the first three years after the first contact. *Schizophrenia Bulletin*, **17**, 421–6.

Muijen, M., Cooney, M., Strathdee, G., *et al.* (1994). Community psychiatric nurse teams: intensive support versus generic care. *British Journal of Psychiatry*, **165**, 211–17.

Netten, A. (1993). Costing informal care. In *Costing Community Care: Theory and Practice*, ed. A. Netten & J. Beecham. Aldershot: Ashgate.

Netten, A. (1994). *Unit Costs of Community Care 1994*. University of Kent at Canterbury: Personal Social Services Research Unit.

Netten, A. & Beecham, J. (1993). *Costing Community Care: Theory and Practice*. Aldershot: Ashgate.

Netten, A. & Smart S. (1993). *Unit Costs of Community Care 1992/1993*. University of Kent at Canterbury: Personal Social Services Research Unit.

North, C. & Ritchie, J. (1993). *Factors Influencing the Implementation of the Care Programme Approach*. London: HMSO.

Ratcliffe, J. (1993). *The Measurement of Indirect Costs and Benefits in Health Care Evaluation: A Critical Review*. Discussion Paper 9. University of Aberdeen: Health Economics Research Unit.

Rice, D.P., Kelman, S. & Miller, L.S. (1992). The economic burden of mental illness. *Hospital and Community Psychiatry*, **43**, 1227–32.

Rossi, G.F. (1990). Principles of surgery for epilepsy. *Acta Neurochirurgica*, Supplement 50, 58–63.

Schneider, J. (1995). Costing the care programme approach. In *Economic Evaluation of Mental Health Care*, ed. M.R.J. Knapp. Aldershot: Ashgate.

Sederer, L., Elsen, S., Dill, D., Grob, M., *et al.* (1992). Case-based re-imbursement for psychiatric hospital care. *Hospital and Community Psychiatry*, **43**, 1120–6.

Silfvenius, H. (1988). Economic costs of epilepsy: treatment benefits. *Acta Neurologia Scandinavica*, **78**, Supplement 117, 136–43.

Stein, L.I. & Test, M.A. (1980). Alternative to mental hospital treatment: conceptual model, treatment program and clinical evaluation. *Archives of General Psychiatry*, **37**, 392–7.

Tarrier, N., Beckett, R., Harwood, S., *et al.* (1993). A trial of two cognitive-behavioural methods of treating drug-resistant residual psychotic symptoms in schizophrenic patients. I. Outcomes. *British Journal of Psychiatry*, **162**, 524–32.

Thornicroft, G. (1991). The concept of case-management for long-term mental illness. *International Review of Psychiatry*, **3**, 125–32.

Weinberger, M., Gold, D.T., Divine, G.W., Cowper, P.A., *et al.* (1993). Expenditures in caring for patients with dementia who live at home. *American Journal of Public Health*, **83**, 338–41.

Weisbrod, B.A. (1979). *A Guide to Benefit Cost Analysis as Seen Through a Controlled Experiment in Treating the Mentally Ill.* Discussion Paper 559-79. University of Wisconsin: Madison Institute for Research on Poverty.

Weisbrod, B.A. (1983). A guide to benefit-cost analysis as seen through a controlled experiment in treating the mentally ill. *Journal of Health Politics, Policy and Law*, **7**, 808–45.

Weisbrod, B.A. & Helming, M. (1980). What benefit cost analysis can and cannot do: the case of treating the mentally ill. In *Evaluation Studies Review Annual*, ed. E. W. Stromsdorfer & G. Farkas. London: Sage.

Weisbrod, B.A. & Schlesinger, M. (1986). Public, private, nonprofit ownership and the response to asymmetric information: the case of nursing homes. In *The Economics of Nonprofit Institutions*, ed. S. Rose-Ackerman. New York: Oxford University Press.

Wiersma, D., Klutter, H., Nierhuis, F., Refine, M., *et al.* (1991). Costs and benefits of day treatment with community care for schizophrenia patients. *Schizophrenia Bulletin*, **17**, 421–6.

Wilkinson, G., Croft-Jeffreys, C., Krekorian, H., *et al.* (1990). QALYs in psychiatric care? *Psychiatric Bulletin*, **14**, 582–5.

Wilkinson, G., Williams, B. & Krekorian, H. (1992). QALYs in mental health: a case study. *Psychological Medicine*, **22**, 725–31.

Williams, A. (1974). The cost benefit approach. *British Medical Bulletin*, **30**, 252–6.

21

Conclusion

GRAHAM THORNICROFT AND HELLE CHARLOTTE KNUDSEN

The preceding chapters in this book have indicated the considerable achievements to date of mental health service research, the shortcomings which remain and the complexities and paradoxes involved in this type of research work, and they allow us to set out an agenda for the future.

In terms of the longer-term timescale, the technical achievements of mental health service research now put us in a unique historical position. There is the possibility that service evaluation can produce firm findings with which to inform mental health service policy and clinical practice. Our predecessors operated to a much greater extent within an informational vacuum when formulating policy and practice guidelines. The availability of research to provide a rational basis, or at least contribution, is a relatively recent phenomenon. In particular we now have good-quality information, although arising too often from small-scale experimental settings, regarding individual patient outcomes in community-orientated systems of care. We have developed in many domains assessment instruments which have undergone rigorous assessment of their psychometric properties, many of which have been developed under the auspices of the WHO Mental Health Division. We have produced more penetrating forms of statistical analysis. In addition, in the research literature we have many examples of excellent clinical practice which should now be subject to detailed research scrutiny and replication, and which should also be subject to rigorous economic evaluation.

A distinct advantage enjoyed for mental health service evaluation, compared with research in other areas of medicine, is that psychiatric services are often informed by a public health perspective. Services are often planned for defined geographical areas, many research workers adopt an epidemiological approach, and this facilitates a population-based assessment of service needs. In specific sites psychiatric case registers have proved an invaluable tool to make such assessments longitudinal, accurate and clinically related. The relatively recent availability and affordability of personal computers has meant that small-scale case registers are now widespread, although very variable in their implementation. The introduction into this field of research of clinical and non-clinical staff with an increasingly high standard of technical training in research design, and statistical analysis, has raised the scientific quality of much work during the last decade.

Research in the field of mental health service evaluation does still demonstrate a number of shortcomings. Within Europe, the large majority of studies are conducted in urban areas and indeed relatively little is known of effective and cost-effective service models for dispersed populations in rural areas. Similarly, service models which may be relevant for the developing world, using very limited staff resources, are also notably absent. Thirdly, the effects which different cultural backgrounds exert upon the service needs and provisions on local sites, even with developed countries, have been insufficiently explored. Fourthly, the published evaluations of services usually use as their subject experimental service models, and little is known about the extent to which such experimental models can be translated into routine clinical practice. A specific concern is the extent to which such community-orientated models are sustainable over a long period of time and, in particular, whether staff morale can be sustained at acceptable levels in non-institutional settings.

There are important aspects of mental health services which have so far been almost entirely neglected by researchers. The area of adverse public and professional attitudes towards the mentally ill, that is the powerful stigma which can affect patients, is relatively little studied. This is especially true in relation to the handicaps which limit the ability of patients to participate in normal social roles. In relation to this, the importance of work and regular structured activities, especially for long-term and more disabled patients, has been subject to remarkably little scrutiny. Also, the impact of local medico-legal arrangements, including provisions for compulsory detention and treatment, in different countries has also remained a research blind-spot. This is true to a large extent also for a full assessment of the views of service users and their carers in assessing service adequacy.

A further area which remains imprecise is the definition of key terms used within mental health services research. It is commonplace to see research reports concerning the 'severely mentally ill', where this phrase has not yet achieved any consensus on its precise definition. In terms of instruments used for assessment, while a number of research domains have been established through precedent and practice, including quality of life, needs assessment, disability, and family burden and care giving, these domains are usually conceptually poorly conceived, and the operational relationships between these domains are largely untested.

Indeed there are a number of aspects of mental illness which render research, as for other chronic disorders, unusually complex compared with more acute medical conditions. Patients suffering from mental disorders frequently have multiple, and severe problems, some of which may be treatment resistant, and which often follow a variable and unpredictable course. Mental disorders are also characterised by their burden upon society as a whole. In Britain, for example, the single diagnostic category of schizophrenia accounts for 9% of all inpatient National Health Service costs, while 9% of the entire health budget is spent upon the treatment of mental disorders. It is therefore clear that because mental disorders occur commonly, and because they together account for a large proportion of all health care costs, that they are an important subject for health service research.

For the future, three issues are of paramount importance. Firstly, the research infrastructure requires continuing development: this will include the development of adequate instruments to measure domains of mental health outcomes, the recruitment and training of a cadre of expert researchers in the field, and clarification to define key terms within the field of research. Secondly, it will be necessary to consolidate international networks of research personnel who can together raise the quality of evaluative research and establish firmer grounds on which to judge how far mental health services succeed in their aims. Thirdly, more solid links need to be cemented into place to connect the triangle between research, policy and practice. Although research affords the opportunity for policy and practice to be underpinned by results of scientific research, very often this contribution is not manifest. The key challenge is to translate the results on the efficacy of specific interventions produced by evaluative research into demonstrated effectiveness in routine clinical settings, so that the scientific contribution will directly contribute towards improved patient treatment and care.

Index

Page numbers in *italic* type refer to illustrations and tables.

For EU product safety concerns, contact us at Calle de José Abascal, 56–1°,
28003 Madrid, Spain or eugpsr@cambridge.org.

www.ingramcontent.com/pod-product-compliance
Ingram Content Group UK Ltd.
Pitfield, Milton Keynes, MK11 3LW, UK
UKHW010853090126
466816UK00011B/207